Traditional, Complementary and Integrative Medicine

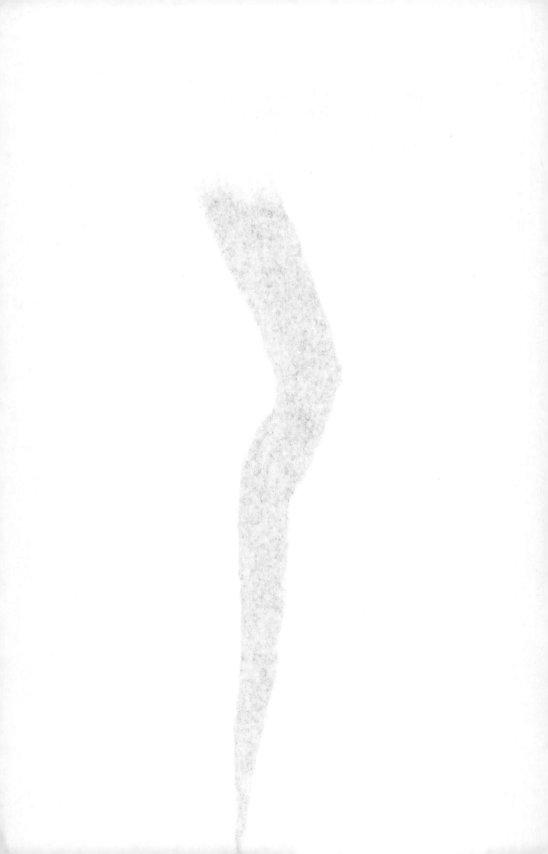

Traditional, Complementary and Integrative Medicine

An International Reader

Editor-in-Chief:
Jon Adams

Co-Editors:
Gavin J. Andrews
Joanne Barnes
Alex Broom
Parker Magin

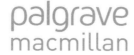

First published 2012 by
PALGRAVE MACMILLAN

Palgrave Macmillan in the UK is an imprint of Macmillan Publishers Limited, registered in England, company number 785998, of Houndmills, Basingstoke, Hampshire RG21 6XS.

Palgrave Macmillan in the US is a division of St Martin's Press LLC, 175 Fifth Avenue, New York, NY 10010.

Palgrave Macmillan is the global academic imprint of the above companies and has companies and representatives throughout the world.

Palgrave® and Macmillan® are registered trademarks in the United States, the United Kingdom, Europe and other countries

ISBN: 978–0–230–23265–5

This book is printed on paper suitable for recycling and made from fully managed and sustained forest sources. Logging, pulping and manufacturing processes are expected to conform to the environmental regulations of the country of origin.

A catalogue record for this book is available from the British Library.

A catalog record for this book is available from the Library of Congress.

10   9   8   7   6   5   4   3   2   1
21   20   19   18   17   16   15   14   13   12

Printed and bound in Great Britain by
CPI Antony Rowe, Chippenham and Eastbourne

For Jack and Maggie Flyght Adams

Contents

List of tables and figures   xiii

Acknowledgements   xiv

Notes on the contributors   xvii

INTRODUCTION   1
Jon Adams, Gavin J. Andrews, Joanne Barnes, Alex Broom and
Parker Magin

**PART A: UTILIZATION: POPULATIONS AND
INDIVIDUALS**   7

SECTION 1: **Profile, demographics and motivations for
complementary and alternative medicine use**   9

Introduction   9
Jon Adams, Gavin J. Andrews, Joanne Barnes, Alex Broom and
Parker Magin

Chapter 1:
The profile of complementary and alternative medicine users and
reasons for complementary and alternative medicine use   11
Gavin J. Andrews, Jon Adams, Jeremy Segrott and Chi Wai Lui

Chapter 2:
Relief, risk and renewal: Mixed therapy regimens in an Australian
suburb   18
Linda Connor

Chapter 3:
Utilizing existing data sets to investigate complementary and
alternative medicine consumption: Cohort studies and
longitudinal analyses   26
David Sibbritt and Jon Adams

SECTION 2: **Complementary and alternative medicine through the life cycle**   33

Introduction   33
Jon Adams, Gavin J. Andrews, Joanne Barnes, Alex Broom and Parker Magin

Chapter 4:
Women's use of complementary and alternative medicine during pregnancy: A critical review of the literature   35
Jon Adams, Chi Wai Lui, David Sibbritt, Alex Broom, Jon Wardle, Caroline Homer, Amie Steel and Shoshannah Beck

Chapter 5:
Complementary and alternative medicine use among infants, children and adolescents   44
Denise Adams, Kathi Kemper and Sunita Vohra

Chapter 6:
'Getting on with life': The experiences of older people using complementary health care   53
Tina Cartwright

SECTION 3: **Traditional, complementary and integrative medicine and disease context**   61

Introduction   61
Jon Adams, Gavin J. Andrews, Joanne Barnes, Alex Broom and Parker Magin

Chapter 7:
Topical and oral complementary and alternative medicine in acne: A consideration of context   63
Parker Magin, Jon Adams, Dimity Pond and Wayne Smith

Chapter 8:
Patient decision making about complementary and alternative medicine in cancer management: Context and process   71
Lynda Balneaves, Laura Weeks and Dugald Seely

Chapter 9:
Mental health and complementary and alternative medicine   79
Jerome Sarris and James Lake

Chapter 10:
Complementary and alternative medicine use among HIV-positive
people: Research synthesis and implications for HIV care 87
Rae Littlewood and Peter Vanable

Chapter 11:
Traditional, complementary and integrative medicine and
well-being 94
Richard Harvey

PART B: PRACTICE, PROVISION AND THE
PROFESSIONAL INTERFACE 103

SECTION 4: **Traditional medicine in context** 105

Introduction 105
*Jon Adams, Gavin J. Andrews, Joanne Barnes, Alex Broom and
Parker Magin*

Chapter 12:
Biopolitics and the promotion of traditional herbal medicine in
Vietnam 107
Ayo Wahlberg

Chapter 13:
The inequalities of medical pluralism: Hierarchies of health,
the politics of tradition and the economies of care in Indian
oncology 116
Alex Broom, Assa Doron and Philip Tovey

Chapter 14:
In the presence of biomedicine: Ayurveda, medical integration
and health seeking in Mysore, South India 125
Tapio Nisula

SECTION 5: **Exploring the complementary and alternative
medicine–conventional medicine interface** 133

Introduction 133
*Jon Adams, Gavin J. Andrews, Joanne Barnes, Alex Broom and
Parker Magin*

Chapter 15:
They don't ask so I don't tell them: Patient–clinician communication
about traditional, complementary and alternative medicine   135
*Brian Shelley, Andrew Sussman, Robert Williams, Alissa Segal and
Benjamin Crabtree on behalf of the RIOS Net Clinicians*

Chapter 16:
The ethics of dietary supplements and natural health products in
pharmacy practice: A systematic documentary analysis   142
Heather Boon, Kristine Hirschkorn, Glenn Griener and Michelle Cali

Chapter 17:
Nostalgic and nostophobic referencing and the authentication
of nurses' use of complementary therapies   150
Philip Tovey and Jon Adams

SECTION 6: Integrative medicine   157

Introduction   157
*Jon Adams, Gavin J. Andrews, Joanne Barnes, Alex Broom and
Parker Magin*

Chapter 18:
Variations in provider conceptions of integrative medicine   159
*An-Fu Hsiao, Gery Ryan, Ronald Hays, Ian Coulter, Ronald Anderson
and Neil Wenger*

Chapter 19:
Which medicine? Whose standard? Critical reflections on medical
integration in China   168
Ruiping Fan and Ian Holliday

Chapter 20:
Complementary and alternative medicine education:
Promoting a salutogenic focus in health care   176
*David Rakel, Mary Guerrera, Brian Bayles, Gautam Desai and
Emily Ferrara*

PART C: KNOWLEDGE PRODUCTION, RESEARCH
DESIGN AND PERSPECTIVES   183

SECTION 7: Evidence, safety and regulation   185

Introduction   185
*Jon Adams, Gavin J. Andrews, Joanne Barnes, Alex Broom and
Parker Magin*

Chapter 21:
The role of evidence in alternative medicine: Contrasting
biomedical and anthropological approaches 187
Christine Barry

Chapter 22:
Researching complementary and alternative treatments:
The gatekeepers are not at home 196
*Vinjar Fønnebø, Sameline Grimsgaard, Harald Walach,
Cheryl Ritenbaugh, Arne Norheim, Hugh MacPherson, George Lewith,
Laila Launsø, Mary Koithan, Torkel Falkenberg, Heather Boon and
Mikel Aickin*

Chapter 23:
Evidence-based complementary and alternative medicine:
Promises and problems 204
Ian Coulter

Chapter 24:
Indirect risks of complementary and alternative medicine 212
Jon Wardle and Jon Adams

Chapter 25:
The liberalization of regulatory structure of complementary and
alternative medicine: Implications for consumers and professions 220
Michael Weir

SECTION 8: **Traditional, complementary and integrative
medicine in perspective** 229

Introduction 229
*Jon Adams, Gavin J. Andrews, Joanne Barnes, Alex Broom and
Parker Magin*

Chapter 26:
The geography of complementary and alternative medicine 231
Gavin J. Andrews, Jeremy Segrott, Chi Wai Lui and Jon Adams

Chapter 27:
Repositioning the role of traditional medicine as essential health
knowledge in global health: Do they still have a role to play? 237
Daniel Hollenberg, David Zakus, Tim Cook and Xue Wei Xu

Chapter 28:
Review of economic methods used in complementary and
alternative medicine   245
Christopher Doran, Dennis Chang, Hosen Kiat and Alan Bensoussan

SECTION 9: Future agendas: Key debates and themes   255

Introduction   255
Jon Adams, Gavin J. Andrews, Joanne Barnes, Alex Broom and
Parker Magin

Chapter 29:
The future of integrative medicine: A commentary on
complementary and alternative medicine and integrative medicine   257
Ian Coulter

Chapter 30:
The challenges of traditional, complementary and integrative
medicine research: A practitioner perspective   266
Jon Wardle and Dugald Seely

Chapter 31:
Research capacity building in traditional, complementary and
integrative medicine: Grass-roots action towards a broader vision   275
Jon Adams, David Sibbritt, Alex Broom, Jon Wardle, Amie Steel,
Vijay Murthy and Jane Daley

Index   283

List of tables and figures

Tables

4.1 Research-based studies on the use of complementary and
alternative medicine in pregnancy, 1999–2008   37

5.1 National community use of paediatric CAM   45

9.1 Future areas of research in CAM and mental health   83

28.1 Findings from literature review of economic methods used in
complementary medicine   248

Figures

5.1 A common-sense guide to CAM treatment recommendations   48

22.1 Research strategies in drug trials and CAM (proposed)   199

Acknowledgements

The editors and publishers wish to thank the following for permission to use copyright material: John Wiley & Sons Ltd (Wiley-Blackwell) for permission to reprint abridged version of Andrews, G., Adams, J. and Segrott, J. (2009) Complementary and alternative medicine (CAM): Production, consumption, research. In T. Brown, S. McLafferty and G. Moon (eds) *A Companion to Health and Medical Geography*. Oxford: Wiley-Blackwell; Elsevier Ltd for permission to reprint abridged version of Connor, L. (2004) Relief, risk and renewal: Mixed therapy regimens in an Australian suburb. *Social Science and Medicine* 59(8): 1695–705; Routledge (Taylor and Francis Ltd) for permission to reprint abridged version of Sibbritt, D. (2006) Utilising and analysing existing datasets for CAM research: A focus upon cohort studies. In J. Adams (ed.) *Researching Complementary and Alternative Medicine*. London: Routledge; American Academy of Pediatrics for permission to reprint extracts from 'Medico-legal and ethical considerations' from Kemper, K., Vohra, S., Walls, R., and the Task force on Complementary and Alternative Medicine and the Provisional Section on Complementary, Holistic, and Integrative Medicine (2008) The use of complementary and alternative medicine in Pediatrics. *Pediatrics* 122: 1374–86 and Figure 5.1 A common-sense guide to CAM treatment recommendations, reproduced with permission from Kemper, K. and Cohen, M. (2004) Ethics meet complementary and alternative medicine: New light on old principles. *Contemporary Pediatrics* 21: 65; John Wiley & Sons Ltd (Wiley-Blackwell) for permission to reprint abridged version of Adams, J., Lui, C., Sibbritt, D., Broom, A., Wardle, J., Homer, C. and Beck, S. (2009) Women's use of complementary and alternative medicine during pregnancy: A critical review of the literature. *Birth* 36(3): 237–45; Elsevier Ltd for permission to reprint abridged version of Cartwright, T. (2007) 'Getting on with life': The experience of older people using complementary health care. *Social Science and Medicine* 64(8): 1692–703; Elsevier Ltd for permission to reprint abridged version of Magin, P., Adams, J., Pond, D. and Smith, W. (2006) Topical and oral CAM in acne: A review of the empirical evidence and a consideration of its context. *Complementary Therapies in Medicine* 14(1): 62–76; Multimed Inc. for permission to reprint abridged version of Balneaves, L., Weeks, L. and Seely, D. (2008) Patient decision-making about complementary and alternative medicine in cancer management: Context and process. *Current Oncology* 15(2): 94–100; Routledge (Taylor and Francis Ltd) for permission to reprint abridged version of Littlewood, R. and Vanable, P. (2008) Complementary and alternative medicine use among HIV-positive people: Research synthesis and implications for HIV care. *AIDS Care* 20(8): 1102–18; Sage Publishing Ltd for permission to reprint abridged version of Wahlberg, A. (2006) Biopolitics and the promotion of traditional herbal medicine in Vietnam. *Health: An Interdisciplinary Journal for the Social Study of Health, Illness and Medicine* 10(2): 123–47; Elsevier Ltd for permission to reprint abridged version of Broom, A., Doron, A. and Tovey, P. (2009) The inequalities of medical pluralism: Hierarchies of health, the politics of tradition and the economies of care in Indian oncology. *Social Science and Medicine* 69: 698–706; Routledge (Taylor and Francis Ltd) for permission to reprint abridged version of Nisula, T. (2006) In the presence of biomedicine: Ayurveda, medical integration and health seeking in Mysore, South India. *Anthropology and Medicine* 13(3): 207–24; American Academy of Family Physicians for permission to reprint abridged version of Shelley, B., Sussman, A., Williams, R., Segal, A. and Crabtree, B. (2009) 'They don't ask me so I don't tell them': Patient–clinician communication about traditional, complementary, and alternative medicine. *Annals of Family Medicine* 7(2): 139–47; John Wiley & Sons Ltd and Royal Pharmacy Society for permission to reprint abridged version of Boon, H., Hirschkorn, K., Greener, G. and Cali, M. (2010) The ethics of dietary supplements and natural health products in pharmacy practice: A systematic documentary analysis. *International Journal of Pharmacy Practice* 17(1): 31–8; Elsevier Ltd for permission to reprint abridged version of Tovey, P. and Adams, J. (2003) Nostalgic and nostophobic referencing and the authentication of nurses' use of complementary therapies. *Social Science and Medicine* 56(7): 1469–80; Elsevier Ltd for permission to reprint abridged version of Hsiao, A., Ryan, G., Hays, R., Coulter, I., Andersen, R. and Wenger, N. (2006) Variations in provider conceptions of integrative medicine. *Social Science and Medicine* 62(12): 2973–87; BMJ Publishing Group for permission to reprint abridged version of Fan, R. and Holliday, I. (2007) Whose medicine? Whose standard? Critical reflections on medical integration in China. *Journal of Medical Ethics* 33: 454–61; Mary Ann Liebert, Inc. for permission to reprint abridged version of Rakel, D., Guerrera, M., Bayles, B., Desai, G. and Ferrara, E. (2008) Complementary and alternative medicine education: Promoting a salutogenic focus in health care. *Journal of Alternative and Complementary Medicine* 14(1): 87–93; Elsevier Ltd for permission to reprint abridged version of Barry, C. (2006) The role of evidence in alternative medicine: Contrasting biomedical and anthropological approaches. *Social Science and Medicine* 62: 2646–57; BioMed Central Ltd for permission to reprint abridged version of Fonnebo, V., Grimsgaard, S., Walach, H., Ritenbaugh, C., Norheim, A., McPherson, H., Lewith, G., Launso, L., Koithan, M., Falkenberg, T., Boon, H. and Aickin, M. (2007) Researching complementary and alternative treatments – the gatekeepers are not at home. *BMC Medical Research Methodology* 7: 7; S. Karger AG Basel for permission to reprint abridged version of Coulter, I. (2007) Evidence based complementary and alternative medicine: Promises and problems. *Forschende Komplementarmedizin* 14: 102–08; John Wiley & Sons Ltd (Wiley-Blackwell) for permission to reprint abridged version of Andrews, G., Adams, J. and

Segrott, J. (2009) Complementary and alternative medicine (CAM): Production, consumption, research. In T. Brown, S. McLafferty and G. Moon (eds) *A Companion to Health and Medical Geography.* Oxford: Wiley-Blackwell; Longwoods Publishing for permission to reprint abridged version of Hollenberg, D., Zakus, D., Cook, T. and Wei Xu, X. (2008) Re-positioning the role of traditional, complementary and alternative medicine as essential health knowledge in global health: Do they still have a role to play. *World Health and Population* 10(4): 62–74; Mary Ann Liebert, Inc. for permission to reprint abridged version of Doran, C., Chang, D., Kiat, H. and Bensoussan, A. (2010) Review of economic methods used in complementary medicine. *Journal of Alternative and Complementary Medicine* 16(5): 591–5. The editors and publishers also wish to thank authors for their permission to reprint their work. Every effort has been made to trace the copyright holders, but if any have been inadvertently overlooked the publishers will be pleased to make the necessary arrangements at the first opportunity.

Notes on the contributors

Editors and contributors of commissioned chapters

Denise Adams is a Research Associate with the CARE Program for Integrative Health and Healing at the University of Alberta, Canada. She holds an Honours degree in Cellular, Molecular and Microbial Biology from the University of Calgary (Canada), and after a career in basic research in a variety of medical fields, she completed a PhD in Public Health Sciences (clinical epidemiology). Her dissertation focused on methodological issues of researching traditional Chinese medicine and was supported by prestigious awards at both provincial and federal levels (Alberta Heritage Foundation for Medical Research Health Research Studentship; Canadian Institute for Health Research Canada Graduate Scholarship Doctoral Award). Her current research interests include the effectiveness and safety of complementary and alternative medicine (CAM) as well as methodologies for clinical trials and systematic reviews. In addition to her research activities, Denise is also a lecturer for the University of Alberta Medical Acupuncture Program (http://cpl.med.ualberta.ca/ Programs/Programs/MAP/Pages/default.aspx) and serves as a reviewer for a number of journals, both CAM and conventional.

Jon Adams is Professor of Public Health at the University of Technology, Sydney, where he leads a national team of 10 CAM researchers and holds a prestigious NHMRC Career Development Fellowship (the only one to be focused on CAM research). Jon is Executive Director of the Network of Researchers in the Public Health of Complementary and Alternative Medicine (NORPHCAM; www.norphcam.org) and a Senior Fellow of the International Brisbane Initiative at the Department of Primary Health Care, University of Oxford. Jon is also National Convenor of the 'Evidence, Research and Policy in Complementary Medicine' Special Interest Group at the Public Health Association of Australia (PHAA), Associate Editor for the peer-reviewed journals *Complementary Therapies in Medicine*, *Journal of Acupuncture and Meridian Studies* and *BMC Complementary and Alternative Medicine*, as well as Regional Co-Editor for the *European Journal of Integrative Medicine*.

Jon has authored over 145 peer-reviewed publications in the last 10 years and he is Editor/Co-Editor of six health research books, including *The Mainstreaming of Complementary and Alternative Medicine: Studies in Social Context* (Routledge), *Complementary and Alternative Medicine in Nursing and Midwifery: Towards a Critical Social Science* (Routledge), *Researching Complementary and Alternative Medicine* (Routledge), *Complementary and*

Integrative Medicine in Primary Health Care (Imperial College Press) and *Evidence-Based Healthcare in Context: Critical Social Science Perspectives* (Ashgate). Jon's current research programme spans a wide range of interests including developing the public health perspective of TCIM, examining CAM in relation to primary health care, rural health, women's health, chronic illness and the wider context of self-care, as well as exploring the potential of traditional medicine in addressing contemporary global health issues.

Gavin J. Andrews is Professor of Social Gerontology and Health Studies, Canada. Gavin was the inaugural Chair of the Department of Health, Aging and Society from 2006–11. A health geographer and predominantly qualitative researcher, Gavin's wide-ranging interests include the dynamics between space/place and complementary medicine, ageing, nursing, specific phobias, fitness, health histories, popular music and primary health care. Much of Gavin's work is positional and considers the development, state of the art and future of his subdiscipline. Gavin's particular interests in complementary medicine include small business entrepreneurship, visualization practices, and the use of music as an everyday practice for well-being. Gavin has published 120 journal articles and book chapters, three journal special editions (two in *Social Science & Medicine*, 2007 and 2009) and three books: *Aging and Place: Perspectives, Policy, Practice* (Routledge); *The Sociology of Aging* (Rawat) and *Primary Health Care: People, Practice, Place* (Ashgate). Gavin is currently preparing another edited book for Ashgate called *Medicinal Melodies: Places of Health and Wellbeing in Popular Music*.

Joanne Barnes is Associate Professor in Herbal Medicines at the School of Pharmacy, University of Auckland, New Zealand. She is an honorary consultant to the World Health Organization's Uppsala Monitoring Centre and a member of its herbal safety signal review panel. Joanne's research interests broadly include the utilization, quality, efficacy, safety and pharmacovigilance of complementary medicines, particularly herbal medicinal products, and the roles and experiences of the pharmacist and other stakeholders in the safe and effective use of complementary medicines. Her work bridges the disciplines of pharmacognosy/natural products, pharmacovigilance/pharmacoepidemiology and pharmacy practice/health services research.

Joanne is Associate Editor of the journal *Phytochemistry Letters* (Elsevier) and a member of the editorial boards of the journals *Drug Safety* (Adis/Wolters Kluwer), *International Journal of Pharmacy Practice* (Pharmaceutical Press) and *Phytotherapy Research* (Wiley), as well as being a member of the international advisory board of *Complementary Therapies in Medicine* (Elsevier). She was Senior Editor of *FACT: Focus on Alternative and Complementary Therapies* (1996–99; Pharmaceutical Press) and Joint Editor-in-Chief of *Complementary Therapies in Medicine* (2003–05; Elsevier). In the last 10 years, Joanne has authored or co-authored over 30 peer-reviewed papers and book chapters and at least 30 other publications in the field of complementary medicines. She has also published three books: two editions of a leading reference text and online publication *Herbal Medicines* (Pharmaceutical Press) as principal author-editor, and *Fundamentals of Pharmacognosy and Phytotherapy* (Churchill Livingstone) as a co-author. She is a registered pharmacist in the UK and New Zealand and is a Fellow of the Linnean Society of London.

Alex Broom is Associate Professor of Sociology and Australia Research Council Future Fellow at the School of Social Science, The University of Queensland, Australia. Alex specializes in the sociology of traditional, complementary and alternative medicine (TCAM) and the sociology of cancer and end-of-life care, and he has led sociological studies of TCAM in Australia, the UK, Brazil, India, Pakistan and Sri Lanka. Alex is currently leading a cross-cultural comparative study of medical pluralism in Australia, India and Brazil and a longitudinal qualitative study of end-of-life care in Australia. Recent co-authored and co-edited books include *Traditional, Complementary and Alternative Medicine and Cancer Care* (Routledge, 2007), *Therapeutic Pluralism* (Routledge, 2008), *Men's Health: Body, Identity and Social Context* (Wiley-Blackwell, 2009), *Health, Culture and Religion in South Asia* (Routledge, 2011) and *Evidence-Based Healthcare in Context: Critical Social Science Perspectives* (Ashgate, forthcoming). Alex is a Visiting Professor at Jawaharlal Nehru University (India) and Brunel University (London), and an Honorary Associate Professor at the University of Sydney (Australia). Alex is also Director of Social Science Research for the Network of Researchers in the Public Health of CAM (www.norphcam.org).

Ian Coulter is a senior health policy analyst at the RAND Corporation, where he holds the Samueli Institute Chair in Policy for Integrative Medicine. Ian is also a Professor at the UCLA School of Dentistry and a Research Professor at the Southern California University of Health Sciences. Ian has more than 20 years of experience conducting both qualitative and quantitative research on chiropractic and has authored or co-authored more than 160 articles and book chapters and two books. Ian was the principal investigator of the Evidence-Based Practice Center for Complementary and Alternative Medicine at RAND, which was funded through the Agency for Healthcare Research and Quality in cooperation with the National Center for Complementary and Alternative Medicine (NCCAM), and he was the Principal Investigator on a case study of integrative medicine, also funded by NCCAM. Ian is currently the Principal Investigator on a US Department of Defense–funded project studying chiropractic in the military, as well as an NCCAM project focusing on assessment of the contextual effects of the health encounter in CAM. Ian received his PhD in sociology from the London School of Economics and Political Science and he is a graduate of the Harvard Institute for Educational Management and the RAND/UCLA Center for Health Policy Study. Ian is a past PEW Fellow and holds an honorary doctorate in humanities.

Jane Daley is a PhD candidate (Gender and Health) at the University of Newcastle, Australia. She also holds a Bachelor of Complementary Medicine from Charles Sturt University, Australia and a Master of Clinical Science from Southern Cross University, Australia. Jane served as an Examiner and Board Director for the National Herbalists Association of Australia (NHAA) for many years and is currently Chair of a subcommittee for the Australian Register of Naturopaths and Herbalists (ARONAH), examining appropriate education standards for Naturopaths and Herbalists in Australia. Jane has published numerous peer-reviewed articles on complementary medicine and is an Editorial Board Member of the *Australian Journal of Medical Herbalism*. Jane has also authored chapters for numerous books including *Naturopathic Clinical Medicine* by Leah Hechtman (Churchill Livingstone), *Clinical Naturopathy: An Evidence-Based Guide to Practice* (Churchill Livingstone) and *Herbs and Natural Supplements: An Evidence-Based Guide* (Churchill Livingstone).

Richard Harvey is an Assistant Professor of Health Education and Holistic Health at San Francisco State University. Richard is a Board Member of the Association for Applied Psychophysiology and Biofeedback, the Biofeedback Society of California and the San Francisco Psychological Association, serves as a Chairperson of the American Public Health Association, Alternative and Complementary Health Practices Special Interest Group and is a representative to the Governing Council of the American Public Health Association. Richard also serves as an Editor for *Psychophysiology Today*, a publication of the Biofeedback Federation of Europe. Before joining the faculty at San Francisco State, Richard was a Research Fellow at the University of California, Irvine Transdisciplinary Tobacco Use Research Center for five years, and collaborated for five years with the University of California, Irvine Counselling Center, where he developed and managed the Biofeedback and Stress Management Program. Richard has published in the fields of biofeedback, stress management, computer-related disorders, tobacco-cessation collaborations and the psychology of hardiness and courage.

Kathi J. Kemper is a Professor in the Departments of Social Science/Health Policy and Pediatrics at Wake Forest University School of Medicine, US. She also holds appointments in Family and Community Medicine, Regenerative Medicine and Bioethics, and is a member of the Comprehensive Cancer Center and the Hypertension and Vascular Research Center. Kathi is also the Caryl J Guth Chair for Complementary and Integrative Medicine, Wake Forest University School of Medicine, Director of the Center for Integrative Medicine, Wake Forest University Baptist Medical Center and Founding Chair of the Section on Complementary and Integrative Medicine, American Academy of Pediatrics. Kathi has more than 100 peer-reviewed research publications and has been the PI for both NIH and Foundation grants. She is recognized internationally as the leading authority on complementary therapies for children, and is frequently consulted by media including the *New York Times*, *Chicago Tribune, Newsweek, ABC News*, the *Wall Street Journal, Readers' Digest, Redbook, First for Women* and *USA Today*.

James Lake is a Board-certified psychiatrist in private practice in Monterey, California. He has chaired symposia and workshops at American Psychiatric Association meetings and other national and international conferences on non-conventional and integrative mental health care. James has served as a Clinical Assistant Professor in the Department of Psychiatry and Behavioral Medicine at Stanford University, and is currently a Visiting Assistant Professor of Medicine at the University of Arizona School of Medicine, Center for Integrative Medicine. He founded and chaired the American Psychiatric Association's Caucus on Complementary, Alternative and Integrative Mental Health Care from 2004 to 2010 and was appointed to a special APA Task Force on CAM and integrative medicine. James is currently Co-Chair of the working group on integrative mental health in the Consortium on Academic Healthcare Centers in Integrative Medicine, and is a founding member and chair of the International Network of Integrative Mental Health.

James has published numerous peer-reviewed articles and chapters on integrative medicine and psychiatry. He contributes a regular column on integrative mental health care to *Psychiatric Times*, and serves on the editorial review boards of *Alternative Therapies in Health and Medicine, Journal of Alternative and Complementary Medicine, Journal of the Association for Advances in Philosophy, Psychiatry and Psychology, and Journal of Clinical Psychiatry*. He is the author or editor of four textbooks on non-conventional mental health care: *Chinese Medical Psychiatry: A Clinical Manual* (with Bob Flaws; Blue Poppy Press, 2000); *Textbook of Integrative Mental Health Care* (Thieme, 2006); *Complementary and Alternative Treatments in Mental Health Care* (co-edited with David Spiegel; American Psychiatric Press, 2007) and *Integrative Mental Health Care: A Therapist's Handbook* (Norton, 2009). Long-standing interests include the role of culture in mental illness, the philosophy and history of medicine, and the role of consciousness and intentionality in healing.

Parker Magin is a general practitioner and is Senior Lecturer and Director, Primary Health Care Research, Evaluation and Development Program, Discipline of General Practice, University of Newcastle, Australia and a Medical Educator, General Practice Training Valley to Coast, Newcastle, Australia. Parker is also a Key Collaborator with the Network of Researchers in the Public Health of Complementary and Alternative Medicine (NORPHCAM), an Affiliated Researcher with the Brain and Mental Health Program, Hunter Medical Research Institute, and a Member of the Royal Australian College of General Practitioners Standing Committee – Research. Parker has authored over 50 peer-reviewed publications in the last six years. A primary research interest has been skin disease in general practice, including the use of CAM therapies for skin diseases. Other areas of research interest are occupational violence in general practice, stroke and cerebral transient ischaemic attacks, and the clinical experiences of general practice vocational trainees.

Vijayendra Murthy is a Postgraduate Research Scholar in Public Health at the University of Newcastle, Australia as well as Educational Consultant, Visiting Lecturer and Honorary Head of Faculty of Ayurvedic Medicine at Wellpark College of Natural Therapies, Auckland, New Zealand. Vijayendra is also a guest lecturer at SDM Hassan Ayurvedic College and Hospital in India and visiting consultant at the Wholistic Medical Centre, Harley Street in London. In addition, he is Chair of the New Zealand Association of Ayurvedic Practitioners and Research Editor for the peer-reviewed journal *Light on Ayurveda: Journal of Health*.

After practising and teaching Ayurveda in India, taking on the roles of Head of Faculty of Ayurvedic Medicine, Research Fellow and Academic Leader at Wellpark College in New Zealand, Vijayendra has taught Diploma and Graduate degree courses in Natural Health as well as Programs in Research Methods. He has been a Panel Member for the New Zealand Qualification Authority accrediting a Bachelor Degree Program in Naturopathy and he is a research collaborator with the Network of Researchers in the Public Health of Complementary and Alternative Medicine (NORPHCAM). Vijayendra has a longstanding interest in integrative approaches to natural health care, which has led him to research the positionality of Ayurveda as a traditional healing modality within western national health care systems.

Jerome Sarris is an NHMRC Clinical Research Fellow at the University of Melbourne, Australia. Jerome moved from clinical practice to academic work, and completed a doctorate at the University of Queensland in the field of psychiatry. He completed his postdoctoral training at the University of Melbourne, Department of Psychiatry; The Centre for Human Psychopharmacology (SUT); and Harvard Medical School (Massachusetts General Hospital). He has a particular interest in mood disorders, anxiety and insomnia research pertaining to complementary and integrative medicine, and in nutraceutical psychopharmacology. Jerome is Co-Editor of *Clinical Naturopathy: An Evidence-Based Guide to Practice*, has over 50 publications, and has published in many eminent psychiatry journals, such as *The Journal of Clinical Psychiatry*, *Psychopharmacology*, *Bipolar Disorders* and *Sleep Medicine Reviews*. Jerome is a founding member and Vice Chair of the International Network of Integrative Mental Health (INIMH).

David Sibbritt is Associate Professor of Biostatistics at the University of Newcastle, Australia. He is Deputy Director of the Network of Researchers in the Public Health of Complementary and Alternative Medicine

(NORPHCAM; www.norphcam.org), Deputy Director of the Centre for Clinical Epidemiology and Biostatistics, University of Newcastle, and a member of the 'Evidence, Research and Policy in Complementary Medicine' Special Interest Group Steering Committee at the Public Health Association of Australia. David is an Associate Editor for the peer-reviewed journal *BMC Health Services Research* and is on the Editorial Board for *Complementary Therapies in Medicine* and the *Journal of Chinese Integrative Medicine*. David has authored over 90 peer-reviewed publications and 50 conference presentations in the last 10 years. His current research interests are predominantly in the public health of CAM, particularly related to women's health. He also has an evolving interest in conducting clinical trials for CAM therapies.

Dugald Seely is a naturopathic doctor and Director of Research at the Canadian College of Naturopathic Medicine (CCNM). Dugald completed his Master's of Science in cancer research from the University of Toronto with a focus on interactions between chemotherapy and natural health products. In his current role as Director of Research, Dugald is the Principal Investigator for a number of clinical trials, and is actively pursuing relevant synthesis research in the production of systematic reviews and meta-analyses. Ongoing projects include three multicentred randomized clinical trials and a comprehensive CIHR synthesis review of natural health products used for cancer. Dugald has published and presented widely and is dedicated to helping build the research capacity of the naturopathic profession. His main interests lie in conducting primary research on complementary therapies used by naturopathic doctors with a focus on integrative cancer care. Dugald is currently a member of Health Canada's Expert Advisory Committee for the Vigilance of Health Products and is a peer reviewer for the Canadian Adverse Reaction Newsletter.

Amie Steel is a Researcher at the University of Technology, Sydney. She is a member of the Network of Researchers in the Public Health of Complementary and Alternative Medicine and co-founder of Embrace Holistic Services (www.embraceholistic.com). Amie is a Board Member of both the Practice Standards Committee for the Australian Register of Naturopaths and Herbalists (www.aronah.org) and the 'Evidence, Research and Policy in Complementary Medicine' Special Interest Group at the Public Health Association of Australia. She is also in clinical practice as a naturopath at Herbs on the Hill (www.herbsonthehill.com.au) in Brisbane, Australia. Amie has authored 12 peer-reviewed publications in the last four years, including contributing to two evidence-based clinical handbooks for complementary medicine. Her current research focus includes a diverse area of complementary medicine including pregnancy and women's health, curriculum content of conventional and complementary medicine courses, integration and regulation of complementary medicine within the wider health system, and the interface between evidence-based medicine and complementary medicine practice.

Sunita Vohra is a pediatrician and clinician scientist, with a Master's degree in clinical epidemiology and fellowship training in clinical pharmacology. A Professor in the Faculty of Medicine and School of Public Health at the University of Alberta, Sunita is the Founding Director of Canada's first academic paediatric integrative medicine programme, the Complementary and Alternative Research and Education (CARE) programme at the Stollery Children's Hospital (www.care.ualberta.ca). She is also the Program Director for Canada's first fellowship programme in paediatric integrative medicine and the Founding Director of the Canadian Pediatric CAM Network (PedCAM) (www.pedcam.ca).

Sunita is recognized as an expert in complementary and alternative medicine (CAM) by Health Canada and has worked with them to identify and mitigate harms related to natural health product use. She is the recipient of a Canadian Institutes of Health Research New Investigator Award and an Alberta Heritage Foundation for Medical Research Health Scholar Award. She was invited to write the Canadian Pediatric Society statement on the use of natural health products in children and was co-principal author of the American Academy of Pediatrics statement on the use of CAM in children. Sunita has authored over 100 peer-reviewed publications and 10 book chapters. Her expertise in CAM has been recognized locally, nationally and internationally and she sits on numerous committees and editorial boards. She is the Vice-Chair for the American Academy of Pediatrics' Section on Complementary and Integrative Medicine and a Co-Convenor for Cochrane Collaboration Adverse Events Methods Group (AEMG). Sunita's research focuses on methodological issues to improve how the safety and effectiveness of CAM is assessed.

Jon Wardle practises as a naturopath in Brisbane, Australia, is an NHMRC Public Health Scholar at the School of Population Health, University of Queensland, Australia and Trans-Pacific Fellow at the School of Medicine, University of Washington, US. Jon is a founding Director of the Network of Researchers in the Public Health of Complementary and Alternative Medicine (NORPHCAM) and is on the editorial board of several journals, including serving as the Editor-in-Chief of the *International Journal of Naturopathic Medicine* and as Associate Editor for the *Foundations of Naturopathic Medicine* project. Jon is Co-Editor of the first evidence-based naturopathic clinical text, *Clinical Naturopathy: An Evidence-Based Guide to Practice* (Churchill Livingstone), which is used as a set naturopathic text in five countries and was recently translated into Spanish. Jon lectures internationally on CAM and has several popular Australian health columns, in addition to his academic publishing endeavours.

Michael Weir is Professor of Law and Associate Dean (Research) of the Law Faculty at Bond University, Australia. Michael has broad professional experience as a solicitor in private legal practice in commercial and property law.

Academically he has published extensively on land law and is a co-author of *Real Property Law in Queensland* (LBC, third edition, 2010). Michael's research interest in complementary medicine and the law is reflected in his authorship of the student textbook *Law and Ethics in Complementary Medicine* (Allen and Unwin, fourth edition, 2011) and the text *Alternative Medicine: A New Regulatory Model* (Bond University Press, 2005).

Introduction

Jon Adams, Gavin J. Andrews, Joanne Barnes,
Alex Broom and Parker Magin

No one paradigm of medicine or system of health care holds a monopoly anywhere in the world and cultures have invariably developed pluralistic ways of understanding health, ill-health, approaches to well-being and forms of treatment. Not only does the social cartography of health and medical care differ across cultures and history, but within such a fluid landscape the borders of what constitutes the 'official', 'legitimate', 'authentic' and 'effective' are also prone to flux. As any rigorous review of contemporary health and health care trends illustrates, what may only recently have been ordained fringe or marginal can soon be seen to occupy a mainstream position.

Within the complex web of health and health care knowledge, technologies, practices and products are the fields of traditional, complementary and integrative medicine (TCIM). These fields do share much common ground, yet they are also in other ways separate and distinct. Furthermore, there is also much heterogeneity within each field and in this sense, the territories addressed by this book are at their core complex and contentious topics (for example, see Chapters 18 and 29 for discussion of the challenges of defining integrative medicine).

Traditional medicine (TM), as defined by the World Health Organization (WHO), refers to 'the sum total of knowledge, skills and practices based on the theories, beliefs and experiences indigenous to different cultures, whether explicable or not, used to maintain health, as well as prevent, diagnose, improve or treat physical and mental illness' (WHO, 2000). A wealth of grey literature has emerged on this topic and the WHO has described aspects of TM in different countries. Nevertheless, the field is relatively under-researched, even in comparison to complementary and alternative medicine (CAM) and integrative medicine (IM). While some ground-breaking empirical fieldwork and scholarship has been undertaken from within anthropology, the field offers a wealth of opportunity for future investigation.

Complementary medicine (otherwise called in this collection complementary and alternative medicine [CAM]) refers to a diverse field of practices, products, knowledge and technologies that are found in late modern societies, many imported with origins in the 'exotic' or 'other' while others have developed domestically. CAM houses a diverse range of modalities, products and practices, including acupuncture, aromatherapy, chiropractic, reflexology,

1

osteopathy, herbalism, homeopathy, naturopathy, massage therapy, vitamins, minerals and supplements, yoga and meditation. Commentators have identified features that do in many cases bind a number of types of CAM (Coulter, 2004) and while different varieties of CAM occupy different positions within the political and cultural landscape (some would argue different stages of mainstreaming), most operate largely outside the mainstay of the public or government-funded health care systems and have traditionally been excluded from the core medical curriculum. Much of CAM is administered and practised in community, self-care settings initiated by the patient within informal networks of carers, friends, family and other significant others, plus also increasingly in consultation with a growing number of therapists in private practice.

Alongside the ranks of CAM practitioners and patient-initiated CAM activity has been another significant development: an increasingly closer interest in and relationship with 'alternatives' from within the conventional medical and health care community. This development has been documented in general practice, nursing and midwifery and among a range of hospital-based specialists and others. There has emerged a climate increasingly sympathetic to therapeutic pluralism and integration. However, not all integration is the same (and here we take a somewhat broad and inclusive approach in keeping with the aim of this book more generally; also see Chapter 29 this collection). It can involve simply a sharing/utilization of different ideas and a willingness to draw on more than one paradigm or system of medicine in health care (not necessarily concurrently). As this model suggests, patients have long been advocates of integration well before practitioners and researchers began to coin the terms 'integrative medicine' or 'integrative health care'.

Integration can also take the form of a more coordinated and specific approach – this is moving into the realms of practitioner cooperation and communication – whereby providers across traditional and complementary paradigms may entertain and establish referrals or even engage in collaborative practice within a common practice setting. This latter feature is not always necessary and a substantial number of conventional health care providers have entered into *direct integrative practice*, whereby one provider practises and utilizes aspects of a range of medicines for the benefit of their patients (Adams, 2004). It is also worth noting that the vast majority of more formal developments in integrative medicine and related scholarship around curriculum development and the like have been led by scholars and practitioners in North America, where the Consortium of Academic Health Centers for Integrative Medicine has been established to advance the principles and practices of integrative health care within academic medical centres across the United States and Canada.

Research developments

The position and profile of the vast landscape of TCIM has led to some exciting developments in the research sphere. Built on some early pioneering work, recent research and interest are fast growing in a range of fields (health economics, health geography, health social science, health psychology, health services research, public health and more). With this expansion the research community around TCIM is maturing and it would appear that there is good reason to remain optimistic.

Advocacy is increasingly being replaced with methodological rigour and disciplinary training in CAM research, although capacity building remains a significant priority for the field (see Chapter 31 in this collection for more details). All disciplines of study with application to health research have a role to play in helping understand TCIM. To argue otherwise, whether from within a discipline (public health for example) or from within the TCIM field itself (even more damaging and counter-productive), is to ignore wider developments in health and medical research; multidisciplinary, multimethod investigation is increasingly the approach of choice. To clarify this position, TCIM should be treated as a substantive topic in its own right (with increasing reach and implications for all involved in health and health care) requiring empirical investigation and critical reflection. This is not to argue for partisan or biased coverage; quite the opposite. The very strength of this approach for TCIM research is that it overcomes some of the previous weaknesses in the field: a lack of good, rigorous design for the understanding of TCIM; a lack of communication between the TCIM field and health researchers versed in mainstream methodology and focused on mainstream topics; and an over-dependence on advocacy and self-interest in justifying TCIM rather than an appeal to empirical, rigorous research findings (a critique equally applicable to many who have attacked these medicines).

The reader collection

The territory addressed in this collection is vast: international in scope, diverse in modality and system, multidisciplinary in methodology and approach, and all in relation to three highly interrelated yet distinct fields of focus. Nevertheless, the collection provides the first wide-ranging overview of contemporary TCIM and its scientific study, highlighting a pathway through understanding and appreciating the significance and insights to be gained from TCIM in a large number of areas, with regard to core issues of importance to many and via the lens of a number of diverse yet complementary methodological and disciplinary viewpoints.

The reader collection can be accessed as a means of efficiently becoming acquainted with a number of core issues and debates taxing these fields (for example with regard to competing debate over what counts as 'evidence' for

TCIM), helping establish an overview of contemporary hotspots for reflection; to provide a perspective on the varied research schools and vast disciplinary approaches to which TCIM is now subject and to which future investigation could or should be directed; and, more simply, to provide an introduction to what is a vast and ever-growing literature on TCIM and TCIM research.

While not claiming to be comprehensive or definitive, this reader constitutes a unique resource for a range of readers. The collection will prove a good resource for postgraduates and other students requiring a far-reaching and thought-provoking collection to help clarify the field and stimulate future prospects for study. Practitioners looking to acquaint themselves with some of the core research issues and approaches available (not only to develop direct research capacity but also to aid in their practice activity) will also gain benefit from this collection. Meanwhile, the book also constitutes a timely resource for researchers currently within or beyond the field.

Despite an emerging field of scholars in TCIM, there is often a lack of coordinated focus and cohesion, which has sometimes led to a lack of appreciation of common interest and purpose. As such, it is worthwhile – essential even – for TCIM researchers to move towards ever closer relations and collaborations across disciplines and methodologies. This book is one particular effort among others to address these challenges and to expose individuals and groups to ideas and perspectives that may as yet be uncharted or have remained beyond consideration in their work to date.

The papers in this reader have been selected and commissioned with regard to a number of criteria: seminal status and/or thought-provoking content and their accessibility to a wider audience beyond disciplinary boundaries. We have also distilled our focus to papers published in the last five years (alongside commissioned pieces, this maintains a contemporary focus while not losing sight of the building blocks of tradition and earlier work). Suggested readings also provide further aids to study and investigation. It is important to note that this collection is a springboard for further review and, while providing an initial and introductory vision and commentary, there is the opportunity for readers to branch off in a multitude of directions to explore the TCIM literature in further depth elsewhere.

The collection has been structured around three overarching parts, each consisting of three interrelated but distinct sections. Part A focuses on TCIM consumption and consumers, while Part B redirects attention to issues of practice, provision and the professional interface and Part C deals with issue around knowledge production, research design and disciplinary perspectives/ contexts (for a more detailed overview of each section and its chapters, see the appropriate section introductions throughout the collection). While individual sections and chapters may in some cases directly address only traditional medicine, complementary and alternative medicine *or* integrative medicine as opposed to all three fields, this is often a reflection of the content within specific areas of study and it is hoped that readers will be able to appropriate interesting themes and ideas to neighbouring fields where relevant.

References

Adams, J. (2004) Demarcating the medical/non-medical border: Occupational boundary-work within GPs' accounts of their integrative practice. In P. Tovey, G. Easthope, and J. Adams (eds) *The Mainstreaming of Complementary and Alternative Medicine: Studies in Social Context*. London: Routledge.

Coulter, I. (2004) Integration and paradigm clash: The practical difficulties of integrative medicine. In P. Tovey, G. Easthope and J. Adams (eds) *The Mainstreaming of Complementary and Alternative Medicine: Studies in Social Context*. London: Routledge.

World Health Organization (2000) *General Guidelines for Methodologies on Research and Evaluation of Traditional Medicine*. Geneva: WHO.

Utilization: Populations and individuals

SECTION 1 Profile, demographics and motivations for
complementary and alternative medicine use   9

SECTION 2 Complementary and alternative medicine
through the life cycle   33

SECTION 3 Traditional, complementary and integrative
medicine and disease context   61

Profile, demographics and motivations for complementary and alternative medicine use

Introduction

Alongside the recent rise in the popularity of CAM (Complementary and Alternative Medicine) has emerged a body of literature examining the exponential growth of CAM consumption. Opening this initial section of the reader, Andrews and colleagues (Chapter 1) provide a brief overview of the findings and trends from the international consumption literature to date. The chapter focuses on prevalence of use, the profile of users and the drivers/motivations for the growth in CAM consumption. As the chapter suggests, while a wealth of data has been collected and analysed on this broad topic, further study is required to better understand different CAM patient journeys through time and space and the motivations of the increasing number of heterogeneous CAM users. The authors also highlight the need to investigate CAM users in a more sophisticated way, being sensitive to variations in the type of modality used, the nature of use and the type of user.

These issues fit well with Chapter 2, in which Connor provides a rich examination of the perspectives and experiences of those embracing 'mixed therapy regimens' in an Australian suburb. This work, drawing on the ethnographic method to explore lay constructions of *therapeutic pluralism* (using multiple types of therapists and therapies at any one time, or moving in serial fashion from one type of therapy to another), alerts us to the importance of appreciating that health service users may not conceptualize the 'field' in terms similar to those of researchers or practitioners. It is telling that the dichotomous model of 'conventional' versus 'complementary' medicine (or other similar titles) was not universally employed by participants in Connor's fieldwork to explain their health care experiences or perceptions. In addition to outlining how sufferers are purposeful and pragmatic in their approach to health-seeking behaviour, Connor also explores possible broader sociological explanations (beyond the epidemiological enquiry outlined in Chapter 1) for why people may be seeking out non-biomedical practitioners and constructing mixed therapy regimens.

Closing this section, Sibbritt and Adams (Chapter 3) return to the CAM use/user literature and draw on their work and that of others to explore a number of challenges and opportunities related to secondary data analyses of existing cohort studies and longitudinal databases. As the authors suggest, researchers can utilize the possible resource of secondary data analyses to help advance CAM consumption research, especially with a view to producing longitudinal analyses charting trends in CAM use.

CHAPTER 1

The profile of complementary and alternative medicine users and reasons for complementary and alternative medicine use

GAVIN J. ANDREWS, JON ADAMS, JEREMY SEGROTT AND
CHI WAI LUI

Introduction

The use of complementary and alternative medicine (CAM) has become a mainstream health care activity in many countries. The rise in prevalence of CAM use over the past decade reflects an epidemiological transition of disease patterns as well as profound transformations in health beliefs and practices in contemporary societies. As a global health trend, the use of CAM plays an increasingly important role in the management of chronic diseases and the promotion of well-being. The rapid increase in the consumption of CAM has generated much concern and discussion among health providers, policymakers and increasingly researchers. Drawing on a wide body of international research, this chapter provides an introduction to the profile of CAM users as well as the reasons people use CAM.

CAM users

The popularity of CAM has grown exponentially over recent years and CAM is now positioned as a major health care resource in most advanced industrial

Source: Andrews, G., Adams, J. and Segrott, J. (2009) Complementary and alternative medicine (CAM): Production, consumption, research. In T. Brown, S. McLafferty and G. Moon (eds) *A Companion to Health and Medical Geography*. Oxford: Wiley-Blackwell. Abridged version reprinted with kind permission of John Wiley & Sons Ltd (Wiley-Blackwell).

societies for both the treatment of illness and the maintenance of well-being (Tovey *et al.*, 2004). Empirical work has identified the use of CAM by a substantial proportion of the general population in a number of countries (Barnes *et al.*, 2004; Adams *et al.*, 2007; Steinsbekk *et al.*, 2007) and analysis suggests that consumers contribute far more financially from their own pocket for CAM than for conventional medicines (MacLennan *et al.*, 2006).

While these and other surveys provide prevalence estimates ranging between 30 and 75 per cent, accurate interpretations and comparisons across surveys are difficult due to variations in CAM definition, question formulation and design rigour (Harris and Rees, 2000). For example, some surveys have reported CAM use over 12-month periods (Adams *et al.*, 2003; Steinsbekk *et al.*, 2007), others lifetime CAM use (Kessler *et al.*, 2001), yet others have begun to produce longitudinal analysis of CAM use over set periods of time (Bair *et al.*, 2002; Sibbritt *et al.*, 2004, Sibbritt *et al.*, 2011). Similarly, whereas some research has reported prevalence rates for consultations with CAM practitioners (Wolsko *et al.*, 2002; Adams *et al.*, 2003), other studies have included the prevalence of such consultations alongside self-prescribed CAM not requiring a practitioner (MacLennan *et al.*, 2006). Geographical variations in CAM definition, as outlined earlier, should also be considered when interpreting such findings (Adams *et al.*, 2004). In addition to prevalence among the general public, work has identified relatively high levels of CAM use among specific patient populations. For example, studies have reported high levels of CAM use among cancer patients (Molassiotis *et al.*, 2005), patients with diabetes (Edge *et al.*, 2002; Yeh *et al.*, 2002) and patients with rheumatism (Rao *et al.*, 1999).

Despite obvious difficulties in comparing prevalence rates across places, populations and cultures, it does appear from the expanding literature that CAM is no longer confined to specific population subsections and minorities, but is a popular treatment choice across society. Nevertheless, much research shows that CAM users are more likely to be female, middle-aged (30–50 years old), have a higher income, have a higher level of education, be in full-time employment and have a poorer health status than non-CAM users. Some work also suggests that CAM users are more likely to reside in non-urban areas than are non-CAM users (Adams *et al.*, 2003). This has prompted some commentators to suggest an urban–rural divide in CAM use. However, further research is required here and at present the use of CAM and its relationship to rural/urban health remains open to conjecture (Adams, 2004).

Research conducted largely in the United States has examined racial/ethnic differences in CAM use, with some revealing a higher level of CAM consumption among non-Hispanic whites relative to minorities (Barnes *et al.*, 2004; Graham *et al.*, 2005; Hsiao *et al.*, 2006). Meanwhile, other work suggests that CAM use is equally prevalent among different racial/ethnic groups (Mackenzie *et al.*, 2003), with different ethnic groups utilizing different CAM modalities, in some cases aligned to cultural traditions (Najm *et al.*, 2003).

As suggested above, the vast majority of CAM consumption data also illustrates that CAM users tend to employ these medicines in conjunction with, and not as a substitute for, conventional health services (Adams, 2004). This finding suggests that consumers do not perceive CAM as being in direct opposition to conventional services, but are instead employing different types of medicines on a more pragmatic basis (Andrews, 2002). Nevertheless, this does not necessarily mean that consumers fail to perceive differences between the two types of medicines, and it may well be that certain features of CAM (not necessarily predominant in conventional medical care) help understand and explain the increasing popularity of CAM with health care consumers.

Why do people use CAM?

Many studies have investigated the reasons people use CAM. Although not always stated in this way, these reasons can be grouped under push factors (from conventional medicine) and pull factors (to CAM). In terms of the former, it is thought that users are effectively pushed towards CAM because they have become dissatisfied with conventional medicine. Various reasons have been given for this, including a lack of confidence in conventional medicine's ability to treat a range of prevalent chronic conditions effectively (Furnham and Forey, 1994; Furnham *et al.*, 1995; Furnham and Kirkcaldy, 1996; McGregor and Peay, 1996), the perceived negative side-effects of drugs and their over-prescribing (Verhoef *et al.*, 1998) and a failure to meet the emotional needs of patients through comfort and support (Peters, 1997).

In terms of pull factors, it is thought that users are pulled towards CAM by a range of factors, including the holistic and personalized nature of many treatments, the greater time spent in consultations, the spiritual dimension to care (Vincent and Furnham, 1996), because CAM is more consistent with many people's personal values and philosophical orientations towards health (Siahpush 1999a, 1999b), because it forms part of a wider identification with an alternative ideology or subculture (Pawluch *et al.*, 1994; Fulder, 1996; Kelner and Wellman, 1997a) and ultimately because it is perceived to work where conventional medicine does not.

Of course, push and pull factors are highly interrelated. For example, a desire for more personal control over treatment can be associated with a perception that conventional medicine disempowers patients whereas CAM empowers them. A desire to engage in a more personalized service in CAM, incorporating a closer and more open form of practitioner–patient relationship, contrasts with a perception that conventional medicine is impersonal and remote. A perceived need to seek 'natural' solutions to health and illness contrasts with a perception that conventional treatments are invasive and involve an unnecessary iatrogenic toll. Also, a need to find responses in CAM for the increasing range of chronic conditions that afflict contemporary populations relates directly to the perception that such conditions are not adequately addressed by the conventional curative model (Millar, 1997; Siahpush, 1998; Bausell *et al.*, 2001; Menniti-Ippolito *et al.*, 2002).

More generally, an added influence, or pathway, to CAM use may also orig-
inate in wider societal change (see Chapter 2 in this collection for further
details). Kelner and Wellman (1997b) argue that the increasing use of CAM
reflects a greater number of 'smart consumers' in western society: more people
who are well informed about health-related issues and who prefer to use their
own personal informed judgement regarding their health and health care.
This, the authors contest, reflects a wider consumer interest in health and
body matters in western society and a pervasive moral duty to act and be well
(Greco, 1993; Conrad, 1994). It is also argued that the media has a part to
play in promoting this consumerist health culture and sustaining the demand
for CAM by providing a wealth of information in popular magazines and
newspapers on diseases and available treatments (Doel and Segrott, 2003).

Some empirical work has helped explore these issues and has begun to test
such hypotheses. However, recent research and commentary suggest that
CAM users need to be investigated in a more sophisticated way that is sensitive
to variations in the type of modality used, the nature of use (whether
prolonged or intermittent and so on) and the type of user (for example across
racial/ethnic, gendered or geographical lines) (Andrews, 2002; Sirois and
Gick, 2002; Adams *et al.*, 2004; Chao *et al.*, 2006; Shmueli and Shuval,
2006). Further empirical research is needed to gain a better understanding of
different CAM patient journeys through time and space and the motivations
of the increasing number of heterogeneous CAM users.

Further reading

Quandt, S.A., Verhoef, M.J., Arcury, T., Lewith, G., Steinsbekk, A., Kristoffersen, A.E.,
Wahner-Roedler, D.L. and Fonnebo, V. (2009) Development of an international
questionnaire to measure use of complementary and alternative medicine
(I-CAM-Q). *Journal of Alternative and Complementary Medicine* 15(4): 331–9.

Sirios, F.M. (2008) Motivations for consulting complementary and alternative medicine practitioners: A comparison of consumers from 1997–8 and 2005. *BMC
Complementary and Alternative Medicine* 8: 16.

References

Adams, J. (2004) Exploring the interface between complementary and alternative
medicine (CAM) and rural general practice: A call for research. *Health and Place*
10: 285–7.
Adams, J., Easthope, G. and Sibbritt, D. (2004) Researching the utilization of complementary and alternative medicine (CAM): Where to from here? *Evidence Based
Integrative Medicine* 1: 169–72.

Adams, J., Sibbritt, D. and Young, A. (2007) Consultations with a naturopath or herbalist: The prevalence of use and profile of users amongst mid-aged women in Australia. *Public Health* 121: 954-7.

Adams, J., Sibbritt, D., Easthope, G. and Young, A. (2003) The profile of women who consult alternative health practitioners in Australia. *Medical Journal of Australia* 179: 297–300.

Andrews, G.J. (2002) Private complementary medicine and older people: Service use and user empowerment. *Ageing and Society* 22: 343–68.

Bair, Y., Gold, E., Greendale, G. *et al.* (2002) Ethnic differences in use of complementary and alternative medicine at midlife: Longitudinal results from SWAN participants. *American Journal of Public Health* 92: 1832–40.

Barnes, P., Powell-Griner, E., McFann, K. and Nahin, R. (2004) *Complementary and Alternative Medicine Use amongst Adults: United States, 2002.* Rockville, MD: Advance Data.

Bausell, R., Lee, W. and Berman, B. (2001) Demographic and health-related correlates of visits to complementary and alternative medical providers. *Medical Care* 39: 190–96.

Chao, M., Wade, C., Kronenberg, F., Kalmuss, D. and Cushman, L. (2006) Women's reasons for complementary and alternative medicine use: Racial/ethnic differences. *Journal of Alternative and Complementary Medicine* 12: 719–22.

Conrad, P. (1994) Wellness as virtue: Morality and the pursuit of health. *Culture, Medicine and Psychiatry* 18: 385–401.

Doel, M.A. and Segrott, J. (2003) Beyond belief? Consumer culture, complementary medicine, and the disease of everyday life. *Environment and Planning D: Society and Space* 21: 739–59.

Edge, L., Zheng, D., Ye, X. and Silverstein, M. (2002) The prevalence and pattern of complementary and alternative medicine use in individuals with diabetes. *Diabetes Care* 25: 324–9.

Fulder, S. (1996) *The Handbook of Alternative and Complementary Medicine.* Oxford: Oxford University Press.

Furnham, A. and Forey, J. (1994) The attitudes, behaviors and beliefs of patients of conventional vs complementary (alternative) medicine. *Journal of Clinical Psychology* 50: 458–69.

Furnham, A. and Kirkcaldy, B. (1996) The health beliefs and behaviors of orthodox and complementary medicine clients. *British Journal of Clinical Psychology* 35: 49–61.

Furnham, A., Vincent, C. and Wood, R. (1995) The health beliefs and behaviors of three groups of complementary medicine and a general practice group of patients. *Journal of Alternative Complementary Medicine* 1: 347–59.

Graham, R., Ahn, A., Davis, R. *et al.* (2005) Use of complementary and alternative medical therapies among racial and ethnic minority adults: Results from the 2002 National Health Interview Survey. *Journal of the National Medical Association* 97: 535–45.

Greco, M. (1993) Psychosomatic subjects and the 'duty to be well': Personal agency within. *Economy and Society* 22: 357–72.

Harris, P. and Rees, R. (2000) The prevalence of complementary and alternative medicine use among the general population: A systematic review of the literature. *Complementary Therapies in Medicine* 8: 88–96.

Hsiao, A., Wong, M., Goldstein, M. *et al.* (2006) Variation in complementary and alternative medicine (CAM) use across racial/ethnic groups and the development of ethnic-specific measures of CAM use. *Journal of Alternative and Complementary Medicine* 12: 281–90.

Kelner, M. and Wellman, B. (1997a) Who seeks alternative health care? A profile of users of five modes of treatment. *Journal of Alternative and Complementary Medicine* 3: 127–40.

Kelner, M. and Wellman, B. (1997b) Health care and consumer choice: Medical and alternative therapies. *Social Science and Medicine* 45: 203–12.

Kessler, R., Davis, R. and Roger, D. (2001) Long-term trends in the use of complementary and alternative medical therapies in the United States. *Annals of Internal Medicine* 135: 262–8.

Mackenzie, E., Taylor, L., Bloom, B., Hufford, D. and Johnson, J. (2003) Ethnic minority use of complementary and alternative medicine (CAM): A national probability survey of CAM utilizers. *Alternative Therapies in Health and Medicine* 9: 50–56.

MacLennan, A., Myers, S. and Taylor, A. (2006) The continuing use of complementary and alternative medicine in South Australia: Costs and beliefs in 2004. *Medical Journal of Australia* 184: 27–31.

McGregor, K. and Peay, E. (1996) The choice of alternative therapy for health care: Testing some propositions. *Social Science and Medicine* 43: 1317–27.

Menniti-Ippolito, F., Gargiulo, L., Bologna, E., Forcella, E. and Raschetti, R. (2002) Use of unconventional medicine in Italy: A nation-wide survey. *European Journal of Clinical Pharmacology* 58: 61–4.

Millar, W. (1997) Use of alternative health care practitioners by Canadians. *Canadian Journal of Public Health* 88: 154–8.

Molassiotis, A., Fernadez-Ortega, P., Pud, G. *et al.* (2005) Use of complementary and alternative medicine in cancer patients: European survey. *Annals of Oncology* 16: 655–63.

Najm, W., Reinsch, S., Hoehler, F. and Tobis, J. (2003) Use of complementary and alternative medicine among the ethnic elderly. *Alternative Therapies in Health and Medicine* 9: 50–57.

Pawluch, D., Cain, R. and Gillet, J. (1994) Ideology and alternative therapy use among people living witrh HIV/AIDS. *Health and Canadian Society* 2: 63–84.

Peters, I. (1997) Clinical supervision for potent practice. *Complementary Therapies in Nursing and Midwifery* 3: 38–41.

Rao, J., Mihiliak, K., Kroenke, K. *et al.* (1999) Use of complementary therapies for arthritis among patients of rheumatologists. *Annals of Internal Medicine* 131: 409–16.

Shmueli, A. and Shuval, J. (2006) Complementary and alternative medicine: Beyond users and non-users. *Complementary Therapies in Medicine* 14: 261–7.

Siahpush, M. (1998) Postmodern values, dissatisfaction with conventional medicine and popularity of alternative therapies. *Journal of Sociology* 34: 58–70.

Siahpush, M. (1999a) Why do people favour complementary medicine? *Australian and New Zealand Journal of Public Health* 23: 266–71.

Siahpush, M. (1999b) Postmodern attitudes about health: A population-based exploratory study. *Complementary Therapies in Medicine* 7: 164–9.

Sibbritt, D., Adams, J. and Young, A. (2004) A longitudinal analysis of mid-aged women's use of complementary and alternative medicine (CAM) in Australia, 1996–1998. *Women and Health* 40: 41–56.

Sibbritt, D., Adams, J. and Lui, C. (2011) Health service utilisation by pregnant women over a seven-year period. *Midwifery* 27(4): 474–6.

Sirois, F. and Gick, M. (2002) An investigation of the health beliefs and motivations of complementary medicine clients. *Social Science and Medicine* 55: 1025–37.

Steinsbekk, A., Adams, J., Sibbritt, D., Jacobsen, G. and Johnsen, R. (2007) A comparison of general practice users, complementary and alternative medicine users, and those who use both. *Scandinavian Journal of Primary Health Care* 25: 86–92.

Tovey, P., Easthope, G. and Adams, J. (eds) (2004) *The Mainstreaming of Complementary and Alternative Medicine: Studies in Social Context.* London: Routledge.

Verhoef, M., Scott, C. and Hilsden, R. (1998) A multi-method research study on the use of complementary therapies among patients with inflammatory bowel disease. *Alternative Therapies in Health and Medicine* 4: 68–71.

Vincent, C. and Furnham, A. (1996) Why do patients turn to complementary medicine? An empirical study. *British Journal of Clinical Psychology* 35: 37–48.

Wolsko, P., Eisenberg, D., Davis, R., Ettner, S. and Phillips, R. (2002) Insurance coverage, medical conditions, and visits to alternative medicine providers: Results of a national survey. *Archives on Internal Medicine* 162: 281–7.

Yeh, G., Eisenberg, D., David, R. and Phillips, R. (2002) Use of complementary and alternative medicine among persons with diabetes mellitus: Results of a national survey. *American Journal of Public Health* 92: 1648–52.

CHAPTER 2

Relief, risk and renewal: Mixed therapy regimens in an Australian suburb

LINDA CONNOR

Introduction

In recent decades, health care has been transformed by the proliferation of non-biomedical therapies that are often referred to in academic literature by such terms as 'alternative' or 'complementary' medicine, or the acronym CAM. However, from the perspective of users, who are often pluralistic and pragmatic in their orientation to healing modalities, 'mixed therapy regimens' is a less dichotomized and more appropriate conceptualization of the process of seeking health care from diverse sources of expertise.

This chapter draws on data collected as part of an ethnographic community-based study of health and illness in an Australian suburb (named 'Oceanpoint' by the research team). Utilizing an inductive approach, the analysis explores the understandings that health care users themselves have of the diverse treatment options available to them.

Mixed therapy regimens in Oceanpoint: An overview

Oceanpoint is a coastal suburb of about 3000 people and approximates the Australian average for many of its sociodemographic indicators (Australian Bureau of Statistics, 2001). The suburb is diverse in terms of socioeconomic strata and household types and a reasonably representative selection of the

Source: Connor, L. (2004) Relief, risk and renewal: Mixed therapy regimens in an Australian suburb. *Social Science and Medicine* 59(8): 1695–1705. Abridged version reprinted with kind permission of Elsevier Ltd.

adult population, by gender, age, occupation, household type and residential location, was achieved (see original paper for more study design details).

In Oceanpoint, it is not uncommon for people to seek treatment from more than one kind of practitioner for the same symptoms, and to visit several kinds of alternative practitioners. In a number of cases, visits to alternative practitioners were made after recommendation from friends and relatives. There were also a number of visits that were prompted either by the recommendation of a doctor or other biomedical health professional, or after approaching a doctor to gain approval prior to alternative therapy. The range of practitioners consulted was diverse and interviewees' own labels for these practitioners have been used.

Lay constructions of therapeutic pluralism

The members of the research team, both GPs and anthropologists, started out with a rough working concept of 'alternative' or 'complementary' medicine. By this we meant those healing modalities that are not part of state-authorized biomedical services, but are offered on a fee-for-service basis by other practitioners with varying types of training and certification. However, we gradually learned from our research that this dichotomous model was not universally used in Oceanpoint. People conceptualized the pluralism that characterizes health services in contemporary suburban Australia in many different ways. This was partly expressed in the terminology they used to refer to the types of therapies available, but unfolded more tellingly in interviews, focus groups and casual conversation, as details of therapy regimens emerged.

Perhaps the only generalization that can be made about residents' utilization of diverse healing resources is that they saw themselves moving among a range of choices. For this reason I have chosen the term 'mixed therapy regimens' to refer to the situation in which people may be using multiple types of therapists and therapies at any one time, or moving in serial fashion from one type of therapy to another.

Issues of legitimacy and effectiveness

How did residents view the legitimacy of alternative therapists? Evaluations of legitimate practice made from within any particular professional knowledge system may not correspond to those of client or patient groups. The scientific legitimacy of a health profession such as biomedicine, and the associated politico-legal legitimacy of practitioners, must contend with the clinical legitimacy of other modalities: the fact that patients experience an improvement in their condition (Willis, 1994: 64). Scientific legitimacy was less important to some Oceanpoint respondents than the felt effectiveness of other practitioners' therapies; clinical legitimacy prevailed.

Effectiveness of treatment figures largely in many people's accounts of practitioners, whether alternative or biomedical. Claire, a 36-year-old small business owner suffering from general lassitude, persevered for weeks with a vile-tasting herbal brew from a Chinese herbalist, but eventually ceased to take it: 'I didn't feel any different.' While acknowledging that such preparations are 'not a sort of a quick fix' and are 'more like a tonic', Claire 'chickened out' because of the unpleasantness of the therapy, which was not proving efficacious. When Garry, a retired storeman aged 62, was asked how he would feel about trying an alternative therapist, he replied:

> Oh, if they work. If you've done everything before and nothing worked and then somebody suggested going to see, like acupuncture and that, yeah. Because my mother's had it, she said it worked.

Most residents profess agnosticism about the knowledge claims of particular therapeutic systems. People evince a preparedness to search for the right therapy when their health problem is refractory to their usual strategies of help seeking, even if this means 'chopping and changing'. They do not in general make a priori judgements about a particular healing modality, preferring to rely on recommendations from trusted members of their social network, and judging effectiveness in terms of their own personal outcome. Speed of relief is an important criterion of efficacy, but not the only one.

The symbolic value of 'natural therapies'

Non-biomedical therapies are frequently described as 'natural', and indeed the term 'natural therapy' in some contexts is used as a synonym for 'alternative medicine'. The term 'natural' seems to imply something about the way in which these therapies work on the body and yet precise mechanisms of action are rarely specified by residents. Rather, 'natural' is often associated with those treatments and medicines that can be used at the discretion of the sufferer. Sometimes it implies therapies with simple ingredients that free the sufferer from the expense of commodified products.

Claire says of her search for relief that took her to the Chinese herbalist:

> I was just feeling tired and run down and sort of looking for something natural that might be able to help my body.

Being 'natural' signifies a lack of danger or risk that renders these therapies more amenable to personal decision making and control rather than professional medical surveillance. One of the most salient threats to their health for Oceanpoint residents was environmental pollution from numerous sources, a form of health threat over which individuals reportedly felt themselves to have very little control. The use of 'natural' therapies can be seen as a counterweight to the diffuse forms of disability and malaise that are often associated with environmental pollution and other threats of modern life, in which the manufactured pharmaceuticals prescribed by doctors are sometimes included.

In many discussions, 'natural therapies' figure as commodities purchased from the health food shop or the therapist's premises. In terms of their action on the body, sufferers value them for their effectiveness in symptom relief, and in this respect they are no different from the way in which biomedical treatments are valued. Also included in the 'natural' category are particular vitamins and herbs that are commonly encountered in residents' therapy regimens. While the definition of a vitamin in nutritional science is quite specific, in residents' accounts there are a whole class of health-giving substances that are often self-administered in a preventive or health-maintaining fashion, which are assimilated to the class of 'vitamin'.

The symbolic value of pharmaceuticals: Toxic therapies

While vitamins are viewed as natural and benign in their action on the body, respondents asserted that the medicines prescribed by biomedical health professionals can have quite opposite effects. Some people voiced a strong critique of drugs and the pharmaceutical industry, as well as the competency and training of biomedical practitioners. Many respondents had stories of friends and relatives whom they considered had suffered some form of damage from prescribed pharmaceuticals. Murray, a 50-year-old school teacher, and his wife Barbara had the following story:

> BARBARA: Well, both Murray's parents, we saw them pumped full of pills, didn't we? And it didn't ultimately help that much except they became dependent on whatever the drugs were.
> MURRAY: Well, that's right, although those –
> BARBARA: Your mother actually – she had so much Indosid she died of a haemorrhaging ulcer.
> INT: Oh, really?
> BARBARA: So we're a bit suspicious about medication, you know.

In the light of opinions such as these, residents' use of vitamins, over-the-counter pharmaceuticals and health food products can be understood as acts of risk avoidance, and of assertion of control over the healing process, although some people with a more stoic disposition may reject these options altogether.

Rather than the biomedical professionals being the reference points in mapping out therapeutic regimens based on prescription pharmaceuticals, relatives and friends, as well as alternative therapists and mass media, have a significant role. The agency of the sufferer and the sufferer's significant others is asserted over and above biomedicine's institutional dominance. In some cases, this involves a 'radical critique' of biomedicine on the basis of criteria such as the purported complicity between doctors and drug companies, or the poor training of doctors. In other cases, patients' agency may also be informed by more personalized resistance; that is, that the drugs haven't worked or have caused intolerable side-effects.

The moral universe of healing

Healing is a moral relationship as well as a technical or social one, invoking judgements of honesty, kindness and integrity. Moral evaluations pervade the accounts of biomedical and non-biomedical ministrations in the previous section. Likewise, residents' descriptions of their encounters with non-biomedical practitioners are sometimes suffused with moral judgements.

Some among the respondents drew on moral discourses of fraud and chicanery in their evaluations of non-biomedical practitioners. Lucy described an iridologist she visited as a 'charlatan' because 'he didn't tell me anything that I hadn't already told him'. Cynthia, who suffered from chronic back pain and other undiagnosed complaints, had been pressured by a friend of her father to visit an alternative therapist whom she described as a 'crazy guru' who used 'electro-magnetic radiation and all this sort of stuff'. Cynthia subsequently embarked on a letter-writing campaign to expose alternative practitioners whom she sees as exploiting desperately ill people with 'all this pseudo-scientific medical hocus-pocus that they sell to people'.

These assertions of fraud and deception point to the more tenuous politico-legal legitimacy of alternative practitioners compared to their biomedical counterparts. In their criticisms of biomedical therapies, respondents drew on moral discourses that challenged doctors' competency and caring rather than imputing dishonesty. Murray, cited earlier, called his doctor a 'bastard' because he did not regard the doctor as properly informing him about the dangerous side-effects of a prescribed medication. Graham (whose case is discussed in more detail in Porteous *et al.*, 2001) suffered from anxiety, headaches, sleeplessness and lassitude and could not work for several months. His initial diagnosis of depression was eventually changed to a number of hormonal, pituitary and viral illnesses. Looking back on his experiences, Graham refers to the early doctors as 'a bunch of donkeys' who 'should have turned around and done it better and done it properly' (Porteous *et al.*, 2001: 334). The perception that some biomedical doctors do not care as much as they should implies a moral judgement about greed and speed that contrasts with attributes of nurturance and insight that some respondents claimed were a strength of alternative treatment.

Conclusion

The growth of therapeutic alternatives in Australia has increased markedly in the past few decades, in keeping with a general diversification and expansion of the capitalist economy in which increasing areas of life, including medicine, are opened up to the forces of commoditization and market competition (Easthope, 1993). Some alternative therapies are supported by private health insurance, to which many Australians do not subscribe. Not too many people complained about the cost of treatment, unless they perceived that it was not effective, although cost may have been a disincentive for those on lower incomes to try it in the first place.

Why do people seek out alternative therapists and construct mixed therapy regimens? One epidemiological answer to this question revolves around the greater prevalence of chronic and functional disorders among the population (or at least those more affluent parts of it) associated with greater longevity, better public health and biomedicine's success in controlling many infectious diseases. Such broadly based generalizations do not have much force in explaining the particularities of residents' views and experiences that we encountered in Oceanpoint. The advantage of the ethnographic method deployed in this study lies in the insights it provides into the nature of residents' agency in the construction of mixed therapy regimens. Sufferers have different reasons at different times for seeking out non-biomedical practitioners, and they are purposeful and pragmatic in doing so. Some have obviously experienced dissatisfaction with biomedical treatments and practitioners, and they construct mixed therapy regimens in the course of their search for relief from the pain and incapacity of various health problems, often combining what they regard as the best (or least harmful) of biomedical and non-biomedical therapies. In this context, mixed therapy regimens can be viewed as a means of undermining the biomedical verification of disease by subjecting such powerful knowledge to the relativizing effects of alternative explanations and treatments.

In striving for wellness, many agents interact. As well as the patient, practitioners and support persons, there is the agency of the illness itself, which can often be experienced as more powerful than all other agents combined, something that has to be 'beaten'. Alternative etiologies, diagnoses and treatments, or, more radical still, alternative epistemologies, may weaken the power of the disease-as-agent over other agents in the process.

Other residents at times seem to be engaged not so much in a battle against powerful disease agents, but rather in the project of remaking the self that Giddens has identified as intrinsic to the 'life politics' of late modernity. He defines 'life politics' as 'a politics of self-actualization in a reflexively ordered environment, where that reflexivity links self and body to systems of global scope' (Giddens, 1991: 214). According to Giddens, part of the reflexive social action in which people engage is the reappropriation of expert knowledge back into the layperson's sphere. This is quite a useful way of understanding the valorization of the 'natural' among the Oceanpoint residents discussed in this chapter, implying as it does elements of healing that are not under the control of the dominant biomedical institutions. Likewise, we can appreciate the particular ways in which people rejected prescription pharmaceuticals as part of their critical stance towards 'expert systems', as these impact directly on the body, and the breakdown of trust in professional knowledge.

Mixed therapy regimens can also be viewed as a defensive response to the experience of living in a 'risk society', in which awareness of hazards and risks created by human agency is a central feature of life (Beck, 1999). Much of the more non-specific use of alternative therapies is directed towards fortifying the body against the hazards of modernity, such as over-work or alienating work, over-use of addictive substances, over-stimulation, and pollution of air, soil, water and food by the products of industrialization.

Thus vitamins and herbs, in their commoditized forms, become constructed as antidotes to hazards both past and future that residents perceive as being otherwise beyond their control, part of a project of resistance to the hazards of modernity carried out at the site of the body. All pluralism involves a politics of therapeutic practices. Sufferers' mixed therapy regimens articulate with diverse and sometimes contradictory relationships of power and authority, able to complement institutional medicine, challenge the premises of its authority and define new arenas of health care.

Further reading

Bishop, F.L., Yardley, L. and Lewith, G. (2008) Treat or treatment: A qualitative study analysing patients' use of complementary and alternative medicine. *American Journal of Public Health* 98(9): 1700–05.

Goldner, M. (2004) Consumption as activism: An examination of CAM as part of the consumer movement in health. In P. Tovey, G. Easthope and J. Adams (eds) *The Mainstreaming of Complementary and Alternative Medicine: Studies in Social Context.* London: Routledge.

Nichol, J., Thompson, E.A. and Shaw, A. (2011) Beliefs, decision-making, and dialogue about complementary and alternative medicine (CAM) within families using CAM: A qualitative study. *Journal of Alternative and Complementary Medicine* 17(2): 117–25.

References

Australian Bureau of Statistics (2001) *Australian Census of Population and Housing.* Canberra: Commonwealth of Australia.

Beck, U. (1999) *World Risk Society.* Cambridge: Polity Press.

Easthope, G. (1993) The response of orthodox medicine to the challenge of alternative medicine in Australia. *Australian and New Zealand Journal of Sociology* 29(3): 289–301.

Giddens, A. (1991) *Modernity and Self-Identity: Self and Society in the Late Modern Age*. Stanford, CA: Stanford University Press.

Porteous, J., Higginbotham, N., Freeman, S. and Conno, L. (2001) Qualitative case-control and case-study designs. In N. Higginbotham, G. Albrecht and L. Connor (eds) *Health Zocial Science: A Transdisciplinary and Complexity Perspective*. Melbourne: Oxford University Press, pp. 304–39.

Willis, E. (1994) *Illness and Social Relations: Issues in the Sociology of Health Care*. St Leonards: Allen and Unwin.

CHAPTER 3

Utilizing existing data sets to investigate complementary and alternative medicine consumption: Cohort studies and longitudinal analyses

DAVID SIBBRITT AND JON ADAMS

Introduction

Health-related data sets resulting from cohort or longitudinal studies (that is, studies where a group of people are followed in terms of their health experiences over many years) are abundant throughout the world. While the research aim and scope of such studies do not necessarily include CAM, some are concerned with CAM-related issues (for instance consultation with a CAM practitioner or consumption of vitamin/mineral/herbal supplements). A focused analysis of CAM users is often neglected in these studies and the potential to explore a rich source of information on CAM use and CAM users frequently remains unexplored (Adams, 2007).

This chapter draws on the experience of the authors in conducting CAM-focused secondary data analysis (SDA) of cohort studies to help describe the advantages and disadvantages of analysing existing longitudinal data sets with a view to CAM use and users.

Source: Sibbritt, D. (2006) Utilising and analysing existing datasets for CAM research: A focus upon cohort studies. In J. Adams (ed.) *Researching Complementary and Alternative Medicine*. London: Routledge. Abridged version reprinted with kind permission of Routledge (Taylor and Francis Ltd).

CAM use and CAM users: Towards longitudinal analyses

There are a considerable number of studies in the literature that have reported primary empirical data with regard to CAM use and CAM users (see Chapter 1 in this collection for more details). In addition to this work there have been a number of studies on CAM use based on secondary data analyses of existing study databases (Adams *et al.*, 2003a, 2009; Sibbritt *et al.*, 2003, 2004, 2011; Steinsbekk *et al.*, 2007, 2008; Sibbritt and Adams 2010), including many studies that have analysed the National Health Interview Survey (NHIS) data conducted in the United States (Kessler *et al.*, 2001; Tindle *et al.*, 2005; Upchurch and Chyu 2005). It is interesting to note that even though these latter studies analyse NHIS data, longitudinal comparisons across the survey time periods have proved difficult due to changes in the wording of questions on CAM use, the sampling strategies and mode of administration (Tindle *et al.*, 2005).

In terms of future directions for CAM use and CAM user research, commentators have highlighted the need for longitudinal (or cohort) analyses to chart the trends in CAM consumption and the need for international comparative analyses to obtain a cross-cultural perspective to health and CAM (Adams *et al.*, 2003a). As such writing highlights, there is a very real and significant role for the use of existing data sets and SDA in CAM consumption research.

Before exploring a number of benefits and challenges of such SDA, it is first necessary to provide a brief overview of the SDA on CAM consumption research that will serve as case studies and help illustrate relevant points later in the chapter.

Background to SDA on CAM consumption: The examples of ALSWH and HUNT

Recent years have seen the analysis of CAM consumption data from two existing cohort studies: the Australian Longitudinal Survey on Women's Health (ALSWH) and the Nord-Trøndelag Health Study (HUNT). Both of these studies are longitudinal in design, are concerned with various health issues and have survey questions that elicit information about participants' CAM consumption. For both cohort studies, a substudy team (including the authors) has initiated and developed SDA for the purposes of examining CAM use and CAM users.

The ALSWH study was designed to investigate multiple factors affecting the health and well-being of women over a 20-year period. Women in three age groups ('young' 18–23, 'mid age' 45–50 and 'older' 70–75 years) were randomly selected from the national Medicare database, with over-representation of women living in rural and remote areas. The baseline survey was conducted in 1996 (n=14779 young, n=14099 mid age, and n=12939 older women). The HUNT study is a population-based study conducted in the Nord-Trøndelag county, located in central Norway. The first phase of this study (HUNT 1) collected information on 74 599 persons aged 20 and older, and was primarily designed to cover four topics (hypertension, diabetes, lung diseases and quality of life). In the second phase (HUNT 2), there were 65 495 participants aged 13 years and over. HUNT 2 used identical or similar questions and assessments of hypertension, diabetes and quality of life as in HUNT 1, but was much more comprehensive, with a wider age range and the collection of more data on each participant, covering an extensive range of health-related topics.

It is important to note that while this chapter focuses on cohort studies, not all SDA relating to CAM consumption is conducted on large cohort datasets. For example, a SDA of CAM use has been undertaken from an original survey designed to measure the supportive care needs of patients with cancer (Girgis *et al.*, 2005). This survey contained questioning in the 'background information' section asking patients about their use of a number of CAM modalities, allowing the creation of a 'CAM user' variable and subsequent modelling employing other variables (for example demographics, health status) measured in the survey instrument (Girgis *et al.*, 2005).

Advantages of utilizing existing cohort study data sets

Perhaps the greatest advantage afforded through analysis of an existing cohort data set for CAM consumption is simply its existence; this is particularly important given the potential difficulty in attracting research funding to undertake large-scale examination of CAM use. This may appear a less than ideal approach, but pre-existing data sets may in many circumstances constitute the only opportunity for CAM consumption and CAM user research. As well as benefits regarding funding, using pre-existing data sets also means that data cleaning (that is, checking for data errors, outliers and so on) and a data dictionary (that is, a database with question details and formats) will both have been completed prior to commencing the substudy – details and procedures that require much time and resource if undertaken as part of the initial design.

There are also some useful statistical advantages in analysing cohort data sets. Typically, the data set will consist of a large sample of participants. This is obviously a design priority for the original researchers in terms of generating adequate statistical power to answer their specific research questions. As such, it is more than likely that there will also be sufficient statistical power to answer CAM-related research questions. These data sets will also tend to have information collected on many variables (including demographic, health status and health service utilization variables), allowing exploration of numerous, wide-ranging factors related to CAM consumption.

Finally, as study designs go, cohort studies are a highly regarded design, especially in comparison to cross-sectional studies (Christie *et al.*, 1990). The major advantage that cohort studies have over cross-sectional studies is that they contain a time component. In cross-sectional studies, measurements are made on an individual at one point in time. Thus, cross-sectional studies can only report the prevalence of a factor of interest (such as CAM use) at a certain time point. In cohort studies, measurements of the same individuals are taken repeatedly over time. This allows investigators to report the prevalence of a factor of interest at several time points, as well as the incidence of a factor of interest and change in a factor of interest over time. It is this last point that is the most appealing: with cohort studies we can characterize the change in a factor of interest (such as CAM use) over time and the factors that influence change. So in terms of CAM use over time, different types of CAM users can be identified: those who consistently use CAM; those who consistently do not use CAM; and those who are intermittent users of CAM. Comparisons of these groups of CAM users and non-users can provide considerable insight into the knowledge about, and reasons for, CAM use over time.

For example, the study by Sibbritt *et al.* (2005) conducted a longitudinal analysis of mid-aged women's consultations with CAM practitioners. The authors were able to report that the growing prevalence of CAM practitioner consultations, from 28 per cent to 29 per cent during the period 1996–98, was deceptive in that this 'snapshot' of CAM users failed to show that the net increase was due to 1058 CAM users in 1996 no longer using CAM in 1998 (CAM relinquishers) and 1146 CAM non-users in 1996 becoming CAM users in 1998 (CAM adopters). Furthermore, this work was able to show that changes in area of residence, use of prescription and non-prescription medications, number of general practitioner (or family doctor) visits and physical health all contributed to the adoption of CAM.

While studies on CAM use/users are beginning to attract some funding and attention (Wider and Ernst, 2003), there remain many gaps in this field (Adams *et al.*, 2003a). As this chapter has illustrated, SDA of pre-existing data sets is certainly one option that should, if possible, be considered by researchers looking to expand and enhance the investigation of CAM use and users. Nevertheless, pre-existing data sets and SDA are not without their challenges and limitations. A number of these limitations – which should be adequately considered by any potential researcher contemplating SDA – are now outlined and discussed below.

Limitations of utilising existing cohort study data sets

One main limitation of using an existing data set to examine CAM use and CAM users is that the definition of CAM may not be ideal. For example, in the baseline ALSWH questionnaire for the mid-age cohort (conducted in 1996), the question relating to CAM was: 'Have you consulted an alternative health practitioner (e.g. herbalist, chiropractor, naturopath, acupuncturist etc.) in the last twelve months for your own health?' In this case, CAM use is defined as consultation with a CAM practitioner, but the definition excludes self-prescribed CAM use (such as vitamin and mineral supplements). Therefore, any prevalence of CAM use identified will be an under-estimate of the true CAM use in the population. In addition, only a few examples of CAM practitioners are provided, thus respondents may vary in the range of thera-pists they include under the heading of 'alternative practitioner'. It is not too surprising that these large cohort studies do not refine definition and nomen-clature regarding CAM; after all, there are often many competing areas for focus and CAM is not necessarily a primary consideration.

Another potential problem that may be encountered when attempting to analyse longitudinal trends in CAM consumption is a changing definition of CAM across different survey periods. For example, consider the wording of the questions used to determine CAM user status for women in the young cohort of the ALSWH study. In time period 1 (1996), the definition of CAM user status is defined by answers to the question: 'How many times have you consulted the following for your own health in the last 12 months? … [includ-ing in a list of practitioners] an 'alternative' health practitioner (e.g. chiroprac-tor, naturopath, acupuncturist, herbalist etc.)?' In time period 2 (1998), this definition of CAM user status has changed somewhat and the question now reads: 'Have you consulted the following people for your own health in the last 12 months? … [including in a list of practitioners] an 'alternative' health practitioner (e.g. naturopath, acupuncturist, herbalist etc.)?' Note that the question in time period 2 does not include chiropractor as an example of an alternative practitioner. In Australia, it has been shown that chiropractors are the most commonly consulted CAM practitioner group (Xue *et al.*, 2007). Given this context, a number of important questions are raised: How impor-tant is it that chiropractor was omitted from the example of CAM practitioners in time period 2? Will subjects consider chiropractors to be alternative health practitioners if they are not included in the list of examples? If there is a decline in the number of subjects who indicate that they consulted a CAM practi-tioner, is it possible to know if there genuinely was a decline in CAM practi-tioner consultation or is the decline due to subjects not considering chiropractors as being alternative health practitioners? In this particular study the change in definition was considered significant enough by the authors to preclude comparisons across the two time periods.

Using an existing data set has another disadvantage in that the reference population may be restricted by the study design; the population to whom the results can be generalized may only be a subset of the community. For example, the ALSWH study was conducted only on women in certain age groups (18–23 years, 45–50 years and 70–75 years) who could speak/read English. In the case of the HUNT study, the population of Nord-Trøndelag county is in many respects a representative sample of the wider Norwegian population with regard to geography, economy, industry, sources of income, age distribution, morbidity and mortality. However, the county lacks a large city, and the level of education and income are somewhat lower than the national average. Nevertheless, it should be noted that these studies do provide some of the largest CAM consumption data and analyses in the world (Adams *et al.*, 2003b) and, as explained earlier, the issue of sample size can in itself be considered a major benefit of conducting such SDA for CAM consumption.

Conclusion

Many health-related data sets, both cross-sectional and longitudinal, do exist around the world and conducting secondary data analyses is relatively easy, can expose early-stage investigators to experienced researchers already involved in the study and can lead to additional analyses. For example, by analysing the ALSWH data with a focus on CAM use, the ALSWH CAM substudy team has been included in ongoing discussions regarding future surveys of the ALSWH cohorts, helping to refine the survey questions and thereby allowing the design of more interesting and pertinent CAM use/user research.

Statistical analyses of pre-existing data sets provide one interesting path to develop the CAM user and CAM consumption research field. Nevertheless, as this chapter suggests, such secondary analysis is not without its own particular difficulties. The definition of CAM users may not be ideal; the definition of CAM users may change over time when the study data is generated from a cohort; and the reference population may be restrictive. However, the advantages usually outweigh the disadvantages in that the data set exists; it may be void of difficulties associated with data collection; and most data errors are typically already cleaned. As such, researchers can utilize the possible resource of SDA to help advance CAM consumption research and to address a broad range of related questions regarding users, nature of use and patterns of use over time.

Further reading

Adams, J. (2007) Restricting CAM consumption research: Denying insights for practice and policy. *Complementary Therapies in Medicine* 15(2): 75–6.

References

Adams, J. (2007) 'Restricting CAM consumption research: Denying insights for practice and policy. *Complementary Therapies in Medicine* 15(2): 75–6.

Adams, J., Easthope, G. and Sibbritt, D. (2003a) Exploring the relationship between women's health and the use of complementary and alternative medicine. *Complementary Therapies in Medicine* 11: 156–8.

Adams, J., Sibbritt, D., Easthope, G. and Young, A. (2003b) The profile of women who use complementary and alternative medicine (CAM) in Australia. *Medical Journal of Australia* 179(6): 297–300.

Adams, J., Sibbritt, D. and Young, A. (2009) A longitudinal analysis of older Australian women's consultations with complementary and alternative medicine (CAM) practitioners, 1996–2005. *Age and Ageing* 38: 93–9.

Christie, D., Gordon, I. and Heller, R. (1990) *Epidemiology: An Introductory Text for Medical and Other Health Science Students.* Kensington: New South Wales University Press.

Girgis, A., Adams, J. and Sibbritt, D. (2005) The use of complementary and alternative therapies by patients with cancer. *Oncology Research* 15: 281–9.

Kessler, R.C., Davis, R.B., Foster, D.F. *et al.* (2001) Long-term trends in the use of complementary and alternative medicine therapies in the United States. *Annals of Internal Medicine* 135(4): 262–8.

Sibbritt, D. and Adams, J. (2010) Back pain amongst 8,910 young Australian women: A longitudinal analysis of the use of conventional providers, complementary and alternative medicine (CAM) practitioners and self-prescribed CAM. *Clinical Rheumatology* 29: 25–32.

Sibbritt, D., Adams, J., Easthope, G. and Young, A. (2003) Complementary and Alternative Medicine (CAM) use among elderly Australian women who have cancer. *Supportive Care in Cancer* 11: 548–50.

Sibbritt, D., Adams, J. and Lui, C. (2011) The prevalence and characteristics of young and mid-age women who use yoga and meditation: Results of a nationally representative survey of 19,209 Australian women. *Complementary Therapies in Medicine* 19(2): 71–7.

Sibbritt, D., Adams, J. and Young, A. (2004) A longitudinal analysis of mid-aged women's use of complementary and alternative medicine (CAM) in Australia, 1996–1998. *Women and Health* 40(4): 41–56.

Steinsbekk, A., Adams, J., Sibbritt, D., Jacobsen, G. and Johnsen, R. (2007) A comparison of general practice users, complementary and alternative medicine users, and those who use both. *Scandinavian Journal of Primary Health Care* 25(2): 86–92.

Steinsbekk, A., Adams, J., Sibbritt, D., Johnsen, R. and Jacobsen, G. (2008) Sociodemographic characteristics and health perceptions among male and female visitors to CAM practitioners in a Norwegian total population study. *Research in Complementary Medicine (Forschende Komplementärmedizin)* 15(3): 146–51.

Tindle, H.A., Davis, R.B., Phillips, R.S. and Eisenberg, D.M. (2005) Trends in use of complementary and alternative medicine by US adults: 1997–2002. *Alternative Therapies in Health and Medicine* 11(1):42–9.

Upchurch, D.M. and Chyu, L. (2005) Use of complementary and alternative medicine among American women. *Women's Health Issues* 15: 5–13.

Wider, B. and Ernst, E. (2003) CAM research funding in the UK: Surveys of medical charities in 1999 and 2002. *Complementary Therapies in Medicine* 11(3):165–7.

Xue, C., Zhang, A.L., Lin, V., Da Costa, C. and Story, D.F. (2007) Complementary and alternative medicine use in Australia: A national population-based survey. *Journal of Alternative and Complementary Medicine* 13(6): 643–50.

Complementary and alternative medicine through the life cycle

Introduction

As Chapter 1 identified, findings from large cohort studies reveal CAM users as more likely to be women than men and CAM does appear to lend itself to a number of women's health issues (including pregnancy, menstruation and menopause). Nevertheless, we still know relatively little about women's use of CAM and this is an area of great potential for the wider CAM research community. Highlighting and also responding to such research gaps in one specific area, Chapter 4 presents a critical review of literature on CAM use during pregnancy. As Adams and colleagues explain, while research activity around CAM use during pregnancy has intensified over recent years, a number of key issues still require in-depth empirical investigation.

One of the limitations of most general CAM consumption studies (as overviewed in Chapters 1 and 3) is their focus on adult use and users. As Adams and colleagues explain (Chapter 5), CAM use among paediatric populations also appears to be increasing and this is indeed an exciting and fruitful topic for future investigation. Adams and colleagues outline the paediatric patient characteristics and reasons for using CAM, as well as exploring some of the medico-legal and ethical considerations arising from such use. Given the lack of spontaneous disclosure about CAM use by families (see Chapter 15 for further discussion of patient–clinician communication about TCIM), the authors highlight the importance of paediatricians enquiring about such use and maintaining their continuing professional development in this growing area of paediatrics.

Another area in which CAM has been identified as holding potential is for treating and coping with chronic illness and other conditions experienced in later life. Recent years have witnessed a boom in trials on the efficacy of CAM with regard to common ageing ailments; this is a clinical evidence base that looks set to continue to grow in the near future. However, in contrast, relatively little research has explored the social and cultural dimensions of CAM use among older people, and this is especially the case with regards to the ways in which older people use CAM to cope with health challenges or disabilities and how they make sense of this consumption in daily life. One exception to this trend has been the research of Cartwright (Chapter 6), who has explored the experiences of older people using complementary health care. As the findings of Cartwright's study reveal, the use of CAM benefits older people's perceptions of quality of life and encourages greater engagement with their health through empowerment.

CHAPTER 4

Women's use of complementary and alternative medicine during pregnancy: A critical review of the literature

JON ADAMS, CHI WAI LUI, DAVID SIBBRITT, ALEX BROOM,
JON WARDLE, CAROLINE HOMER, AMIE STEEL AND
SHOSHANNAH BECK

Introduction

Women are leading CAM consumption trends (Adams *et al.*, 2003b) and much potential appears to exist for these products and therapies for women's health (Adams et al., 2004, 2003a), including for use during pregnancy. Although the evidence base for efficacy of CAM use in the gestation period is gradually emerging (Smith and Cochrane, 2009), understanding is lacking about the pattern of use of this kind of treatment in pregnancy. This chapter presents a critical review of literature on CAM use during pregnancy, focusing on both over-the-counter treatment and therapy/practitioner-based therapies.

Methods

A search of research articles between 1999 and 2008 was conducted on MEDLINE, CINAHL, AMED and Maternity and Infant Care, using a range of relevant keywords. The search was confined to peer-reviewed articles published in English and containing an abstract (for more details of the methods

Source: Adams, J., Lui, C., Sibbritt, D., Broom, A., Wardle, J., Homer, C. and Beck, S. (2009) Women's use of complementary and alternative medicine during pregnancy: A critical review of the literature. *Birth* 36(3): 237–45. Abridged version reprinted with kind permission of John Wiley & Sons Ltd (Wiley-Blackwell).

employed, see the original paper). In total, 24 articles reporting findings from 21 empirical studies (three research projects were reported by more than one article) met the selection criteria. A summary of the basic details of these research-based studies is presented in Table 4.1. The table also reports the coverage of these studies with respect to four key themes: user prevalence and profile; motivation and condition of use; perception and self-reported evaluation; and referral and information sources. These four key themes were identified from the content of the 24 articles reviewed.

Results

User prevalence and profile

The studies reported a wide variation in the use of CAM during pregnancy. The prevalence rate of those 14 studies that had relatively large sample sizes (n>200) ranged from 1 to 87 per cent (with 9 falling between 20 and 60 per cent). Differences in definition of CAM, research design and focus on different time frames of pregnancy are factors that may contribute to the disparity. Although such differences make it difficult to compare findings across studies, most of the research concluded that consumption of CAM was common among pregnant women.

Use of various CAM therapies was reported, including acupuncture/ acupressure, aromatherapy, massage, yoga, homeopathy and chiropractic care (Table 4.1). The most frequently used herbal medicines during pregnancy were ginger, raspberry leaf and echinacea. Evidence also shows that many pregnant women had used more than one complementary product or service.

Consistent with the findings on user characteristics of CAM more generally (Adams *et al.*, 2003b), women who are older, have higher education and income and report more physical symptoms are more likely to use CAM during their pregnancy. Previous or habitual use of CAM (Hollyer *et al.*, 2002; Lapi *et al.*, 2008), primiparity (Forster *et al.*, 2006), not smoking (Forster *et al.*, 2006) and planning a natural birth (Hepner *et al.*, 2002) were also factors found to be associated with consumption of CAM.

Motivation and condition of use

The studies reported that CAM was used for relief of stress and pregnancy-related complaints, as preparation for labour and for general health benefits during pregnancy. Two studies (Hollyer *et al.*, 2002; Wang *et al.*, 2005) specifically examined the use of CAM for reducing nausea and vomiting and low-back pain during pregnancy.

Review findings suggest that CAM was used consistently throughout the three trimesters of pregnancy. For those who stopped using a complementary product or service during pregnancy, the most commonly cited reason was a

Table 4.1 Research-based studies on the use of complementary and alternative medicine in pregnancy, 1999–2008

Author/year	Country	Focus of study	CAM modality	Method	Sample characteristics	I	II	III	IV
Byrne et al., 2002	Australia	Prevalence and attitude towards CAM use	Herbal preparations, aromatherapy oils, homeopathic preparations, flower essences, therapeutic oils, antioxidants and other dietary supplements	Interview with standard questionnaire	n = 48 Patients of antenatal wards	√	√	√	×
Calvert and Steen, 2007 **Steen and Calvert, 2007**	UK	Use and impact of CAM during childbirth on women and their birth partners	Self-administered homeopathic kit (10 remedies)	Semi-structured questionnaire and follow-up interview	n = 19 (women only) Women with an expected date of delivery within the study period	√	×	√	√
Chuang et al., 2007	Taiwan	Prevalence and related factors of CAM use	Chinese herbal medicine	Interview with structured questionnaire	n = 1783 Postpartum women (6 months after their deliveries) identified in national birth registration	√	√	×	×
Forster et al., 2006	Australia	Prevalence and attitude towards CAM use	Herbal and vitamin supplements	Self-administered questionnaire	n = 588 Patients (36–38 weeks' gestation) of antenatal clinic/birth centre	√	√	√	√
Furlow et al., 2008	US	Physicians' and patients' attitude towards CAM	Various, including movement therapies, biofeedback, acupuncture and yoga	Survey	n = 480 (women only) Obstetric patients of a health care centre	√	√	×	√
Gaffney and Smith, 2004	Australia	Attitude towards CAM use	Various, including vitamins, herbal therapies and massage	Interview with structured questionnaire	n = 220 Patients (≥36 weeks' gestation) of an antenatal clinic	√	√	√	×

Themes

continued overleaf

Table 4.1 continued

Author/year	Country	Focus of study	CAM modality	Method	Sample characteristics	Themes* I	II	III	IV
Glover et al., 2003	US	Use of OTC and herbal medicine in rural area	OTC and herbal prescriptions	Repeated interviews with structured questionnaire over 26 months	n = 578 (with 2086 interviews) Patients from outreach clinic or medical centre	✓	✓	×	×
Hepner et al., 2002	US	Prevalence and attitude towards CAM use	23 commonly used herbal remedies plus others named by the participants	Self-administered questionnaire	n = 734 Hospital patients expected to deliver within 20 weeks	✓	✓	✓	✓
Hollyer et al., 2002	Canada	Pattern of CAM use and efficacy for reducing nausea and vomiting	Various, including ginger, acupressure and vitamins	Telephone survey	n = 70 Users of a hotline on nausea and vomiting during pregnancy	✓	✓	✓	✓
Holst et al., 2008	Sweden	Prevalence and pregnancy outcome of herbal drug use	Various, including iron-rich herbs, ginseng, valerian and echinacea	Analysis of birth register	n = 860 215 Records of birth register (usage refers to first trimester only)	✓	✓	×	×
Hope-Allan et al., 2004	Australia	Attitude towards CAM use	Acupuncture	Self-administered questionnaire	n = 37 Patients of an antenatal clinic	✓	✓	✓	✓
Lapi et al., 2008	Italy	Usage, attitude towards and knowledge of CAM drugs	Herbal and natural products, including almond oil, propolis, fennel and mauve	Interview with structured questionnaire	n = 150 Patients (in third trimester) of gynaecology wards	✓	✓	✓	✓
Maats and Crowther, 2002	Australia	Use of OTC and herbal medicine	Vitamin, mineral and herbal supplements	Interview with structured questionnaire	n = 211 Patients (≥26 weeks' gestation) of an antenatal clinic	✓	✓	×	×

Study	Country	Aim	CAM type	Method	Sample	I	II	III	IV
Nordeng and Havnen, 2004; Nordeng and Havnen, 2005	Norway	Prevalence, attitude towards and knowledge of CAM use	Herbal medicine	Interview with structured questionnaire	n = 400 Patients (Norwegian only) who gave birth in a local hospital	✓	✓	✓	✓
Ong et al., 2005	Hong Kong	Prevalence and attitude towards CAM use	Chinese herbal medicine	Self-administered questionnaire	n = 593 Patients of a postnatal ward	✓	✓	×	×
Pinn and Pallett, 2002	Australia	Prevalence and attitude towards CAM use	Herbal medicine	Self-administered questionnaire	n = 305 Patients (16–24 weeks' gestation) of an antenatal clinic	✓	✓	×	×
Refuerzo et al., 2005	US	Prevalence and attitude towards CAM use	OTC and herbal medicine	Self-administered questionnaire	n = 418 Postpartum women before hospital discharge	✓	✓	×	×
Skouteris et al., 2008	Australia	Prevalence and attitude towards CAM use	Various, including massage, vitamins, meditation, yoga and aromatherapy	Self-administered questionnaire	n = 321 Pregnant women in a local community	✓	✓	✓	×
Tsui et al., 2001	US	Prevalence and attitude towards CAM	Dietary supplements	Survey	n = 150 Patients from two birth clinics	✓	✓	×	✓
Wang et al., 2005	US	Pattern of CAM use and efficacy (among women and providers) on reducing low-back pain	Various, including massage, yoga and chiropractic	Survey	n = 950 (women only) Patients of local antenatal clinics	✓	✓	✓	×
Westfall, 2003; Westfall, 2004	Canada	Prevalence and attitude towards CAM use	Herbal medicine	In-depth interview	n = 27 Patients in their third trimester recruited from local midwives' offices or maternal care programmes	✓	✓	✓	✓

* I = User prevalence/profile; II = Motivation/condition of use; III = Perception/self-reported evaluation; IV = Referral and information source. CAM = complementary and alternative medicine; OTC = over-the-counter medicine.

concern about side-effects on the foetus (Tsui et al. 2001; Maats and Crowther, 2002). A lack of information about product safety and advice from a doctor were also reasons given for relinquishing CAM use (Tsui *et al.*, 2001; Hepner *et al.*, 2002).

Perception and self-reported evaluation

Most users regarded CAM as more natural, safe and/or having at least equal efficacy when compared with medical prescriptions for pregnancy and related symptoms (Hollyer *et al.*, 2002; Westfall, 2003; Gaffney and Smith, 2004; Lapi *et al.*, 2008). Many women expressed a greater comfort with using herbal than pharmaceutical drugs. Concurrently, evidence also shows that only small proportions of these women had much knowledge of (Nordeng and Havnen, 2005), or were able to correctly classify, the complementary products they consumed (Lapi *et al.*, 2008). This finding is of concern given that a substantial proportion of women using CAM may be using herbal drugs that may be harmful or provide no information on safety (Nordeng and Havnen, 2004).

When asked about the effectiveness of CAM, many participants intimated some benefit or perceived the intervention to be helpful. Many women in particular endorsed these products or practices for allowing them a more 'active role' in maintaining their health (Hollyer *et al.*, 2002; Gaffney and Smith, 2004).

Referral and information sources

The most common source of referral for CAM use was friends and family (Hepner *et al.*, 2002; Hollyer *et al.*, 2002; Nordeng and Havnen, 2004; Furlow *et al.*, 2008), whereas medical professionals and allied health care practitioners played a relatively insignificant role in referral to complementary treatment (Nordeng and Havnen, 2004; Forster *et al.*, 2006; Furlow *et al.*, 2008). In contrast, allied health professionals and pharmacists remained important as a source for advice on CAM use (Tsui *et al.*, 2001; Nordeng and Havnen, 2005). Print media and the internet were also common channels through which women gained information about complementary treatment (Tsui *et al.*, 2001; Hope-Allen *et al.*, 2004; Furlow *et al.*, 2008).

Discussion

Research examining the use of CAM during pregnancy has intensified over recent years. Nevertheless, this review has identified several gaps in the scientific literature. Although preliminary prevalence and profile data on this topic have begun to emerge, many studies to date have failed to use large-scale samples and much opportunity remains for larger, nationally representative studies to identify prevalence and profile data on a broader scale. In addition, researchers also need to understand the changes in types of product or therapy used during the three trimesters of pregnancy and the considerations behind such trends.

Moreover, the need to explore the lived experience of CAM use in pregnancy is urgent. Survey design or analysis of official records was used in 19 of the 21 studies included in this review, providing a relatively broad snapshot of consumption patterns of CAM. However, these survey instruments provide little insight into the process and logic of women's decision making and the nature of communication about CAM between different stakeholders (such as practitioners and family).

Such work should also be accompanied by in-depth examination of how pregnant women perceive and experience the risks and benefits of using CAM, and the ways in which their consumption may be influenced and shaped by biographical and cultural details. These types of data would be invaluable to maternity care providers who seek a better understanding of the use of CAM and its potential associated risks during pregnancy.

A more detailed understanding of trends in consumption of CAM between pregnancies also requires further attention. Information is lacking about any changes in the use of CAM or of a particular therapy or medicine during the three trimesters of pregnancy. Other future research should examine the experience of CAM use among different ethnic groups during pregnancy (within a particular country or across cultures). In addition, attention needs to be focused on the therapeutic encounter with respect to the use of CAM in maternity care. An exploration of communication and interaction between women and service providers and how this evolves over time provides a significant opportunity for researchers to situate women's use of CAM for pregnancy within wider organizational, professional and cultural contexts.

Further reading

Sibbritt, D., Adams, J. and Lui, C. (2011) Health service utilisation by pregnant women over a seven-year period. *Midwifery* 27(4): 474–6.

Smith, C. and Cochrane, S. (2009) Does acupuncture have a place as an adjunct treatment during pregnancy? A review of randomized controlled trials and systematic reviews. *Birth* 36(3): 246–53.

References

Adams, J., Easthope, G. and Sibbritt, D. (2003a) Exploring the relationship between women's health and the use of complementary and alternative medicine. *Complementary Therapies in Medicine* 11: 156–68.

Adams, J., Easthope, G. and Sibbritt, D. (2004) Researching the utilisation of complementary and alternative medicine (CAM): Where to from here? *Evidence Based Integrative Medicine* 1(3): 169–72.

Adams, J., Sibbritt, D., Easthope, G. and Young, A. (2003b) The profile of women who consult alternative health practitioners in Australia. *Medical Journal of Australia* 179: 297–300.

Beal, M.W. (1998) Women's use of complementary and alternative therapies in reproductive health care. *Journal of Nurse Midwifery* 43(3): 224–34.

Byrne, M.J., Semple, S.J. and Coulthard, K.P. (2002) Complementary medicine use during pregnancy: Interviews with 48 women in a hospital antenatal ward. *Australian Pharmacist* 21(12): 954–9.

Calvert, J. and Steen, M. (2007) Homeopathic remedies for self-administration during childbirth. *British Journal of Midwifery* 15(3): 159–65.

Chuang, C.-H., Hsieh, W.-S., Guo, Y.L. *et al.* (2007) Chinese herbal medicines used in pregnancy: A population-based survey in Taiwan. *Pharmacoepidemiology and Drug Safety* 16(4): 359–472.

Forster, D.A., Denning, A. and Wills, G. *et al.* (2006) Herbal medicine use during pregnancy in a group of Australian women. *BMC Pregnancy and Childbirth* 6: 21.

Furlow, M.L., Patel, D.A., Sen, A. and Liu, J.R. (2008) Physician and patient attitudes towards complementary and alternative medicine in obstetrics and gynecology. *BMC Complementary and Alternative Medicine* 8: 35.

Gaffney, L. and Smith, C. (2004) The views of pregnant women towards the use of complementary therapies and medicines. *Birth Issues* 13(2): 43–50.

Glover, D.D., Amonkar, M., Rybeck, B.F. and Tracy, T.S. (2003) Prescription, over-the-counter, and herbal medicine use in a rural, obstetric population. *American Journal of Obstetrics and Gynecology* 188(4): 1039–45.

Hepner, D.L., Harnett, M., Segal, S. *et al.* (2002) Herbal medicine use in parturients. *Anesthesia and Analgesia* 94(3): 690–93.

Hollyer, T., Boon, H., Georgousis, A. *et al.* (2002) The use of CAM by women suffering from nausea and vomiting during pregnancy. *BMC Complementary and Alternative Medicine* 2: 5.

Holst, L., Nordeng, H. and Haavik, S. (2008) Use of herbal drugs during early pregnancy in relation to maternal characteristics and pregnancy outcome. *Pharmacoepidemiology and Drug Safety* 17(2): 151–9.

Hope-Allan, N., Adams, J., Sibbritt, D. *et al.* (2004) The use of acupuncture in maternity care: A pilot study evaluating the acupuncture service in an Australian hospital antenatal clinic. *Complementary Therapies in Nursing and Midwifery* 10(4): 229–32.

Lapi, F., Vannacci, A., Moschini, M. *et al.* (2008) Use, attitudes and knowledge of complementary and alternative drugs (CADs) among pregnant women: A preliminary survey in Tuscany. *Evidence Based Complementary and Alternative Medicine* 0: nen031v1–nen031.

Maats, F.H. and Crowther, C.A. (2002) Patterns of vitamin, mineral and herbal supplement use prior to and during pregnancy. *Australian and New Zealand Journal of Obstetrics and Gynaecology* 42(5): 494–6.

Nordeng, H. and Havnen, G.C. (2004) Use of herbal drugs in pregnancy: A survey among 400 Norwegian women. *Pharmacoepidemiology and Drug Safety* 13(6): 371–80.

Nordeng, H. and Havnen, G.C. (2005) Impact of socio-demographic factors, knowledge and attitude on the use of herbal drugs in pregnancy. *Acta Obstetricia et Gynecologica Scandinavica* 84(1): 26–33.

Ong, C.O., Chan, L.Y., Yung, P.B. *et al.* (2005) Use of traditional Chinese herbal medicine during pregnancy: A prospective survey. *Acta Obstetricia et Gynecologica Scandinavica* 84(7): 699–700.

Pinn, G. and Pallett, L. (2002) Herbal medicine in pregnancy. *Complement Therapies in Nursing and Midwifery* 8(2): 77–80.

Refuerzo, J.S., Blackwell, S.C., Sokol, R.J. *et al.* (2005) Use of over-the-counter medications and herbal remedies in pregnancy. *American Journal of Perinatology* 22(6): 321–4.

Skouteris, H., Wertheim, E.H., Rallis, S. *et al.* (2008) Use of complementary and alternative medicines by a sample of Australian women during pregnancy. *Australian and New Zealand Journal of Obstetrics and Gynaecology* 48(4): 384–90.

Smith, C. and Cochrane, S. (2009) Does acupuncture have a place as an adjunct treatment during pregnancy? A review of randomized controlled trials and systematic reviews. *Birth* 36(3): 246–53.

Steen, M. and Calvert, J. (2007) Self-administered homeopathy part two: A follow-up study. *British Journal of Midwifery* 15(6): 359–65.

Tsui, B., Dennehy, C.E. and Tsourounis, C. (2001) A survey of dietary supplement use during pregnancy at an academic medical center. *American Journal of Obstetrics and Gynecology* 185(2): 433–7.

Wang, S., DeZinno, P., Fermo, L. *et al.* (2005) Complementary and alternative medicine for low-back pain in pregnancy: A cross-sectional survey. *Journal of Alternative and Complementary Medicine* 11(3): 459–64.

Westfall, R.E. (2003) Herbal healing in pregnancy: Women's experiences. *Journal of Herbal Pharmacotherapy* 3(4): 17–39.

Westfall, R.E. (2004) Use of anti-emetic herbs in pregnancy: Women's choices, and the question of safety and efficacy. *Complementary Therapies in Nursing and Midwifery* 10(1): 30–36.

Complementary and alternative medicine use among infants, children and adolescents

DENISE ADAMS, KATHI KEMPER AND SUNITA VOHRA

Introduction

Complementary and alternative medicine (CAM) use by infants, children and young people is considerable around the world. In this chapter, we explore rates and patterns of CAM use, patient characteristics and reasons for CAM use, as well as medico-legal and ethical considerations.

Rates and patterns of CAM use among paediatric populations

Use of CAM therapies by children and adolescents appears to be increasing, both in the community at large as well as in specific patient populations. A 2004 Australian health survey estimated annual paediatric use at 18.4 per cent (Smith and Eckert, 2006). A community survey in the United States in 2007 reported annual paediatric use of 11.8 per cent (Barnes *et al.*, 2008), up from 2 per cent in 1996 (Davis and Darden, 2003). The most commonly used CAM therapies are listed in Table 5.1.

In outpatient care settings, paediatric CAM use ranges from 20 to 40 per cent, while use in children with recurrent, chronic or incurable conditions can be much higher (Crawford *et al.*, 2006; McCann and Newell, 2006; Kemper *et al.*, 2008; Robinson *et al.*, 2008; Post-White *et al.*, 2009), including asthma (Reznik *et al.*, 2002; Braganza *et al.*, 2003; Dinkevich *et al.*, 2003), neurological or developmental disorders (Hurvitz *et al.*, 2003; Levy and Hyman, 2003; Soo *et al.*, 2005; Harrington *et al.*, 2006; Adams *et al.*, 2009), cancer (Kelly *et al.*, 2000; Kemper and Wornham, 2001; Neuhouser *et al.*, 2001; Sencer and Kelly, 2007), gastrointestinal disorders (Day, 2002; Day *et al.*, 2004; Vlieger

Table 5.1 National community use of paediatric CAM

Study	Type of CAM used
Barnes *et al.* (2008), USA	Non-vitamin, non-mineral, natural health products or dietary supplements (3.9%)
	Chiropractic or osteopathic manipulation (2.8%)
	Deep breathing exercises (2.2%)
	Yoga (2.1%)
	Homeopathic treatment (1.3%)
	Visits to traditional healers (1.1%)
	Massage (1.0%)
	Meditation (1.0%)
Smith and Eckert (2006), Australia	Chiropractic (34%)
	Herbal medicine (34%)
	Massage (21%)
	Aromatherapy (16%)
	Special diets (15%)

et al., 2008; Wong *et al.*, 2008) and juvenile rheumatoid arthritis (Hagen *et al.*, 2003).

Studies in patient populations have commonly used the therapies listed in Table 5.1, as well as acupuncture, aromatherapy, folk/home remedies, naturopathy, prayer/faith healing/spirituality, reflexology, relaxation and vitamins/minerals (Crawford *et al.*, 2006; Hughes and Wingard, 2006; Sawni *et al.*, 2007; Adams *et al.*, 2009; Post-White *et al.*, 2009). The concurrent use of conventional medicines and CAM is not uncommon in paediatric populations (McCann and Newell, 2006). Data from the 2007 US community survey demonstrated that CAM use increased with the use of prescription medicine in the previous three months (Birdee *et al.*, 2010). A recent study reported that 20 per cent of paediatric patients in a Canadian emergency room used CAM and prescription medication concurrently (Goldman *et al.*, 2008), while a recent survey in Canadian paediatric outpatient clinics identified 46.1 per cent of patients reporting using CAM at the same time as conventional medicine (Adams *et al.*, 2009).

Despite such popularity of use, CAM disclosure rates to physicians vary among paediatric populations, with rates as low as 23 per cent (Robinson and McGrail, 2004). Furthermore, research shows that fewer than half of paediatric oncologists routinely enquire about their patients' use of CAM (Roth *et al.*, 2009).

Given the prevalence rates for CAM use among paediatric populations, the supplementary nature of much of this use (alongside conventional treatments) and the potential for polypharmacy if all treatments are not sufficiently coordinated, it is imperative that health care providers communicate openly with families regarding potential and identified CAM use.

Paediatric patient characteristics and reasons for using CAM

The 2007 US community survey determined that paediatric CAM use (excluding vitamins and minerals) significantly increased with increasing parent education and use of CAM by a parent, and was significantly more likely in certain geographical regions and with certain medical conditions (Birdee *et al.*, 2010). CAM use was also found to be significantly more likely among adolescents aged 12–17 years than younger children aged 5–11 years or pre-school children aged 0–4 years (Barnes *et al.*, 2008). Use in specific adolescent populations can be much higher, as with homeless adolescents, where use has been reported as high as 70 per cent (Breuner *et al.*, 1998).

Previous studies in paediatric populations have reported that CAM use in children is more likely if they are consulting their paediatrician for an illness, take medication on a regular basis or have ongoing medical problems (Pitetti *et al.*, 2001). However, its relationship to other factors, including parental income, parental education level, child's gender, child's age, family ethnicity, insurance coverage and usual source of care, has varied (Pitetti *et al.*, 2001; Crawford *et al.*, 2006; McCann and Newell, 2006; Sencer and Kelly, 2007; Robinson *et al.*, 2008).

Reasons for CAM use most commonly include hearing that a particular treatment was considered effective; personal recommendation of family or friend/word of mouth; long-lasting medical problems; cultural tradition/ values; and the need for more personal attention. While dissatisfaction with conventional medicine was listed, a more common reason for use was fear of adverse effects from drugs (Smith and Eckert, 2006; Sawni *et al.*, 2007; Robinson *et al.*, 2008).

Medico-legal and ethical considerations

Medico-legal

CAM poses a challenging risk-management issue, with the potential for either a medical malpractice lawsuit, disciplinary proceedings from state licensing boards, or fraud and abuse actions from federal or state regulators (Cohen and Kemper, 2005; Sheldon, 2006). The use of some types of CAM in adults has been judicially held to be below the standard of care constituting medical negligence (*Johnson v TBME*, 2003); that is, use of complementary therapies in and of itself does not constitute negligence. In terms of practising within the standard of care, more clinicians are willing to offer CAM, and more insurers are willing to pay for it (Nedrow, 2006).

US clinicians need to be aware of individual state laws relating to CAM, because medicine is regulated by state rather than federal laws (Cohen, 2002).

In its database of closed paediatric malpractice claims from 1985–2005, the Physicians Insurers Association of America reported that the average indemnity payment for all CAM claims was \$358 333, which was 37.1 per cent higher than the average for all paediatric claims (\$261 321) (PIAA, 2006). A proposed risk-management model limits liability for the use of CAM if the physician is recommending, accepting or avoiding CAM depending on the availability of evidence relating to safety and/or efficacy (Cohen, 2005).

Some CAM modalities may need to be included in discussions about informed consent for treatment. The informed consent process may potentially require a discussion about the possible risks of CAM, notwithstanding the ability of a patient to acquire CAM without the involvement of the paediatrician (for example through dietary supplements and their interaction with prescribed medication). Case law has placed a burden on clinicians at least to discuss viable options for treatment even though he or she may be unwilling to offer the therapy (*Matthies v Mastromonaco*, 1998).

Paediatricians need to be aware of the use of alternative therapies as a substitute for conventional medical care for children with life-threatening conditions and of whether they believe such treatment is reportable under state abuse and neglect laws. Another legal duty of paediatricians relates to the assurance that seeking reimbursement for CAM therapy does not trigger a potential violation of fraud and abuse laws for therapy deemed 'medically unnecessary'. It is prudent to be cautious about any representations or guarantees.

Ethics

There are several ethical challenges to integrating CAM into mainstream paediatric practice. There is a lack of systematic paediatric education about the safety and effectiveness of CAM therapies; uncertainty about the scope of practice, licensing requirements and credentialling of non-physician CAM providers; concerns about patient safety and legal liability when recommending CAM therapies or therapists; and uncertainty about how to translate principles of medical ethics into CAM (Kemper and Cohen, 2004).

The first guideline for ethical practice is to seek reliable, evidence-based information about the safety and effectiveness of specific therapies and therapists. Indeed, the 2001 AAP policy statement 'Counseling Families Who Choose Complementary and Alternative Medicine for Their Child with Chronic Illness or Disability' recommended that paediatricians seek information, evaluate the scientific merits of specific therapeutic approaches and identify risks or potential harmful effects (AAP, 2001).

It is also prudent to apply common sense to balancing risks and benefits when making therapeutic decisions (see Figure 5.1). The specific ethical questions in clinical practice vary in different clinical situations. If a therapy is both safe and effective, the paediatrician is ethically obligated to recommend and encourage its use, as he or she would for any other such therapy in conventional care.

Is the therapy effective?		
	Yes	No
Is the therapy safe? Yes	Recommend	Tolerate
No	Monitor closely or discourage	**Discourage**

Figure 5.1 A common-sense guide to CAM treatment recommendations

Source: Kemper, K. and Cohen, M. (2004) Ethics meet complementary and alternative medicine: New light on old principles. *Contemporary Pediatrics* 21: 65.

Factors to be included in a risk/benefit analysis when considering CAM therapies include the severity and acuteness of illness; curability with conventional care; degree of invasiveness; toxicities and adverse effects of conventional treatment; quality of evidence for efficacy and safety of the complementary therapy; and the family's understanding of the risks and benefits of CAM treatment, voluntary acceptance of those risks, and persistence of intention to use CAM therapy (Cohen, 2005). Thus, the level of evidence required for evaluating efficacy can be small when there is little to no risk of harm from a therapy, especially when other therapies are likely to be futile. Likewise, the level of evidence for efficacy required to endorse a particular complementary therapy would be quite high when that therapy is risky and safer, more effective therapies are available.

Situation-specific variables can also affect ethical decision making. Situation-specific variables include the patient's and parents' personal beliefs, cultural values and practices and therapeutic goals; the type and severity of illness; and the lack of efficacy and safety data in a specific patient. Even when such data are known for other populations, application of population data to individual paediatric patients requires inference and implies some degree of uncertainty. The tolerance of the patient, family and clinician for uncertainty varies from one situation to another (Cohen, 2005).

Finally, clinicians should be aware of the four basic principles of biomedical ethics: (1) respect for patients' autonomy; (2) non-maleficence (avoiding harm); (3) beneficence (putting the patient's interest and well-being first); and (4) justice (fairness in providing access to essential care) (Cohen, 2005).

Conclusions

Paediatricians and other clinicians who care for children have the responsibility to advise and counsel patients and families about relevant, safe, effective and age-appropriate health services (conventional or CAM). Survey research shows that 73 per cent of paediatricians agree that it is their role to provide patients/families with information about all potential treatment options for the patient's condition, and 54 per cent agree that paediatricians should consider the use of all potential therapies, not just those of conventional medicine, when treating patients (Kemper *et al.*, 2004). Because most families use CAM services without spontaneously reporting this use to their clinician, paediatricians can best provide appropriate advice and counselling if they regularly enquire about all the therapies the family is using to help the child (Prussing *et al.*, 2004; Sibinga *et al.*, 2004).

Paediatricians should seek continued and updated knowledge about the therapeutic options available to their patients (including CAM) and about the specific services used by individual patients, in order to ensure that issues of the safety, appropriateness and advisability of CAM can be addressed. Only then can paediatricians appreciate the concerns of their patients and families and offer them the thoughtful and knowledgeable guidance they may require.

Further reading

Bishop, F., Prescott, P., Chan, Y.K. *et al.* (2010) Prevalence of complementary medicine use in pediatric cancer: A systematic review. *Pediatrics* 125(4): 768–76.

Robinson, N., Lorenc, A. and Blair, M. (2009) Developing a decision-making model on traditional and complementary medicine use for children. *European Journal of Integrative Medicine* 1(1): 43–50.

Sidora-Arcoleo, K., Yoos, H.L., Litzman, H., McCullen, A. and Anson, E. (2008) Don't ask, don't tell: Parental non-disclosure of complementary and alternative medicine and over-the-counter medication use in childrens' asthma management. *Journal of Pediatric Health Care* 22(4): 221–9.

References

Adams, D., Bateman, J., Mittra, D. *et al.* (2009) Complementary and alternative medicine: A survey of its use in pediatric neurology. *North American Research Conference on Complementary and Integrative Medicine: Alternative Therapies in Health and Medicine* 15(3): s134.

Adams, K.E., Cohen, M.H., Eisenberg, D. and Jonsen, A.R. (2002) Ethical considerations of complementary and alternative therapies in conventional medical settings. *Annals of Internal Medicine* 137(8): 660–64.

American Academy of Pediatrics, Committee on Children with Disabilities (2001) Counseling families who choose complementary and alternative medicine for their child with chronic illness or disability [published correction appears in *Pediatrics* 2001, 108: 507]. *Pediatrics* 107(3): 598–601.

Ball, S.D., Kertesz, D. and Moyer-Mileur, L.J. (2005) Dietary supplement use is prevalent among children with a chronic illness. *Journal of the American Dietetic Association* 105(1): 78–84.

Barnes, P.M., Bloom, B. and Nahin, R.L. (2008) Complementary and alternative medicine use among adults and children: United States, 2007. *National Health Statistics Reports* 10: 1–23.

Birdee, G.S., Phillips, R.S., Davis, R.B. and Gardiner, G. (2010) Factors associated with pediatric use of complementary and alternative medicine. *Pediatrics* 125: 249–56.

Braganza, S., Ozuah, P.O. and Sharif, I. (2003) The use of complementary therapies in inner-city asthmatic children. *Journal of Asthma* 40(7): 823–7.

Breuner, C.C., Barry, P.J. and Kemper, K.J. (1998) Alternative medicine use by homeless youth. *Archives of Pediatrics and Adolescent Medicine* 152(11): 1071–5.

Cohen, M.H. (2002) Legal issues in complementary and integrative medicine: A guide for the clinician. *Medical Clinics of North America* 86(1): 185–96.

Cohen, M.H. (2005) Legal issues in caring for patients with kidney disease by selectively integrating complementary therapies. *Advances in Chronic Kidney Disease* 12(3): 300–11.

Cohen, M.H. and Kemper, K.J. (2005) Complementary therapies in pediatrics: A legal perspective. *Pediatrics* 115(3): 774–80.

Crawford, N.W., Cincotta, D.R., Lim, A. and Powell, C.V.E. (2006) A cross-sectional survey of complementary and alternative medicine use by children and adolescents attending the University Hospital of Wales. *BMC Complementary and Alternative Medicine* 6(1): 16.

Davis, M.P. and Darden, P.M. (2003) Use of complementary and alternative medicine by children in the US. *Archives of Pediatrics and Adolescent Medicine* 157(4): 393–6.

Day, A. (2002) Use of complementary and alternative therapies and probiotic agents by children attending gastroenterology outpatient clinics. *Journal of Paediatrics and Child Health* 38: 343–6.

Day, A.S., Whitten, K.E. and Bohane, T.D. (2004) Use of complementary and alternative medicines by children and adolescents with inflammatory bowel disease. *Journal of Paediatrics and Child Health* 40(12): 681–4.

Dinkevich, E., Sass, P., Pereira, L., Asimolowo, O., Glater, L. and Rao, M. (2003) Complementary and alternative medicine use by African-American and Caribbean-American children with asthma [abstract 1068]. *Pediatric Research* 53(suppl): 188A.

Goldman, R.D., Rogovik, A.L., Lai, D. and Vohra, S. (2008) Potential interactions of drug–natural health products and natural health products–natural health products among children. *Journal of Pediatrics* 152(4): 521–6.

Hagen, L.E., Schneider, R., Stephens, D., Modrusan, D. and Feldman, B.M. (2003) Use of complementary and alternative medicine by pediatric rheumatology patients. *Arthritis and Rheumatism* 49(1): 3–6.

Harrington, J.W., Rosen, L., Garnecho, A. and Patrick, P.A. (2006) Parental perceptions and use of complementary and alternative medicine practices for children with autistic spectrum disorders in private practice. *Journal of Developmental and Behavioral Pediatrics* 27(2 suppl): S156–S161.

Hughes, S.C. and Wingard, D.L. (2006) Children's visits to providers of complementary and alternative medicine in San Diego. *Ambulatory Pediatrics* 6(5): 293–6.

Hurvitz, E.A., Leonard, C., Ayyangar, R. and Nelson, V.S. (2003) Complementary and alternative medicine use in families of children with cerebral palsy. *Developmental Medicine and Child Neurology* 45(6): 364–70.

Johnson v Tennessee Board of Medical Examiners, 2003 Tenn App Lexis 226.

Kelly, K.M., Jacobson, J.S., Kennedy, D.D., Braudt, S.M., Mallick, M. and Weiner, M.A. (2000) Use of unconventional therapies by children with cancer at an urban medical center. *Journal of Pediatric Hematology/Oncology* 22(5): 412–16.

Kemper, K.J. and Cohen, M.H. (2004) Ethics meet complementary and alternative medicine: New light on old principles. *Contemporary Pediatrics* 21(3): 61–72.

Kemper, K.J. and O'Connor, K.G. (2004) Pediatricians' recommendations for complementary and alternative medical (CAM) therapies. *Ambulatory Pediatrics* 4(6): 482–7.

Kemper, K.J., Vohra, S. and Walls, R. (2008) The use of complementary and alternative medicine in pediatrics. *Pediatrics* 122(6): 1374–86.

Kemper, K.J. and Wornham, W.L. (2001) Consultations for holistic pediatric services for inpatients and outpatient oncology patients at a children's hospital. *Archives of Pediatrics & Adolescent Medicine* 155(4): 449–54.

Levy, S.E. and Hyman, S.L. (2003) Use of complementary and alternative treatments for children with autistic spectrum disorders is increasing. *Pediatric Annals* 32(10): 685–91.

Matthies v Mastromonaco, 310 NJ Super 572 (App Div 1998), cert granted 1998; 156 NJ 406.

McCann, L.J. and Newell, S.J. (2006) Survey of paediatric complementary and alternative medicine use in health and chronic illness. *Archives of Disease in Childhood* 91(2): 173–4.

Nedrow, A. (2006) Status of credentialing alternative providers within a subset of US academic health centers. *Journal of Alternative and Complementary Medicine* 12(3): 329–35.

Neuhouser, M.D., Patterson, R.E., Schwartz, S.M., Hedderson, M.M., Bowen, D.J. and Standish, L.J. (2001) Use of alternative medicine by children with cancer in Washington state. *Preventive Medicine* 33(5): 347–54.

Physician Insurers Association of America (2006) *Risk Management Review: Pediatrics.* Rockville, MD: Physician Insurers Association of America.

Pitetti, R., Singh, S., Hornak, D., Garcia, S.E. and Herr, S. (2001) Complementary and alternative medicine use in children. *Pediatric Emergency Care* 17(3): 165–9.

Post-White, J., Fitzgerald, M., Hageness, S. and Sencer, S.F. (2009) Complementary and alternative medicine use in children with cancer and general and specialty pediatrics. *Journal of Pediatric Oncology Nursing* 26: 7–15.

Prussing, E., Sobo, E.J., Walker, E., Dennis, K. and Kurtin, P.S. (2004) Communicating with pediatricians about complementary/alternative medicine: perspectives from parents of children with Down syndrome. *Ambulatory Pediatrics* 4(6): 488–94.

Reznik, M., Ozuah, P.O., Franco, K., Cohen, R. and Motlow, F. (2002) Use of complementary therapy by adolescents with asthma. *Archives of Pediatrics and Adolescent Medicine* 156(10): 1042–4.

Robinson, N., Blair, M., Lorenc, A., Gully, N., Fox, P. and Mitchell, K. (2008) Complementary medicine use in multi-ethnic paediatric outpatients. *Complementary Therapies in Clinical Practice* 14: 17–24.

Robinson, A. and McGrail, M.R. (2004) Disclosure of CAM use to medical practitioners: A review of qualitative and quantitative studies. *Complementary Therapies in Medicine* 12: 90–98.

Roth, M., Lin, J., Kim, M. and Moody, K. (2009) Pediatric oncologists' views toward the use of complementary and alternative medicine in children with cancer. *Journal of Pediatric Hematology/Oncology* 31(3): 177–82.

Sawni, A., Ragothaman, R., Thomas, R.L. and Mahajan, P. (2007) Use of complementary/alternative therapies among children attending an urban pediatric emergency department. *Clinical Pediatrics* 46(1): 36–46.

Sencer, S.F. and Kelly, K.M. (2007) Complementary and alternative therapies in pediatric oncology. *Pediatric Clinics of North America* 54(6): 1043–60.

Sheldon, T. (2006) Dutch doctors suspended for use of complementary medicine. *British Medical Journal* 332(7547): 929.

Sibinga, E.M., Ottolini, M.C., Duggan, A.K. and Wilson, M.H. (2004) Parent/pediatricians communication about complementary and alternative medicine use for children. *Clinical Pediatrics* 43(4): 367–73.

Smith, C. and Eckert, K. (2006) Prevalence of complementary and alternative medicine and use among children in South Australia. *Journal of Paediatrics and Child Health* 42: 538–43.

Soo, I., Mah, J.K., Barlow, K., Hamiwka, L. and Wirrell, E. (2005) Use of complementary and alternative medical therapies in a pediatric neurology clinic. *Canadian Journal of Neurological Sciences* 32(4): 524–8.

Vlieger, A.M., Blink, M., Tromp, E. and Benninga, M.A. (2008) Use of complementary and alternative medicine by pediatric patients with functional and organic gastrointestinal diseases: Results from a multicenter survey. *Pediatrics* 122(2): e446–51.

Wong, A.P., Clark, A.L., Garnett, E.A. *et al.* (2008) Use of complementary medicine in pediatric patients with inflammatory bowel disease: Results from a multicenter survey. *Journal of Pediatric Gastroenterology and Nutrition* 48: 55–60.

CHAPTER 6

'Getting on with life': The experiences of older people using complementary health care

TINA CARTWRIGHT

Introduction

There are very few studies that have explored the use of CAM in older people. This omission is surprising in light of our increasingly ageing society and the high incidence of multiple chronicity in the older population. Notwithstanding the substantial cost of providing health care to this age group, the complex health care needs of older patients make it difficult to provide a comprehensive care package that incorporates physical, social and emotional well-being (Adams *et al.*, 2001). It has therefore been suggested that CAM can provide an important adjunct to orthodox medicine (OM) in enhancing quality of life in the ageing population, in addition to reducing health care costs (Dossey, 1997; Willison and Andrews, 2004).

Nevertheless, there is a lack of research into the experiences of CAM use among older people, and particularly among older people of mixed ethnic and social backgrounds. Further research is clearly needed to elucidate the meaning of complementary health care for older people and understand how treatment impacts on physical and mental health and well-being. The aim of the study reported here was to explore the experiences of older people using subsidised complementary health care. Semi-structured interviews were conducted with 17 regular attendees of a single centre offering low-cost complementary health care to the over-60s in London, UK (for further details of methods, see original paper).

Source: Cartwright, T. (2007) 'Getting on with life': The experience of older people using complementary health care. *Social Science and Medicine* 64(8): 1692–703. Abridged version reprinted with kind permission of Elsevier Ltd.

Study results

The majority of participants suffered from chronic degenerative complaints for which OM offered limited effective treatment, and CAM was perceived as providing highly beneficial adjunct care. The core of participants' experiences of complementary health care were organized around 'getting on with life'. The importance of keeping active and being 'able to do your normal things' was central to participants' sense of independence and well-being.

> [I] don't expect to live forever mind you, but you like to know if you're going to live, at least do something with it, not just sit there as if you're gone if you know what I mean! (Peter, 66 years; shiatsu for spondylitis)

Maintenance of activity and social participation were crucial to participants and there was a strong sense of continuing despite the difficulties created by painful conditions. Indeed, there was a sense of being stronger than the disease and 'not giving in', since this was perceived as instigating a downward spiral of further disability. Factors that restricted 'normal' functioning, such as pain and impaired mobility, were therefore met with considerable concern and anxiety, since they posed a direct challenge to the individual's sense of self.

The challenges posed by illness to notions of self were further evidenced by the way in which most participants contextualized their health through social and personal comparisons. In many cases, there were evident incongruences between participants' perceptions of themselves and their actual physical state ('I shouldn't be like this', James). Frequent reference was made to past and possible selves, relating to the loss of previous capabilities, as well as projections about possible negative selves that had apparently been averted by using complementary medicine.

> I would definitely have been in a wheelchair if it hadn't been for the acupuncture and then coming on to here. (George, 84 years; acupuncture for osteoarthritis)

Using complementary health care was therefore viewed within the context of the broad goal of keeping active and maintaining everyday activities, and treatment success was primarily evaluated in terms of its impact on physical functioning. Several subordinate themes emerged from the data relating to the quality of care and the experience of the treatment process itself.

Whole package care

The holistic nature of care provided by the centre was alluded to by all participants. The highly personalized care provided by the centre was greatly valued by all participants and frequently contrasted with the impersonal experiences of OM.

It is two separate entities ... [in OM] they have too many people to be taking care of so they cannot give the right care they should give to everybody because they have a very limited time for individuals ... you can't compare the two. (Sarah, 63 years; osteopathy for osteoarthritis)

The 'personal touch' related not only to the well-documented individualized nature of CAM treatment, but more broadly at the overall care package, which was seen to make the entire process of seeking care a positive one, from arranging an appointment to visiting the centre and receiving treatment.

Relationships with both the practitioner and other members of the centre were valued for their therapeutic and social functions. Participants discussed the importance of discussing feelings and concerns within a supportive and non-judgemental environment. While this applied to both complementary and orthodox approaches, it was recognized that the opportunities for the talking component of therapy were more limited within OM, where 'doctors have not got the time for these sorts of things now' (Cath).

Treatment impact

Since participants' overall goal was to maintain 'normal' functioning, perceived physiological effects were most salient to their accounts of treatment experiences and outcomes. Additionally, experiences of complementary health care were inevitably considered within the context of the broader illness experience, which included a recognition that allopathic medicine offered little hope in terms of treatment for chronic complaints such as osteoarthritis – 'there's nothing they can give you for it really' (Cath). All participants had experienced some relief of symptoms through using CAM, and several had permanent improvement of either their main condition or a secondary complaint. Similarly, although improvements in mobility were generally temporary, they enabled a short-term return to pre-illness functioning, which allowed participation in everyday activities as well as a sense of being 'free' from the physical limitations of debilitating conditions.

Although less dramatic than symptom alleviation and improvements in mobility, relaxation was valued for its inherently positive effects as well as for its impact on pain relief and stress reduction. Thus, the relaxing nature of treatments made participants more aware of the relationship between mental and physical states and facilitated coping with the physical consequences of their condition.

I think it's been very beneficial because apparently unbeknown to me, the stress I was obviously feeling was manifesting itself in knots in my shoulders and the two young ladies have been massaging me, they both said the same thing, that these knots need breaking down which is what they've been doing, and it's been very good indeed, and it does make you feel more relaxed when you've been there as well I think. (Brenda)

While participants primarily emphasized the impact of treatment on their physical complaints, the psychological effects of treatment were recognized as playing a role in the healing process and contributing to overall well-being.

Gaining a sense of control

Dealing with chronic, often degenerative illness raised several issues of control for participants. On the one hand, most participants felt that OM offered little personal control, either in terms of involvement or choice. In contrast, CAM offered empowerment by encouraging patients to participate in their health through lifestyle changes and by providing a safe environment in which they felt confident to ask questions and address their health concerns – 'they help you to live a better life' (Susana).

> She tells me how to how to do a bit of exercises indoors, how to help yourself (…) You don't want somebody to keep giving you orders. (Fatma)

The potential to make decisions (even choosing to stop treatment) and the empowering nature of adequate explanation were particularly salient for those with negative experiences of OM (one third of participants). Several participants discussed incidences in which they had either not been fully informed about their condition or their treatment requests had been ignored, resulting in a loss of confidence in allopathic medicine.

In contrast, participants' discourses regarding complementary health care demonstrated a sense of ownership over both the treatment process and the centre itself – 'we're all friendly, we all get on well with one another' (Jane). Additionally, treatment was perceived as providing a crucial sense of control over pain and symptoms. This had a significant impact on the core theme of 'getting on with life', since the unpredictability and uncontrollability of symptoms were linked with reductions in activities (such as leaving the house), as well as heightened anxiety. The sense of control that arose as a result of successful treatment was therefore important in alleviating participants' fear and anxieties, which in turn facilitated a return to 'normal' functioning.

> You're dead scared in case you can't move. I've got no fear now of it seizing up, that was my main fear. (Peter, 66 years; shiatsu for spondylitis)

Beliefs about treatment

All participants strongly advocated the use of complementary health care, irrespective of prior beliefs and experience. While several participants described their initial scepticism of CAM, confidence and faith in the treatment developed for all participants through continued use of CAM, from both personal experiences and observations of treatment effects on others.

A contrast was drawn between the holistic and natural approach of CAM and the reductionist and chemical approach of OM. This was closely related to participants' causal explanations of illness and the importance placed on treating the underlying cause of illness through readjustment of the body.

> The whole, holistic idea that your body is being treated, the whole body is being treated as well, and the mind and the (...) you know, that is what I like about it and also not having chemicals ... I don't really like chemical medicines, I know I have to take them but I would like to be totally un-chemical! (Rosemary)

Participants attempted to control their medication usage and avoid 'overdoing it', reflecting a wider concern with long-term medication use and dependency. Despite the fact that CAM was repeatedly described as more harmonious with the body, several participants applied similar means of control to their use of CAM, such as stopping treatment when they felt better in order to allow 'the body to try to get back to normal' (Jane). Although perceived as 'two separate entities', both orthodox and complementary medicines were seen as necessary for the maintenance of health; the importance of allopathic medication in managing pain and symptoms was readily acknowledged. Additionally, in several cases CAM was seen to augment OM, particularly through supporting recovery from operations.

> The recovery from the hip operations was absolutely fantastic, I used to come here and they used the needles and things and I think myself, if I hadn't have been coming here for the acupuncture I would have been like a lot of people – 'hip operations are no good'. (George)

Discussion

Access to complementary health care was highly valued by the older people in this study, both in terms of the physical benefits received from treatment and the overall package of care provided by a highly personalized service. Despite coming from a range of social and cultural backgrounds, the way in which treatment was evaluated was remarkably congruent across participants and related to wider concerns about getting older and coping with ill-health. The primary focus was 'getting on with life' and maintaining physical and social functioning within the constraints imposed by chronic conditions. Consequently, the effects of treatment that were most valued were those that improved mobility and reduced pain; however, the more subtle psychological effects on well-being were equally apparent and interacted with physical outcomes, particularly with regard to pain.

Treatment was perceived within the overall context of health enablement: CAM facilitated everyday functioning in several ways and thereby had both direct and indirect effects on health and well-being. First, CAM had a positive impact on physical functioning and mobility, key dimensions of quality of life in older people (Farquhar, 1995). Secondly, treatment contributed to a more positive psychological profile by reducing anxiety and encouraging a more optimistic outlook. Thirdly, participants felt empowered by CAM, since it encouraged a more active and participatory role in their health (Conway and Hockey, 1998; Andrews, 2002). Additionally, the holistic nature of the treatment resulted in attention to psychosocial issues that might impede everyday living (for instance independent bathing) but were not necessarily directly related to health.

The significance of this underlying theme can be viewed within the wider context of the individual's construal of the self. Maintenance of the self was central to older people's perceptions of quality of life, and was directly challenged by the experience of ageing and illness. Participants' accounts of treatment were therefore linked in a wider illness narrative that included past health history and experiences, as well as aspirations about the future such as maintaining energy and mobility. Complementary health care played a significant role in the way older people coped with the consequences of ill-health, particularly in dealing with health-related anxiety.

Research has consistently shown independence, mobility and active engagement with life to be important criteria for wellness in older people (Bryant *et al.*, 2001; Willison and Andrews, 2004; Borglin *et al.*, 2005). Chronic disease cannot be cured, but treatment can minimize the impact of disease on functioning and quality of life. OM is increasingly recognizing the importance of tailored collaborative care and patient participation for managing chronic illness (Von Korff *et al.*, 2002; Hunkeler *et al.*, 2006); CAM may be an additional tool in the effective management of chronic illness in older people with complex health needs. In addition to alleviating symptoms and facilitating mobility, the current study supports findings in the wider literature that the use of CAM benefits older people's perceptions of quality of life and encourages greater engagement with their health through empowerment.

Further reading

Adams, J., Lui, C. and McLaughlin, D. (2009) The use of complementary and alternative medicine in later life. *Reviews in Clinical Gerontology* 19: 227–36.

Andrews, G.J. (2003) Placing the consumption of private complementary medicine: Every-day geographies of older people's use. *Health and Place* 9: 337–49.

References

Adams, L., Gatchel, R. and Gentry, C. (2001) Complementary and alternative medicine: Applications and implications for cognitive functioning in elderly populations. *Alternative Therapies in Health and Medicine* 7(2): 52–61.

Andrews, G. (2002) Private complementary medicine and older people: Service use and user empowerment. *Ageing and Society* 22(3): 343–68.

Borglin, G., Edberg, A. and Hallberg, I.R. (2005) The experience of quality of life among older people. *Journal of Ageing Studies* 19: 201–20.

Bryant, L., Corbett, K. and Kutner, J. (2001) In their own words: A model of healthy aging. *Social Science & Medicine* 53: 927–41.

Conway, S. and Hockey, J. (1998) Resisting the 'mask' of old age? The social meaning of lay health beliefs in later life. *Ageing and Society* 18(4): 469–94.

Dossey, B. (1997) Complementary and alternative therapies for our ageing society. *Journal of Gerontology & Nursing* 23(19): 45–51.

Farquhar, M. (1995) Older people's definitions of quality of life. *Social Science & Medicine* 10(41): 1439–46.

Hunkeler, E., Katon, W., Tang, L. *et al.* (2006) Long term outcomes from the IMPACT randomised trial for depressed elderly patients in primary care. *British Medical Journal* 332: 259–63.

Von Korff, M., Glasgow, R.E. and Sharpe, M. (2002) Organising care for chronic illness. *British Medical Journal* 325: 92–4.

Willison, K. and Andrews, G. (2004) Complementary medicine and older people: Past research and future directions. *Complementary Therapies in Nursing and Midwifery* 10: 80–91.

Traditional, complementary and integrative medicine and disease context

Introduction

The rise of TCIM has been broad and far-reaching, not only in terms of prevalence and users, but also with regard to impact and influence on areas of health care and treatment such as cardiovascular medicine, diabetes and obesity. In this section of the reader authors examine the impact and influence, opportunities and challenges posed by TCIM in relation to a number of practice areas, including skin disease (acne), cancer care, mental health and care for people living with HIV.

In Chapter 7, Magin and colleagues review the empirical evidence for the efficacy of CAM in acne. The authors suggest that while anecdotally the use of CAM in acne may be common, the empirical evidence for their use is often lacking and some of the existing evidence is compromised by lack of methodological rigour. As this chapter concludes, a number of wider factors also influence CAM use for acne, and empirical trials are required to establish both efficacy and adverse effect profiles of CAM acne therapies.

One area where CAM has received substantial attention and where integration into mainstream care has increasingly taken place is in cancer care. As with more general CAM consumption, CAM use in cancer care is often patient led and one area of significance for practitioners and academics alike is the decision-making process via which patients decide to use or not use CAM treatments. In response to this brief, Balneaves and colleagues (Chapter 8) draw on previous decision-making models to provide a summary of the main stages within the CAM decision-making process, illustrating how decisions about CAM are dynamic entities requiring attention by health professionals throughout cancer patients' illness.

Traditional medicines have long treated mental disorders (often conceived in different ways) and there is a newly evolving paradigm within mental health care that appears to be moving away from a reductive, symptom-focused model dominated by pharmacotherapy towards a more integrated, biopsychosocial model that is possibly more favourable to CAM use. In Chapter 9,

Sarris and Lake overview the current state of evidence for CAM in psychiatry and propose a number of areas in which future examination of CAM within mental health care may hold potential. Similarly, with regard to care for people living with HIV, Littlewood and Vanable (Chapter 10) provide a critical review of research investigating CAM use and discuss the implications of their findings for the provision of conventional HIV care more generally.

Yet, given the holistic orientation of much TCIM, including an emphasis on healing and prevention rather than simply addressing a set of symptoms (see Chapter 20 for a discussion of such qualities in relation to CAM within the medical curriculum), it is important to acknowledge and investigate the potential of TCIM for broader understandings of well-being. In Chapter 11, Harvey explores this terrain, arguing that TCIM practices (such as biofeedback) enhance advice giving in support of finding meaning and increasing well-being. Such themes of prevention and well-being are also closely interwoven with the development of a more formal public health perspective around TCIM (see Chapter 27 for relevant discussion with respect to the potential of traditional medicine in primary health care in low-income countries).

CHAPTER 7

Topical and oral complementary and alternative medicine in acne: A consideration of context

PARKER MAGIN, JON ADAMS, DIMITY POND AND
WAYNE SMITH

Introduction

Acne is 'one of the commonest diseases to afflict humanity' (Chan and Rohr, 2000), overall prevalence in adolescents being 23–85 per cent (Lello *et al.*, 1995; Kilkenny *et al.*, 1998; Smithard *et al.*, 2001).

Complementary and alternative medicines (CAM) are employed by a substantial number of patients with skin diseases. For example, in the United States 6.7 per cent of people who reported having skin diseases in the past 12 months reported having used alternative therapy, and 2.2 per cent saw an alternative practitioner for their condition (Eisenberg *et al.*, 1998).

For acne, however, there is no available data on the prevalence of use of CAM. A systematic review of CAM usage in dermatological patients (Ernst, 2000b) found studies of CAM use in psoriasis, atopic eczema, melanoma and unselected dermatological outpatients, but not in acne. While there is no data regarding prevalence of usage, a large number of CAM therapies have been advocated for, or were noted to be used in treatment of, acne. These include a range of topical essential oils/aromatherapy, topical plants/herbs, ingested plants/herbs, homeopathy, Indian ayurvedic therapy (oral or topical), Asian topical therapies (multiple plant ingredients), ingested or topical inhibitors of 5 alpha-reductase, miscellaneous topical applications, and ingested vitamins and minerals (see Magin *et al.*, 2006 for a comprehensive list).

Source: Magin, P., Adams, J., Pond, D. and Smith, W. (2006) Topical and oral CAM in acne: A review of the empirical evidence and a consideration of its context. *Complementary Therapies in Medicine* 14(1): 62–76. Abridged version reprinted with kind permission of Elsevier Ltd.

A narrative systematic review illustrates that while a great number and range of CAM therapies are advocated (and are presumably being widely used) in the management of acne, empiric evidence for their use is, in most cases, lacking (Magin *et al.*, 2006). Some of the existing evidence is compromised by lack of methodological rigour. The observation that research into the efficacy of essential oils used for skin diseases is 'superficial, with a tendency to be anecdotal' (Walsh, 1996) could apply to CAM acne therapies generally. Other studies that have been quoted as showing efficacy – including studies of tea tree oil (Bassett *et al.*, 1990) and gluconolactone (Hunt and Barnetson, 1992) – in fact show that their overall efficacy is less than the orthodox first-line acne topical therapy of 5% benzoyl peroxide. Studies from dermatological practice of 70% glycolic acid (Kim *et al.*, 1999) and 14% gluconolactone (Hunt and Barnetson, 1992) may be of very limited relevance as these concentrations far exceed those of available over-the-counter fruit acid acne creams (which typically have 'concentrations not exceeding 8%'; Taffe, 1997). Despite this, available evidence suggests that anti-acne properties are biologically plausible for many advocated CAM therapies. Adverse effects are established for many CAM acne therapies. But, almost universally, the efficacy, and efficacy versus adverse effect profiles, of CAM acne therapies remain uncertain.

In this chapter we examine the context of acne therapy with CAM modalities: evidence for CAM effects on the known aetiological factors in acne, and for adverse effects of CAM acne therapies.

The context of empirical evidence for the efficacy of CAM in acne

Despite the very limited methodologically high-level evidence for the efficacy of CAM in acne (Magin *et al.*, 2006), it is necessary to examine the context of this evidence before reaching conclusions about the pragmatic use of CAM in acne.

Mechanism of action and the potential for adverse effects

Acne aetiology is multifactorial. Demonstrated aetiological factors are genetic, increased sebum production (influenced by endogenous androgens), follicullar hyper-keratinization, skin colonization with Propionibacterium acnes, and inflammation (Gollnick, 2003). Orthodox medical therapies address at least one of these pathogenic mechanisms (excepting genetic susceptibility) (Gollnick, 2003). CAM acne therapies have also been proposed as addressing infection, inflammation, hyperkeratinization, sebum activity and androgenicity.

Antimicrobial properties of CAM acne therapies

Although topical and systemic antibiotics in acne therapy also exert their effects through other mechanisms such as anti-inflammatory properties, antibacterial activity against P. acnes, the organism implicated in acne pathogenesis, is an important attribute. The essential oils of tea tree, basil, lemon, orange, pettigrain, pumpkin, juniper, lavender, patchouli, sandalwood and geranium (Deans and Ritchie, 1987; Carson and Riley, 1994; Hammer *et al.*, 1999; Orafidiya *et al.*, 2001) have all been found to have in vitro antibacterial effects, and the antibacterial properties of essential oils have been proposed as a rationale in their use in acne (Bensouilah, 2002). Nevertheless, in the absence of demonstrated efficacy against P. acnes, such evidence would appear tenuous. Carson and Riley (1994) have reported having demonstrated antibacterial action of tea tree oil against P. acnes, but have not published full details of their findings. Kuroyanagi *et al.* (1999) have demonstrated Sophora flavescens to have both in vitro antibacterial activity against P. acnes and antiandrogen activity. Kampo products have been found in vitro to inhibit the growth of P. acnes and to reduce P. acnes lipase activity (Higaki *et al.*, 1998).

Anti-inflammatory properties of CAM acne therapies

Anti-inflammatory properties are prominent attributes of many orthodox medical acne treatments, including adapalene, oral antibiotics and isotretinoin (Cunliffe and Shuster, 1969). CAM acne therapies for which in vivo skin anti-inflammatory properties have been demonstrated are basil, tea tree oil, Aloe vera and witch hazel (Singh *et al.*, 1996; Vazquez *et al.*, 1996; Reynolds and Dweck, 1999; Brand *et al.*, 2002). In vitro inhibition of inflammation has also been demonstrated for tea tree oil (Hart *et al.*, 2000), Jumi-haidoku-to (Higaki *et al.*, 2000) and linoleic acid (Akamatsu *et al.*, 1990).

Anti-androgenic properties of proposed CAM acne therapies

Anti-androgens (especially cyproterone acetate) (Gruber *et al.*, 1998) are often used in the orthodox medical therapy of acne in females. Impatiens balsamina, green tea, Artocarpus incisus, Alpinia officinarum and Sophora flavescens (Liao and Hiipakka 1995; Kuroyanagi *et al.*, 1999; Ishiguro *et al.*, 2000; Kim *et al.*, 2003; Shimizu *et al.*, 2000) have all been found to have antiandrogen activity in vitro and have, on this basis, been proposed as acne therapies, although no clinical trials are apparent.

Linoleic acid and comedogenicity of sebum

Similarly, studies of the linoleic acid composition of comedones and the skin of subjects with acne and non-acne controls have suggested that linoleic acid-deficient skin may be comedone prone (Morello *et al.*, 1976; Wertz *et al.*, 1985).

Adverse effects of CAM acne therapies

Adverse effects of CAM acne therapies have been demonstrated for tea tree oil (Knight and Hausen, 1994; Soderberg *et al.*, 1996; Bassett *et al.*, 1990; Jancin, 2002; Wabner, 2002), lemon peel oil (Cardullo *et al.*, 1989; Jancin, 2002; Wabner, 2002), orange peel oil (Cardullo *et al.*, 1989), rosemary, eucalyptus oil, juniper oil and chamomile (Jancin, 2002), sandalwood, geranium oil, lavender oil and rose oil (Ernst 2000a; Bleasel *et al.*, 2002), black cumin oil (Ernst, 2000a) and gluconolactone (Hunt and Barnetson, 1992). The toxicities demonstrated were in vivo – contact dermatitis (Cardullo *et al.*, 1989; Knight and Hausen, 1994; Bleasel *et al.*, 2002; Jancin, 2002) and irritation (Bassett *et al.*, 1990; Hunt and Barnetson, 1992) – and in vitro – cytotoxic effects (Soderberg *et al.*, 1996). Of note in the cited studies is that only in two was the finding of adverse effects found in a clinical study of treatment of acne; and in both of these, for tea tree oil (Bassett *et al.*, 1990) and gluconolactone (Hunt and Barnetson, 1992), the skin irritation produced was less than for the benzoyl peroxide solution used as comparator in the studies.

An Indian study of facial massage (which often involved application of witch hazel face packs) reported adverse effects of witch hazel-induced allergic contact dermatitis (patch testing diagnosed) and of acneiform eruptions (Khanna and Gupta, 2002). The acneiform eruptions were primarily nodular and comedonal, and biopsies revealed inflammatory and granulomatous changes (Khanna and Gupta, 1999).

Oral Vitamin A in acne treatment is associated with headaches, nausea and dry skin (Labadarios *et al.*, 1987). Also of concern is adulteration of CAM acne therapies with orthodox medical therapies. Chinese herbal dermatological creams have been found to be adulterated with potent topical corticosteroids (Allen and Parkinson, 1990; O'Driscoll *et al.*, 1992; Graham-Brown *et al.*, 1994; Wood and Wishart, 1997; Keane *et al.*, 1999; Ramsay *et al.*, 2003), as have topical dead sea extracts (Broberg *et al.*, 2003) and oral herbal dermatological preparations (Hughes *et al.*, 1994). Potent topical steroids may seemingly suppress acne in the short term through anti-inflammatory properties, but have the potential to cause 'steroid acne' (Kelly, 1996) and perioral dermatitis (White, 1996).

Discussion

The wider perspective: Other factors in the use of CAM in acne

A far greater range of CAM therapies than those in the literature may be being used in practice. As Dattner (2003) points out, many systems of traditional medicine, unlike western medicine, 'have cosmologies for choosing herbs which are based on the characteristics of the given patient' rather than their diagnosis. Furthermore, it is possible (if not probable) that over-the-counter

CAM-containing skin-care products are used 'generically' by some consumers; that is, for any skin condition, including acne. Illustrating this point is the large number of phytotherapies in one ethnopharmacognostic survey found to be used for reddened skin, as a facial 'skin toner', to treat facial skin inflammation, to 'smooth' facial skin and 'to clean the skin' (Pieroni *et al.*, 2004). Also, most individuals with acne do not see a doctor regarding their acne (Emerson and Strauss, 1972) and, of those who use CAM for skin conditions, most self-access it rather than visiting a CAM practitioner (Eisenberg *et al.*, 1998). The 'incorporation of herbs into cosmetic and over-the-counter skin preparations has already assumed the force of a whirlwind' (Dattner, 2003). It is likely that this has resulted in a large and unsystematic range of extant acne therapies, easily accessible to acne sufferers and very unlikely to be subjected to empirical scrutiny.

Conclusions

Anecdotally the use of CAM in acne may be common, but evidence of its prevalence is lacking. CAM dermatological therapies appear to be more commonly used than the frequency with which CAM practitioners are consulted for dermatological conditions, but specific data on the use of acne therapies and CAM practitioners for acne are not available. Empirical evidence for the efficacy of CAM therapies in acne is not strong, but for many therapies efficacy is biologically plausible. Empirical trials are required to establish both efficacy and adverse effect profiles of CAM acne therapies.

Further reading

Fuhrmann, T., Smith, N. and Tausk, F. (2010) Use of complementary and alternative medicine among adults with skin disease: Updated results from a national study. *Journal of the American Academy of Dermatology* 63(6): 1000–05.

Magin, P. and Adams, J. (2007) Complementary and alternative medicines: Use in skin diseases. *Expert Review in Dermatology* 2(1): 41–9.

References

Akamatsu, H., Komura, J., Miyachi, Y., Asada, Y. and Niwa, Y. (1990) Suppressive effects of linoleic acid on neutrophil oxygen metabolism and phagocytosis. *Journal of Investigative Dermatology* 95(3): 271–4.

Allen, B.R. and Parkinson, R. (1990) Chinese herbs for eczema. *Lancet* 336: 177.

Bassett, I.B., Pannowitz, D.L. and Barnetson, R.S. (1990) A comparative study of tea-tree oil versus benzoylperoxide in the treatment of acne. *Medical Journal of Australia* 153(8): 455–8.

Bensouilah, J. (2002) Aetiology and management of acne vulgaris. *International Journal of Aromatherapy* 12(2): 99–104.

Bleasel, N., Tate, B. and Rademaker, M. (2002) Allergic contact dermatitis following exposure to essential oils. *Australasian Journal of Dermatology* 43(3): 211–13.

Brand, C., Townley, S.L., Finlay-Jones, J.J. and Hart, P.H. (2002) Tea tree oil reduces histamine-induced oedema in murine ears. *Inflammation Research* 51(6): 283–9.

Broberg, A., Gruvberger, B. and Isaksson, M. (2003) Dead Sea extract sold under-the-counter. *British Journal of Dermatology* 149(1): 206–07.

Cardullo, A.C., Ruszowski, A.M. and De Leo, V.A. (1989) Allergic contact dermatitis resulting from sensitivity to citrus peel, geraniol, and citral. *Journal of the American Academy of Dermatology* 21: 395–7.

Carson, C.F. and Riley, T.V. (1994) The antimicrobial activity of tea tree oil. *Medical Journal of Australia* 160(4): 236.

Chan, J. and Rohr, J. (2000) Acne vulgaris: Yesterday, today and tomorrow. *Australasian Journal of Dermatology* 41(Suppl): S69–S72.

Cunliffe, W.J. and Shuster, S. (1969) Pathogenesis of acne. *Lancet* 1(7597): 685–7.

Dattner, A.M. (2003) From medical herbalism to phytotherapy in dermatology: Back to the future. *Dermatologic Therapy* 16(2): 106–13.

Deans, S.G. and Ritchie, G. (1987) Antibacterial properties of plant essential oils. *International Journal of Food Microbiology* 5: 165–80.

Eisenberg, D.M., Davis, R.B., Ettner, S.L. *et al.* (1998) Trends in alternative medicine use in the United States, 1990–1997: Results of a follow-up national survey. *Journal of the American Medical Association* 280: 1569–75.

Emerson, G.W. and Strauss, J.S. (1972) Acne and acne care: A trend survey. *Archives of Dermatology* 105(3): 407–11.

Ernst, E. (2000a) Adverse effects of herbal drugs in dermatology. *British Journal of Dermatology* 143(5): 923–9.

Ernst, E. (2000b) The usage of complementary therapies by dermatological patients: A systematic review. *British Journal of Dermatology* 142(5): 857–61.

Gollnick, H. (2003) Current concepts of the pathogenesis of acne. *Drugs* 63(15): 1579–96.

Graham-Brown, R.A., Bourke, J.F. and Bumphrey, G. (1994) Chinese herbal remedies may contain steroids. *British Medical Journal* 308(6926): 473.

Gruber, D.M., Sator, M.O., Joura, E.A., Kokoschka, E.M., Heinze, G. and Huber, J.C. (1998) Topical cyproterone acetate treatment in women with acne: A placebo-controlled trial. *Archives of Dermatology* 134(4): 459–63.

Hammer, K.A., Carson, C.F. and Riley, T.V. (1999) Antimicrobial activity of essential oils and other plant extracts. *Journal of Applied Microbiology* 86(6): 985–90.

Hart, P.H., Brand, C., Carson, C.F., Riley, T.V., Prager, R.H. and Finlay-Jones, J.J. (2000) Terpinen-4-ol, the main component of the essential oil of Melaleuca alternifolia (tea tree oil), suppresses inflammatory mediator production by activated human monocytes. *Inflammation Research* 49(11): 619–26.

Higaki, S., Kitagawa, T., Kagoura, M., Morohashi, M. and Yamagishi, T. (2000) Relationship between Propionibacterium acnes biotypes and Jumi-haidoku-to. *Journal of Dermatology* 27(10): 635–8.

Higaki, S., Morimatsu, S., Morohashi, M. and Yamagishi, T. (1998) The anti-lipase activity of shiunko on Propionibacterium acnes. *International Journal of Antimicrobial Agents* 10(3): 251–2.

Hughes, J.R., Higgins, E.M. and Pembroke, A.C. (1994) Oral dexamethasone masquerading as a Chinese herbal remedy. *British Journal of Dermatology* 130(2): 261.

Hunt, M.J. and Barnetson, R.S. (1992) A comparative study of gluconolactone versus benzoyl peroxide in the treatment of acne. *Australasian Journal of Dermatology* 33(3): 131–4.

Ishiguro, K., Oku, H. and Toyonari, K. (2000) Testosterone 5alpha-reductase inhibitor bisnapthoquinone derivative from Impatiens balsamina. *Phytotherapy Research* 14: 54–6.

Jancin, B. (2002) Cross-sensitivity common in tea tree oil allergy. *Skin and Allergy News* 33(3): 38.

Keane, F.M., Munn, S.E., du Vivier, A.W., Taylor, N.F. and Higgins, E.M. (1999) Analysis of Chinese herbal creams prescribed for dermatological conditions. *British Medical Journal* 318(7183): 563–4.

Kelly, P.A. (1996) Acne and related disorders. In M. Sams and P.J. Lynch (eds) *Principles and Practice of Dermatology*. New York: Churchill Livingstone, pp. 801–18.

Khanna, N. and Gupta, S. (1999) Acneiform eruptions after facial beauty treatment. *International Journal of Dermatology* 38(3): 196–9.

Khanna, N. and Gupta, S. (2002) Rejuvenating facial massage – a bane or boon? *International Journal of Dermatology* 41(7): 407–10.

Kilkenny, M., Merlin, K., Plunkett, A. and Marks, R. (1998) The prevalence of common skin conditions in Australian school students: 3. acne vulgaris. *British Journal of Dermatology* 139: 840–45.

Kim, S.W., Moon, S.E., Kim, J.A. and Eun, H.C. (1999) Glycolic acid versus Jessner's solution: Which is better for facial acne patients? *Dermatologic Surgery* 25: 270–73.

Kim, Y.U., Son, H.K., Song, H.K., Ahn, M.J., Lee, S.S. and Lee, S.K. (2003) Inhibition of 5alpha-reductase activity by diarylheptanoids from Alpinia officinarum. *Planta Medica* 69(1): 72–4.

Knight, T.E. and Hausen, B.M. (1994) Melaleuca oil (tea tree oil) dermatitis. *Journal of the American Academy of Dermatology* 30(3): 423–7.

Kuroyanagi, M., Arakawa, T., Hirayama, Y. and Hayashi, T. (1999) Antibacterial and antiandrogen flavonoids from Sophora flavescens. *Journal of Natural Product* 62(12): 1595–9.

Labadarios, D., Cilliers, J., Visser, L. *et al.* (1987) Vitamin A in acne vulgaris. *Clinical & Experimental Dermatology* 12(6): 432–6.

Lello, J., Pearl, A., Arroll, B., Yallop, J. and Birchall, N.M. (1995) Prevalence of acne vulgaris in Auckland senior high school students. *New Zealand Medical Journal* 108(1004): 287–9.

Liao, S. and Hiipakka, R.A. (1995) Selective inhibition of steroid 5 alpha-reductase isoenzymes by tea epieatechin-3-gallate and epigallaeatechin-3-gallate. *Biochemical and Biophysical Research Communications* 214(3): 833–8.

Magin, P.J., Adams, J., Pond, C.D. and Smith, W. (2006) Topical and oral CAM in acne: A review of the empirical evidence and a consideration of its context. *Complementary Therapies in Medicine* 14: 62–76.

Morello, A.M., Downing, D.T. and Strauss, J.S. (1976) Octadecadienoic acids in the skin surface lipids of acne patients and normal subjects. *Journal of Investigative Dermatology* 66(5): 319–23.

O'Driscoll, J., Burden, A.D. and Kingston, T.P. (1992) Potent topical steroid obtained from a Chinese herbalist. *British Journal of Dermatology* 127(5): 543–4.

Orafidiya, L.O., Oyedele, A.O., Shittu, A.O. and Elujoba, A.A. (2001) The formulation of an effective topical antibacterial product containing Ocimum gratissimum leaf essential oil. *International Journal of Pharmaceutics* 224(1–2): 177–83.

Pieroni, A., Quave, C.L., Villanelli, M.L. *et al.* (2004) Ethnopharmacognostic survey on the natural ingredients used in folk cosmetics, cosmeceuticals and remedies for healing skin diseases in the inland Marches, Central-Eastern Italy. *Journal of Ethnopharmacology* 91: 331–44.

Ramsay, H.M., Goddard, W., Gill, S. and Moss, C. (2003) Herbal creams used for atopic eczema in Birmingham, UK illegally contain potent corticosteroids. *Archives of Disease in Childhood* 88(12): 1056–7.

Reynolds, T. and Dweck, A.C. (1999) Aloe vera leaf gel: A review update. *Journal of Ethnopharmacology* 68(1–3): 3–37.

Shimizu, K., Fukuda, M., Kondo, R. and Sakai, K. (2000) The 5 alpha-reductase inhibitory components from heartwood of Artocarpus incisus: Structure-activity investigations. *Planta Medica* 66(1): 16–19.

Singh, S., Majumdar, D.K. and Rehan, H.M. (1996) Evaluation of anti-inflammatory potential of fixed oil of Ocimum sanctum (Holybasil) and its possible mechanism of action. *Journal of Ethnopharmacology* 54(1): 19–26.

Smithard, A., Glazebrook, C. and Williams, H.C. (2001) Acne prevalence, knowledge about acne and psychological morbidity in mid-adolescence: A community-based study. *British Journal of Dermatology* 145: 274–9.

Soderberg, T.A., Johansson, A. and Gref, R. (1996) Toxic effects of some conifer resin acids and tea tree oil on human epithelial and fibroblast cells. *Toxicology* 107(2): 99–109.

Taffe, A.M. (1997) Acne treatment: A comprehensive review of pharmacotherapy. *Lippincott's Primary Care Practice Dermatology* 1(1): 70–87.

Vazquez, B., Avila, G., Segura, D. and Escalante, B. (1996) Antiinflammatory activity of extracts from Aloe vera gel. *Journal of Ethnopharmacology* 55(1): 69–75.

Wabner, D. (2002) The peroxide value – a new tool for the quality control of essential oils. *International Journal of Aromatherapy* 12(3): 142–4.

Walsh, D. (1996) Using aromatherapy in the management of psoriasis. *Nursing Standard* 11(13–15): 53–6.

Wertz, P.W., Miethke, M.C., Long, S.A., Strauss, J.S. and Downing, D.T. (1985) The composition of the ceramides from human stratum corneum and from comedones. *Journal of Investigative Dermatology* 84(5): 410–12.

White, J.W. (1996) Localised eczematous disease. In M. Sams and P.J. Lynch (eds) *Principles and Practice of Dermatology*. New York: Churchill Livingstone, pp. 441–54.

Wood, B. and Wishart, J. (1997) Potent topical steroid in a Chinese herbal cream. *New Zealand Medical Journal* 110: 420–21.

CHAPTER 8

Patient decision making about complementary and alternative medicine in cancer management: Context and process

LYNDA BALNEAVES, LAURA WEEKS AND DUGALD SEELY

Introduction

Individuals living with cancer have varying needs regarding their preferred level of involvement in treatment decisions and, correspondingly, vary in the way in which they can best be supported by health professionals during the decision-making process (Davison *et al.*, 2002). Although previous research has provided insight into the decision-support strategies required by patients faced with conventional treatment decisions, its applicability to patients making decisions about complementary and alternative medicine (CAM) is questionable.

Most Canadian cancer patients use CAM at some point during their illness (Eng *et al.*, 2003; Balneaves *et al.*, 2006). It is therefore essential that oncology health professionals understand and acknowledge the unique contexts and processes that influence treatment decisions specific to CAM for each patient. This acknowledgement is especially important given the emerging field of integrative oncology in North America, in which evidence-based CAM is gradually being integrated into mainstream cancer care (Deng *et al.*, 2007). Decision-support strategies that facilitate patients' informed

Source: Balneaves, L., Weeks, L. and Seely, D. (2008) Patient decision-making about complementary and alternative medicine in cancer management: Context and process. *Current Oncology* 15(2): 94–100. Abridged version reprinted with kind permission of Multimed Inc.

use of CAM and full disclosure of CAM use with health professionals are essential for the safe integration of CAM with conventional cancer care (see Chapter 15 in this collection for more discussion on disclosure with health professionals).

Research in Canada has resulted in the development of several models that capture the complex interplay between key personal, social and cultural factors and the cognitive processes that underlie the CAM decision-making process (Montbriand, 1995; Truant and Bottorff 1999; Boon *et al.*, 1999, 2003; Balneaves *et al.*, 2007). Although these models have been limited mainly to breast and prostate cancer and have yet to be empirically tested, they provide health professionals with insight into the experiences of patients making CAM decisions, and highlight moments during the cancer trajectory when patients may possibly benefit most from decision support.

Here we begin our discussion by highlighting the highly complex, dynamic and individualized nature of CAM decisions, which results from the unique personal, social and cultural contexts in which these decisions are embedded. We then draw on previous decision-making models and provide a summary of the main stages within the CAM decision-making process. This overview emphasizes the iterative nature of the CAM decision-making process and how it unfolds across the cancer trajectory.

The context of CAM decisions

The decision about whether to use CAM, and, if so, the type or types of CAM employed, is influenced throughout the cancer trajectory by a myriad of factors: sociodemographic and disease-related, psychological and social.

Sociodemographic and disease-related factors

At a basic level, specific demographic factors have been found to be associated with CAM use, including age (younger), sex (women) and socioeconomic status (higher education and income). Despite an increasing number of private health insurance plans providing coverage for specific CAM practices, many patients do not have access to such plans and, for those who do, many CAM practices remain uncovered. As a result, the decision to use CAM can be an expensive undertaking for many patients, particularly those who are on disability as a result of their illness.

It is also imperative to acknowledge the important influence that ethnicity may have on CAM use. Alongside many communities in developing countries, a growing number of immigrants and Aboriginal peoples in western societies rely on traditional medical systems for their primary source of health care. As a result, many cancer patients arrive at initial consultations already acquainted with CAM therapies that are not considered 'alternative' within their ethno-cultural community.

Increased CAM use has also been related to disease characteristics. CAM use has been observed to be higher in breast and prostate cancer populations than in populations with other cancer diagnoses (Kimby *et al.*, 2003), which may be a consequence of the proactive nature of these patient groups with regard to advocacy and self-care. Cancer patients with advanced disease have also been found to have a heightened interest in CAM (Broom and Tovey, 2007).

Lastly, CAM that requires intensive time and energy, such as restrictive diets or frequent visits to a practitioner, may be impractical for patients undergoing active cancer treatment, particularly for those experiencing fatigue or other debilitating physical or psychological symptoms.

Psychological factors

For many individuals, the initial decision to explore CAM arises from a strong internal locus of control; that is, the tendency to attribute event outcomes to one's own control (Rotter, 1966) and a desire to be an active participant in treatment decisions (Davidson *et al.*, 2005). For some patients, CAM may also provide the hope and optimism required to cope with the cancer journey (Singh *et al.*, 2005). For others, their fears about death and dying may motivate their search for treatment options beyond conventional cancer care (Rakovitch *et al.*, 2005).

Social factors

It is important to recognize how the personal and psychological factors associated with CAM use are also embedded within a larger social context that legitimizes and reinforces the exploration and use of many CAM therapies. For example, the increasing tendency of cancer patients to consider CAM as a treatment option during their illness may reflect the currently persistent postmodern ideals of individualism, consumerism and holism (Leis *et al.*, 2010). In addition, an individual's understandings of what constitutes appropriate treatment and how it can best be achieved are derived not only from personal experience, but also through social interaction and interface with popular culture, most notably the mass media (Lupton, 1994). Information about CAM is increasingly available and accessible through media sources (Weeks *et al.*, 2007), which lend visibility and perceived legitimacy to this group of therapies and practices.

Furthermore, male and female cancer patients both describe family members, friends and fellow cancer survivors to be highly influential in their CAM decisions (Öhlèn *et al.*, 2006; Evans *et al.*, 2007b). Members of a patient's social network can take on a variety of decision-support roles depending on a patient's diagnosis and stage of illness, and the nature of their relationship with the patient (Öhlèn *et al.*, 2006).

The CAM decision-making process

Unlike the many rational treatment decision-making models presented within the health care literature, CAM decision making has been described as a dynamic and iterative process that is highly variable across individuals (Balneaves *et al.*, 2007). Despite its complex, non-linear and individualized nature, some common stages of the CAM decision-making process can be explicated.

Taking stock of treatment options

Research has shown that the CAM decision-making process begins immediately following a diagnosis of cancer. Despite being emotionally overwhelmed by the news of their diagnosis, most cancer patients are eager to learn about the full spectrum of treatment options and often do not distinguish between conventional and complementary therapies (Truant and Bottorff, 1999). At the time of diagnosis, cancer patients are particularly interested in CAM therapies that will enhance the effectiveness of their conventional treatment protocols and mediate potential side-effects, such as fatigue, nausea and vomiting, and anxiety (Balneaves *et al.*, 2007). However, the already complex decision about whether to use CAM is challenged by concerns held by some patients and their health professionals regarding the potential risks posed by inappropriate CAM use (Singh *et al.*, 2005; Balneaves *et al.*, 2007).

Gathering and evaluating CAM information

During the initial phase of taking stock of available treatment options and identifying a personal interest in CAM, cancer patients begin to gather and evaluate information about the possible role of CAM in their cancer experience. Because the decision-making process is dependent on unique contextual factors, the process of gathering and evaluating information is highly variable across individuals.

For some cancer patients, particularly those who feel overwhelmed by their diagnosis, the information-gathering and evaluation phase is a passive process in which they seek information only about CAM therapies with which they have had previous experience or which are recommended by a trusted health professional, family member or friend (Truant and Bottorff, 1999; Balneaves *et al.*, 2007). Other cancer patients take on a more active role in which they engage in an extensive and iterative information-seeking and evaluation process related to a diverse range of CAM therapies. This process often continues throughout their cancer journey and is revisited at key milestones, such as at the end of conventional treatment and at diagnosis of recurrence (Evans *et al.*, 2007b). For these individuals, the search for CAM information is motivated by their information needs, including the potential risks and benefits of CAM use, the likelihood of negative interactions of specific CAM therapies (typically natural health products) with conventional treatments, the appropriate timing of CAM use in the cancer trajectory, and the availability and financial cost of specific therapies (Truant and Bottorff, 1999; Balneaves *et al.*, 2007).

The type of evidence privileged by cancer patients in making CAM decisions varies widely and includes professional advice, the scientific literature, anecdotes about CAM use from social networks and the media, the internet and previous personal CAM experiences (Balneaves *et al.*, 2007; Evans *et al.*, 2007b). As a result, patients seek information about CAM from a multitude of sources, although there seems to be a preference to seek assistance from trusted individuals who are perceived as credible (for instance oncologists or regulated CAM practitioners) (Balneaves *et al.*, 2007; Roberts *et al.*, 2005).

The information-gathering and evaluation phase can be an anxiety-provoking experience. Some individuals are able to control the amount of information they obtain about CAM by restricting their search to a limited number of therapies or by avoiding certain resources, such as the internet, but others report feeling overwhelmed by the amount of CAM information they acquire (Truant and Bottorff, 1999; Balneaves *et al.*, 2007). Some patients struggle to make sense of the contradictory information that often exists about CAM (Balneaves *et al.*, 2007; Evans *et al.*, 2007a) and report being particularly distressed about the lack of consensus between and among CAM and conventional health professionals regarding the implications of CAM use. This conflict causes profound anxiety in some cancer patients, who are fearful of making the 'wrong' treatment decision with potentially serious consequences regarding their survival.

Making a CAM decision

How cancer patients ultimately reach a decision about CAM varies considerably between individuals and along the cancer trajectory. This complex process, previously labelled 'bridging the gap' (Balneaves *et al.*, 2007), involves cancer patients attempting to make sense of the disparate advice and information identified about CAM while reflecting on their personal beliefs about cancer, treatment and healing.

Previous work has identified three different types of CAM decision. First, individuals in the midst of conventional treatment who are experiencing high anxiety and conflict often 'take it one step at a time' and postpone their CAM decisions to when they have more energy to reflect on a broader spectrum of treatments. This delay is particularly evident in patients who have received limited support from their oncology health professionals in the CAM decision-making process. The CAM chosen by these patients are typically those that fall within the realm of supportive care (such as massage or relaxation therapy) and have been associated with positive psychosocial outcomes (Balneaves *et al.*, 2007).

Secondly, cancer patients who have a high level of trust in the conventional health care system engage in a 'playing it safe' decision-making process in which the advice of their oncologists is privileged throughout the cancer trajectory. Only CAM therapies that can be easily incorporated into their conventional treatment protocol are chosen. Frequently, these patients perceive their cancer diagnosis to be 'too serious to play around with' and are hesitant to use any therapies that may negatively interact with their conventional treatment (Montbriand, 1995; Balneaves *et al.*, 2007).

In contrast, a third group of cancer patients is able to 'bring it all together' and make treatment decisions that incorporate CAM as part of their treatment plan with minimal conflict and anxiety. These individuals often report having a life-long commitment to CAM use that precedes their diagnosis, and believe that CAM is natural, supportive of the body's innate ability to heal and better able than conventional care alone to address physiological and psycho-social needs holistically (Evans *et al.*, 2007b).

It is important to note, however, that some patients have described feeling 'pushed' towards CAM care during their cancer journey as a result of their beliefs about conventional cancer treatments being 'toxic', 'poisonous' or immunosuppressive (Singh *et al.*, 2005). Still others have turned towards CAM because of their dissatisfaction with conventional care, including the quality and frequency of interactions with health professionals, the adverse effects of conventional treatment and their experiences with ineffective therapies (Singh *et al.*, 2005; Hann *et al.*, 2006; Evans *et al.*, 2007b).

Revisiting the CAM decision

As patients move through the cancer trajectory and reach the end of their conventional treatment protocol, many revisit the decisions they made regarding CAM use following their diagnosis and during adjuvant treatment. For some individuals, this reflection is a consequence of feeling as if they have 'fallen off the cliff' as they lose the frequent contact they have had with their oncology health professionals during active treatment (Boyd, 2007). Adding CAM to their health care repertoire allows these individuals to feel as if they are 'still doing something' and helping their bodies recover from the trauma of chemotherapy and radiation.

Cancer patients also revisit their CAM decisions in response to new information received regarding disease progression and prognosis (Balneaves *et al.*, 2007). The identification of a recurrence or metastases can lead some individuals to return to the decision-making process and reconsider the CAM therapies they had initially chosen. Others interpret disease progression as a sign of ineffectiveness, resulting in the discontinuation or significant alteration of their CAM regimen. Conversely, results suggestive of remission or tumour regression can encourage some individuals to maintain or increase their use of CAM.

CAM research is providing new data on the efficacy and safety of specific CAM on an almost daily basis. This information is rapidly translated to cancer patients and oncology health professionals through the media, scientific journals and research-based databases. For individuals for whom scientific evidence is an important consideration in their treatment decisions, such information may encourage the exploration of promising CAM therapies or a withdrawal from products or practices suggested to be ineffective or potentially harmful (Balneaves *et al.*, 2007).

Conclusion

CAM decisions are highly individualized, complicated and multifaceted, and involve dynamic processes that vary throughout the cancer trajectory. The decision to use or not use CAM is one that leads cancer patients to reflect on their unique personal and social context and to ponder how CAM may fit with their values, beliefs and specific health care needs. Decisions about CAM are not static; rather, they are dynamic entities that require assessment and follow-up by health professionals throughout a patient's illness.

Further reading

Broom, A. and Adams, J. (2009) Discussing complementary and alternative medicine with cancer patients: Challenges for the clinical encounter, professional education and multi-disciplinary teamwork in oncology. *Health: An Interdisciplinary Journal for the Social Study of Health, Illness and Medicine* 13(3): 317–36.

Smithson, J., Paterson, C., Britten, N., Evans, M. and Lewith, G. (2010) Cancer patients' experiences of using complementary therapies: Polarization and integration. *Journal of Health Services Research and Policy* 15(2): 54–61.

References

Balneaves, L.G., Bottorff, J.L., Hislop, T.G. and Herbert, C. (2006) Levels of commitment: Exploring complementary therapy use by women with breast cancer. *Journal of Alternative and Complementary Medicine* 12: 459–66.

Balneaves, L.G., Truant, T.L., Kelly, M., Verhoef, M.J. and Davison, B.J. (2007) Bridging the gap: Decision-making processes of women with breast cancer using complementary and alternative medicine (CAM). *Supportive Care in Cancer* 15: 973–83.

Boon, H., Brown, J.B., Gavin, A., Kennard, M.A. and Stewart, M. (1999) Breast cancer survivors' perceptions of complementary/alternative medicine (CAM): Making the decision to use or not. *Qualitative Health Research* 9: 639–53.

Boon, H., Brown, J.B., Gavin, A. and Westlake, K. (2003) Men with prostate cancer: Making decisions about complementary/alternative medicine. *Medical Decision Making* 23: 471–9.

Boyd, D.B. (2007) Integrative oncology: The last ten years – a personal retrospective. *Alternative Therapies in Health and Medicine* 13: 56–64.

Broom, A. and Tovey, P. (2007) The dialectical tension between individuation and depersonalization in cancer patients' mediation of complementary, alternative and biomedical cancer treatments. *Sociology* 41: 1021–39.

Davidson, R., Geoghegan, L., McLaughlin, L. and Woodward, R. (2005) Psychological characteristics of cancer patients who use complementary therapies. *PsychoOncology* 14: 187–95.

Davison, B.J., Gleave, M.E., Goldenberg, S.L., Degner, L.F., Hoffart, D. and Berkowitz, J. (2002) Assessing information and decision preferences of men with prostate cancer and their partners. *Cancer Nursing* 25: 42–9.

Deng, G.E., Cassileth, B.R., Cohen, L. *et al.* (2007) Integrative oncology practice guidelines. *Journal of the Society for Integrative Oncology* 5: 65–84.

Eng, J., Ramsum, D., Verhoef, M., Guns, E., Davison, B.J. and Gallagher, R. (2003) A population based survey of complementary and alternative medicine use in men recently diagnosed with prostate cancer. *Integrative Cancer Therapies* 2: 212–16.

Evans, M.A., Shaw, A.R., Sharp, D.J. *et al.* (2007a) Men with cancer: Is their use of complementary and alternative medicine a response to needs unmet by conventional care? *European Journal of Cancer Care* 16: 517–25.

Evans, M., Shaw, A., Thompson, E.A. *et al.* (2007b) Decisions to use complementary and alternative medicine (CAM) by male cancer patients: Information-seeking roles and types of evidence used. *BMC Complementary and Alternative Medicine* 7: 25.

Hann, D., Allen, S., Ciambrone, D. and Shah, A. (2006) Use of complementary therapies during chemotherapy: Influence of patients' satisfaction with treatment decision making and the treating oncologist. *Integrative Cancer Therapies* 5: 224–31.

Kimby, C.K., Launso, L., Henningsen, I. and Langgaard, H. (2003) Choice of unconventional treatment by patients with cancer. *Journal of Alternative and Complementary Medicine* 9: 549–61.

Leis, A., Sagar, S., Verhoef, M.J., Balneaves, L.G., Seely, D. and Oneschuk, D. (2010) Shifting the paradigm: From complementary and alternative medicine to integrative oncology. In J.M. Elwood and S.B. Sutcliffe (eds) *Cancer Control*. New York: Oxford University Press.

Lupton, D. (1994) Theoretical perspectives on medicine and society. In D. Lupton (ed.) *Medicine as Culture*. London: Sage, pp. 5–21.

Montbriand, M.J. (1995) Decision tree model describing alternate health care choices made by oncology patients. *Cancer Nursing* 18: 104–17.

Öhlén, J., Balneaves, L.G., Bottorff, J.L. and Brazier, A.S. (2006) The influence of significant others in complementary and alternative decisions by cancer patients. *Social Science & Medicine* 63: 1625–36.

Rakovitch, E., Pignol, J.P., Chartier, C. *et al.* (2005) Complementary and alternative medicine use is associated with an increased perception of breast cancer risk and death. *Breast Cancer Research and Treatment* 90: 139–48.

Roberts, C.S., Baker, F., Hann, D. *et al.* (2005) Patient–physician communication regarding use of complementary therapies during cancer treatment. *Journal of Psychosocial Oncology* 23: 35–60.

Rotter, J.B. (1966) Generalized expectancies for internal versus external control of reinforcement. *Psychological Monographs* 80: 1–28.

Singh, H., Maskarinec, G. and Shumay, D.M. (2005) Understanding the motivation for conventional and complementary/alternative medicine use among men with prostate cancer. *Integrative Cancer Therapies* 4: 187–94.

Truant, T. and Bottorff, J.L. (1999) Decision making related to complementary therapies: A process of regaining control. *Patient Education and Counseling* 38: 131–42.

Weeks, L., Verhoef, M. and Scott, C. (2007) Presenting the alternative: Cancer and complementary and alternative medicine in the Canadian print media. *Supportive Care in Cancer* 15: 931–8.

CHAPTER 9

Mental health and complementary and alternative medicine

JEROME SARRIS AND JAMES LAKE

Introduction

For millennia, traditional medicine systems have used a variety of natural products and therapeutic arts to treat mental disorders. Many traditional systems of medicine treated mental disorders in an energetic or spiritual model, and often sufferers were viewed as being affected by a spiritual force (especially in cases of psychosis). The modern field of complementary and alternative medicine (CAM) and psychiatry has evolved significantly from its folkloric roots, and its present use is prevalent among sufferers of mental disorders (Wu *et al.*, 2007; Sarris *et al.*, 2010b).

This chapter gives an overview of the current state of evidence for CAM in the mental health field and explores the present paradigm in mental health care, which appears to be undergoing a shift from a reductive, symptom-focused and pharmacotherapy-dominated approach to a more integrated, biopsychosocial model. The chapter concludes with a discussion of emerging areas of CAM research and clinical application in mental health. Only minor emphasis is placed on a review of clinical evidence, as this has been extensively covered in many other publications. Here we focus on exploring the future of CAM practice within mental health care.

Evolving paradigms in mental health care

Understandings of the neurochemical and psychological mechanisms underlying both normal brain functioning and mental illness continue to change at a rapid rate; this points to the limitations of current explanatory models in the neurosciences and psychiatry. The conceptual framework employed in contemporary biomedical psychiatry is an eclectic mix of disparate theories. However, there is still no falsifiable theory of mental illness causation. An adequate theory of mental illness causation will require novel research methodologies and advances in functional brain imaging, genetics and molecular biology that can elucidate complex relationships between the biological, electromagnetic and possibly quantum-level activity of the brain and body, and discrete cognitive, affective or behavioural symptoms. Future theories will take into account both classically described biological factors (that is, neurophysiological and immunological functioning) as well as non-classical phenomena, including the postulated role of macroscopic coherent quantum fields in neuronal activity underlying human consciousness (Penrose, 1994).

Complexity theory, which regards living systems from the perspective of non-linear dynamics, may be increasingly used in biomedicine to characterize symptom patterns as novel 'emergent' properties of the brain–body (Bak, 1996). Conventional biomedical psychiatry is beginning to acknowledge the role of complex relationships between genetic and biochemical individuality in the pathogenesis of mental illness. Recent findings suggest that complex interactions between immune functioning, neurotransmitters and hormones are coupled to depressed mood, anxiety and other mental and emotional symptoms (Neimssen and Kern, 2007). Progress in functional brain imaging, including positron emission tomography (PET), single photon emission computed tomography (SPECT) and functional magnetic resonance imaging (fMRI), may eventually permit quantitative analysis of complex relationships between neurotransmitter systems and neuroendocrinological factors associated with mental illness, resulting in more effective and more individualized pharmacological treatments of mental disorders (Bandettini, 2009). Future research findings in the neurosciences and medicine may lead to advances in understanding of normal human consciousness and, by extension, mental illness. Advances in clinical biomedicine may confirm some conventional theories of mental illness causation while refuting others. Emerging paradigms may contribute to future theories of brain function, leading to more complete understandings of the biological, energetic, informational and possibly spiritual causes or 'meanings' of mental illness.

Practitioners of many traditional systems of medicine argue that illness, health and healing can be more completely understood within conceptual frameworks that differ in fundamental ways from the empiricism of allopathic medicine. For example, in traditional Chinese medicine and Ayurveda, symptoms are interpreted as imbalances of postulated energetic principles. In this model, the causes of mental illness cannot be described in simple causal terms according to the accepted dogma of biomedicine. Emerging models like complexity theory and quantum field theory (QFT) may be consistent with the 'energetic imbalances' postulated by Ayurveda and other non-western systems of medicine. The disparate viewpoints of conventional allopathic medicine and highly evolved non-western healing traditions call for conceptual bridges between different systems of medicine and practical strategies for integration.

Current evidence of CAM in psychiatry

Over the past two decades a marked increase has occurred in research in both conventional and complementary medicine in the field of psychiatry. The most highly researched natural products (NPs) include St John's wort, L-tryptophan, omega-3 and S-adenosyl methionine (SAMe) for depression; kava for anxiety disorders; ginkgo and bacopa for cognitive deficits; valerian for sleep disorders; nutrients such as zinc and iron for ADHD; and traditional Chinese medicines, amino acids and antioxidants to enhance the efficacy of mood stabilizers and antipsychotics in bipolar disorder and schizophrenia (Sarris *et al.*, 2010a; Sarris and Byrne, 2011; Larzelere *et al.*, 2010). An abundance of gold-standard randomized controlled trials (RCTs) have shown support for these natural medicines, apart for mixed evidence for ginkgo and valerian. In respect to therapies, acupuncture has demonstrated evidence for mood, anxiety and sleep disorders, while being ineffective in bipolar disorder (Samuels *et al.*, 2008; Dennehy *et al.*, 2009). Yoga and Tai Chi have been found to have beneficial effects on mood, anxiety and sleep, especially in ageing populations (Gooneratne, 2008; Larzelere *et al.*, 2010). Homeopathy to date has not been sufficiently assessed in psychiatric application, although its individualized approach makes it a better candidate for outcome-focused research rather than research of a standardized prescription. Recent research is now validating the importance of a nutrient-rich healthy diet in benefiting mood, with epidemiological evidence revealing that better-quality nutrition equals better mental health (Jacka *et al.*, 2010). Emerging research is also showing that exposure to nature (green space) also has a potent beneficial effect on mental well-being (Barton and Pretty, 2010).

A novel research project from Canada in the area of holistic practice provides a template for future research. The first trial of naturopathic care (NC) for anxiety was conducted, consisting of a multicomponent intervention. The 12-week RCT compared NC to standardized psychotherapy and deep breathing in 81 working people with moderate to severe anxiety (Cooley *et al.*, 2009). Participants in the NC group received dietary counselling, deep breathing relaxation techniques, a standard multivitamin and the anxiolytic herbal medicine withania (300 mg twice a day). The control intervention received psychotherapy, matched deep breathing relaxation techniques and herbal placebo tablets. The study results reveal a significant reduction in anxiety, concentration, fatigue and overall quality of life in favour of NC. The significance of this study is that multicomponent naturopathic practice used for mental disorders can be as effective, if not more so, than standard therapy, and can be researched in a methodologically rigorous manner. Taking all of the above detailed evidence together, CAM in the form of natural products, therapies or whole-system practice is increasingly being validated by modern research.

Future directions for CAM and mental health

Mental health care is at a crossroads. While pharmaceutical research in the area of psychopharmacology has flourished over the past half-century, the evidence in respect of improved outcomes and increased remission of mental disorders has been underwhelming. In light of the billions invested in new drugs, mental disorders remain prevalent and are still inadequately treated by pharmacotherapy monotherapy approaches. Certainly, there are for example strengths in the application of certain synthetic pharmacotherapies (for example mood stabilizers for bipolar disorder, antipsychotics for schizophrenia and psychotic disorders, benzodiazepines for acute anxiety and insomnia, and antidepressants for severe depression) (Sarris *et al.*, 2010a). Nevertheless, many of these drugs have common side-effects and in some cases only partial benefit is derived, with persistent frank or subclinical symptoms being maintained. While it is unwise and fallacious to advocate CAM as the sole solution, a future mainstream direction of research and clinical practice may involve an evidence-based combination of orthodox and traditional medicine in the form of integrative models.

As detailed in Table 9.1, a number of potential future focuses exist for CAM in the field of psychiatry. A much-needed future focus of research and clinical application is in the integrated approach to treatment of mental health disorders via biopsychosocial models. One of the future paradigm shifts required is the exploration of 'whole-person' research (Verhoef and Vanderheyden, 2007). In the area of psychiatry and CAM research, this relates to exploring the quantitative effects (on established psychiatric scales) and qualitative experiences (personal benefits, unknown effects, adverse reactions); the use of an individually tailored multiple-component intervention, which essentially studies the 'art' of CAM as much as the science (that is, outcome-focused exploration of the practice of therapies such as naturopathy); and the interrelationship between systems (such as the effect of CAM psychopharmacology on other physiology such as digestion, metabolism, cardiovascular system; or vice versa, the effect of these systems on mental health).

Research of novel botanical medicines is in its infancy, and it remains to be seen which plants are going to be the 'next St John's wort'. In the area of depression, likely candidates include rhodiola (Panossian *et al.*, 2010), saffron (Akhondzadeh *et al.*, 2005) and happy bark (Kim *et al.*, 2007). Nutrient research in psychiatry is also evolving, with many positive studies demonstrating psychotropic effects as monotherapies or adjuvants (Sarris *et al.*, 2009). The area of adjuvant natural product research combines nutrients or botanicals with conventional pharmacotherapies to improve efficacy and potentially reduce side-effects by allowing less medication to be used. For example, this has been demonstrated as effective in many studies that have shown increased effects from SAMe, folic acid, L-tryptophan and omega-3 with antidepressants in depression (Sarris *et al.*, 2009); and n-acetly cysteine, magnesium, folic acid and amino acids in bipolar disorder (Sarris *et al.*, 2010a).

Table 9.1 Future areas of research in CAM and mental health

Area	Potential application
Integrative psychiatry	Combining the best evidence from conventional medicine, CAM therapies and NPs, psychological interventions and lifestyle modification in an integrative approach
Whole-person, practice-focused research	A movement towards studying the 'practice of CAM' rather than a reductive focus on NP monotherapies; this may scientifically validate CAM therapies. Incorporation of qualitative research in RCTs can explore personalized experiences in addition to gathering quantitative data
Adjuvancy studies	The majority of adjuvancy studies provide positive evidence of the use of NPs to increase the efficacy of psychopharmaceuticals. More NPs can be studied in this area to aid in providing increased beneficial effects
Novel herbal medicines	Our planet contains many unexplored plant medicines that have the potential to be the 'next St John's wort'. Recent examples include saffron, rhodiola and happy bark
Novel uses of nutrients	As our understanding of pathophysiology improves, we can apply particular nutrients to modulate specific neurochemical imbalances
Research of synergistic nutrient formulations	Moving away from monotherapies, synergistic NP formulations are likely to have greater pharmacodynamic effects
Pharmacogenomics	This involved discovering which NPs are beneficial for individuals according to their neurochemistry. Also, if they are poor or fast drug metabolizers (CYP450 polymorphisms), the dose can be adjusted to suit the person
Epigenetics	This is validating the effects of NPs on inhibiting harmful genes being activated and promoting beneficial gene expression
Neuroimaging	As technology increases and costs are reduced, this can be applied to observe the effect of CAM therapies and NPs on brain function

A paradigm change that needs to occur in respect to research into nutrients involves a greater understanding and utilization of 'synergy' between nutrients (Sarris *et al.*, 2009). This is often ignored by the mainstream in a quest for the 'reductive silver bullet'. Future studies involving nutrients should adopt synergistic formulae of nutrients, as they always act in concert, for example SAMe, folic acid and B12 in the 'one-carbon cycle' that is important for stable mood (Williams *et al.*, 2005).

A novel area of emerging significance in medicine is genetics. This includes the specific areas of pharmacogenomics and epigenetics. Pharmacogenomics involves the identification of genetic differences between individuals (polymorphisms), which may affect either how the pharmacotherapy (herbal, nutrient or drug) is metabolized (via CYP P450 polymorphisms) (Preskorn, 2006) or whether any differences occur in pharmacodynamic activity via differences in neurochemistry. These genetic differences in individuals may affect monoamine production, receptor binding or transporter activity, all of which provide differing responses to medications. Examples of polymorphisms that may be assessed in the future include serotonin transporter SLC 6A4 (for anti-depressant CAMs, for example St John's wort), noradrenaline (NET) and dopamine (D2) receptors (for cognitive enhancers, for example ginkgo), GABA transporters and receptors (for anxiolytic CAMs, for example kava) and APOE (for antidementic CAMs, for example bacopa) (Preskorn, 2006; Bellgrove and Mattingley, 2008; Horstmann and Binder, 2009; Ulrich-Merzenich *et al.*, 2009;). Epigenetics is an emerging area of research whereby interventions can be tested for their effect on gene expression (Kirk *et al.*, 2008). To date only a handful of studies exist observing the effect that natural products can have on inhibiting or triggering the expression of particular genes. Future research in this area is promising, with the potential to demonstrate quantifiable genetic effects from natural products as either monotherapies or multicomponent formulations, such as TCM herbal formulae.

A final area of potential that has been pursued over the last decade to quantify the effects of acupuncture is the use of neuroimaging techniques. In the area of psychiatry these techniques are valuable to observe the effects of substances on brain waves (electroencephalography, EEG), cerebral blood flow (fMRI) and activation of brain function (PET) (Bandettini, 2009). Future application of these techniques may provide hard biological evidence of the effects of various NPs, and potentially can show an effect physiologically before it manifests as a psychological change in the individual. Examples using NPs could include showing an increase in pre-frontal cortex activity in ADHD, cognitive deficit and depression; and limbic/hippocampal effects in anxiety disorders.

Conclusion

The future of the field of CAM in mental health appears to be positive, with emerging evidence of efficacy and safety, its increasing integrative mainstream clinical use, and the evolving application of various technologies to provide validation. To illustrate the growth of this field we note the two recent over-prescribed integrative mental health conferences (in Europe and the United States) that clearly demonstrate an interest from clinicians, particularly when married with the public usage data and increased research (publications indexed in this area have grown over 50 per cent in the last five years). A manifestation of this evolving interest in the area of CAM and mental health is the creation of the International Network of Integrative Mental Health (INIMH, see website at www.INIHM.org), which was formed in Phoenix, USA in 2009 to create a vibrant network of clinicians, researchers and public health advocates to advance the research, education and practice of an evidence-based, integrative, whole-person approach to mental health. The future challenge is to assist in evolving a paradigm in which this approach is the norm and not the exception.

Further reading

Lake, J. (2006) *Textbook of Integrative Mental Health Care.* New York: Thieme Medical Publishers.

Sarris, J. (2007) Herbal medicines in the treatment of psychiatric disorders: A systematic review. *Phytotherapy Research* 21(8): 703–16.

Sarris, J., Kavanagh, D.J. and Byrne, G.J. (2009) Adjuvant use of nutritional and herbal medicines with antidepressants, mood stabilizers and benzodiazepines. *Journal of Psychiatric Research* 44: 32–41.

Ulrich-Merzenich, G. (2007) Application of the '-omic-'technologies in phytomedicine. *Phytomedicine* 14(1): 70–82.

Werneke, U., Turner, T. and Priebe, S. (2006) Complementary medicines in psychiatry: Review of effectiveness and safety. *British Journal of Psychiatry* 188: 109–21.

References

Akhondzadeh, S., Tahmacebi-Pour, N., Noorbala, A.A. *et al.* (2005) Crocus sativus L. in the treatment of mild to moderate depression: A double-blind, randomized and placebo-controlled trial. *Phytotherapy Research* 19: 148–51.

Bak, P. (1996) *How Nature Works: The Science of Self-Organised Criticality.* New York: Copernicus.

Bandettini, P.A. (2009) What's new in neuroimaging methods? *Annals of the New York Academy of Sciences* 1156: 260–93.

Barton, J. and Pretty, J. (2010) What is the best dose of nature and green exercise for improving mental health? A multi-study analysis. *Environmental Science and Technology* 44: 3947–55.

Bellgrove, M.A. and Mattingley, J.B. (2008) Molecular genetics of attention. *Annals of the New York Academy of Sciences* 1129: 200–12.

Cooley, K., Szczurko, O., Perri, D. *et al.* (2009) Naturopathic care for anxiety: A randomized controlled trial. *PLoS One* 4: e6628.

Dennehy, E.B., Schyer, R., Bernstein, I.H. *et al.* (2009) The safety, acceptability, and effectiveness of acupuncture as an adjunctive treatment for acute symptoms in bipolar disorder. *Journal of Clinical Psychiatry* 70: 897–905.

Gooneratne, N.S. (2008) Complementary and alternative medicine for sleep disturbances in older adults. *Clinics in Geriatric Medicine* 24: 121–38.

Horstmann, S. and Binder, E.B. (2009) Pharmacogenomics of antidepressant drugs. *Pharmacology and Therapeutics* 124: 57–73.

Jacka, F.N., Pasco, J.A., Mykletun, A. *et al.* (2010) Association of western and traditional diets with depression and anxiety in women. *American Journal of Psychiatry* 167(3): 305–11.

Kim, J.H., Kim, S.Y., Lee, S.Y. and Jang, C.G. (2007) Antidepressant-like effects of Albizzia julibrissin in mice: Involvement of the 5-HT1A receptor system. *Pharmacology Biochemistry and Behavior* 87: 41–7.

Kirk, H., Cefalu, W.T., Ribnicky, D., Liu, Z. and Eilertsen, K.J. (2008) Botanicals as epigenetic modulators for mechanisms contributing to development of metabolic syndrome. *Metabolism* 57: S16–23.

Larzelere, M.M., Campbell, J.S. and Robertson, M. (2010) Complementary and alternative medicine usage for behavioral health indications. *Primary Care* 37: 213–36.

Neimssen, T. and Kern, S. (2007) Psychoneuroimmunology – cross-talk between the immune and nervous systems. *Journal of Neurology* 255: 309–10.

Panossian, A., Wikman, G. and Sarris, J. (2010) Rosenroot (Rhodiola rosea): Traditional use, chemical composition, pharmacology and clinical efficacy. *Phytomedicine* 17: 481–93.

Penrose, R. (1994) *Shadows of the Mind: A Search for the Missing Science of Consciousness*. Oxford: Oxford University Press.

Preskorn, S.H. (2006) Pharmacogenomics, informatics, and individual drug therapy in psychiatry: Past, present and future. *Journal of Psychopharmacology* 20: 85–94.

Samuels, N., Gropp, C., Singer, S.R. and Oberbaum, M. (2008) Acupuncture for psychiatric illness: A literature review. *Behavioral Medicine* 34: 55–64.

Sarris, J. and Byrne, G. (2011) A systematic review of insomnia and complementary medicine. *Sleep Medicine Reviews* 15(2): 99–106.

Sarris, J., Kavanagh, D. and Byrne, G. (2010a) Adjuvant use of nutritional and herbal medicines with antidepressants, mood stabilizers and benzodiazepines. *Journal of Psychiatric Research* 44: 32–41.

Sarris, J., Robins Wahlin, T.B., Goncalves, D.C. and Byrne, G.J. (2010b) Comparative use of complementary medicine, allied health, and manual therapies by middle-aged and older Australian women. *Journal of Women and Aging* 22: 273–82.

Sarris, J., Schoendorfer, N. and Kavanagh, D. (2009) Major depressive disorder and nutritional medicine: A review of monotherapies and adjuvant treatments. *Nutrition Reviews* 67: 125–31.

Ulrich-Merzenich, G., Panek, D., Zeitler, H., Wagner, H. and Vetter, H. (2009) New perspectives for synergy research with the 'omic'-technologies. *Phytomedicine* 16: 495–508.

Verhoef, M. and Vanderheyden, L. (2007) Combining qualitative methods and RCTs in CAM intervention research. In J. Adams (ed.) *Researching Complementary and Alternative Medicine*. London: Routledge.

Williams, A.L., Girard, C., Jui, D., Sabina, A. and Katz, D.L. (2005) S-adenosylmethionine (SAMe) as treatment for depression: A systematic review. *Clinical and Investigative Medicine* 28: 132–9.

Wu, P., Fuller, C., Liu, X. *et al.* (2007) Use of complementary and alternative medicine among women with depression: Results of a national survey. *Psychiatric Services* 58: 349–56.

Complementary and alternative medicine use among HIV-positive people: Research synthesis and implications for HIV care

RAE LITTLEWOOD AND PETER VANABLE

Introduction

On average, published research indicates that 60 per cent of HIV-positive (HIV+) individuals use CAM to treat HIV-related health concerns (for example Mikhail *et al.*, 2004). In the context of conventional HIV care, where survival depends on proper use of and adherence to highly active antiretroviral treatment (HAART) (Lohse *et al.*, 2007), the potential for CAM use to interfere with such treatment success is a pressing concern. Indeed, use of certain types of CAM may compromise the efficacy of HAART as a result of an unanticipated drug interaction or side-effect of CAM (Ernst, 2002; Hennessy *et al.*, 2002). The potential for adverse outcomes may be amplified when HIV+ patients do not disclose their CAM use to their primary HIV care providers or when patients' preferences for CAM interfere with the uptake of conventional HIV treatments (Kremer *et al.*, 2006). Prior to HAART, research investigating CAM use among HIV+ patients focused on describing the prevalence and types of CAM used and characterizing HIV+ CAM users on a range of demographic, biomedical and psychosocial indices. More recently, CAM research has expanded to focus on patients' reasons for using CAM and to address how CAM is incorporated into conventional HIV care.

Source: Littlewood, R. and Vanable, P. (2008) Complementary and alternative medicine use among HIV-positive people: Research synthesis and implications for HIV care. *AIDS Care* 20(8): 1102–18. Abridged version reprinted with kind permission of Routledge (Taylor and Francis Ltd).

To characterize the factors associated with CAM use and synthesize the literature on the potential impact of CAM use on HIV care, we conducted a critical review of research investigating CAM use among people living with HIV. To date, only one review on CAM use among HIV+ individuals has been conducted (Wootton and Sparber, 2001). Since the publication of Wootton and Sparber's review, an additional 22 studies of CAM use have been published characterizing the demographic, biomedical, psychosocial and health behaviur correlates of CAM use. In addition to providing a concise synthesis of research dating back to the early stages of the HIV epidemic, important conceptual and methodological limitations in this literature are identified and implications of review findings for the provision of conventional HIV care are discussed.

Method

Literature available in MEDLINE and PsychINFO was searched using a number of relevant keywords; 78 English-language articles published in peer-reviewed journals were screened for inclusion. Studies were included if they assessed HIV+ patients' use of CAM using qualitative or quantitative methodology and defined CAM use as a purposeful action taken to treat, cope with or alleviate HIV symptoms or side-effects of conventional HIV treatment. Studies exploring CAM use not specifically directed at treatment of HIV and studies examining the efficacy of CAM were excluded. According to these criteria, 40 studies were included.

Review findings

Review findings are organized as follows. First, we describe the demographic, biomedical and psychosocial correlates of CAM use among HIV+ individuals. Second, a synthesis of research describing HIV+ patients' reasons for using CAM is provided. Third, we review literature investigating whether HIV+ patients' use of CAM interferes with conventional HIV care.

Demographic correlates of CAM use

Our review indicates that CAM use among HIV+ people is disproportionately higher among Caucasians as compared to minority respondents (Suarez and Reese 1997, 2000; Smith *et al.*, 1999; Wutoh *et al.*, 2001; Risa *et al.*, 2002; Hsiao *et al.*, 2003), men who have sex with men as compared to respondents of other sexual orientations (Smith *et al.*, 1999; Suarez and Reese, 2000; Bica *et al.*, 2003; Hsiao *et al.*, 2003; London *et al.*, 2003), individuals with more education (Ostrow *et al.*, 1997; Fairfield *et al.*, 1998; Smith *et al.*, 1999; de Visser and Grierson, 2002; Bica *et al.*, 2003; Chang *et al.*, 2003; Colebunders *et al.*, 2003; Hsiao *et al.*, 2003; Mikhail *et al.*, 2004; Tsao *et al.*, 2005) and those who have higher incomes (Ostrow *et al.*, 1997; Bica *et al.*, 2003; London *et al.*, 2003). This pattern of findings suggests that CAM use is more likely among individuals who have greater education and financial resources (for discussion of predictors of CAM use generally, see Chapter 1).

Health-related correlates of CAM use

Research examining the relationship between CAM use and health status indicates that HIV+ individuals who have been diagnosed with AIDS (Jernewall *et al.*, 2005), experienced symptoms of HIV (Suarez *et al.*, 1996; Knippels and Weiss, 2000; Mikhail *et al.*, 2004) or have longer disease duration (Anderson *et al.*, 1993; Colebunders *et al.*, 2003; Mikhail *et al.*, 2004; Woolridge *et al.*, 2005) are more likely to use CAM than healthier individuals or those with shorter disease duration. In addition, several studies indicate that CAM use is associated with greater HIV-symptom severity (Ostrow *et al.*, 1997; Chang *et al.*, 2003) and a higher degree of disability (Burg *et al.*, 2005; Woolridge *et al.*, 2005). Taken together, these findings suggest that patients who have experienced HIV-related symptoms are most likely to pursue CAM, presumably to alleviate such symptoms.

Psychosocial correlates of CAM use

Research seeking to determine whether HIV+ CAM users differ from non-users with respect to depressive symptomology and coping approaches has yielded mixed findings. In relation to psychological adjustment, only one study found higher levels of distress among CAM users as compared to non-users (Risa *et al.*, 2002). There is more evidence to suggest that CAM use is associated with fewer depressive symptoms (Suarez and Reese, 2000) and better mental health (Sugimoto *et al.*, 2005). Several studies suggest that CAM use is associated with the employment of more adaptive approaches to coping with HIV-related stressors, including problem-focused coping, seeking social support and turning to religion (Suarez and Reese, 1997, 2000; Knippels and Weiss, 2000). In addition, HIV+ CAM users are more likely than non-users to appraise HIV as a controllable stressor (Suarez and Reese, 1997, 2000).

Reasons for CAM use among HIV+ people

Sixteen of the reviewed studies assessed HIV+ patients' reasons for using CAM. HIV+ patients report that they use CAM primarily for practical reasons: to alleviate HIV symptoms and HAART side-effects and to improve quality of life. For some HIV+ people, CAM offers a means of addressing their concerns with conventional treatment and engaging in health care practices that align with their health beliefs. To clarify why some HIV+ patients use CAM whereas others do not, quantitative research into the relationship between CAM use and patients' reasons for CAM use is needed.

HAART adherence and CAM use

Seven studies have evaluated the association between CAM use and adherence. Two studies identified an association between CAM use and treatment non-adherence. Jernewall *et al.* (2005) found that users of 'Latino CAM' (that is, traditional healing practices in Latino culture) were less likely to attend medical appointments and had lower rates of HAART adherence for the previous three days. In addition, users of plant-based remedies had lower rates of adherence to HAART (Jernewall *et al.*, 2005). More recently, HIV+ women who reported using orally administered CAM to treat their HIV were more likely to report missing at least one dose of their prescribed HIV medications in the past 30 days (Owen-Smith *et al.*, 2007). The remaining studies found no differences in HAART adherence between CAM users and non-users.

Attitudes towards conventional medicine and the decision to use CAM

Early in the HIV epidemic, research suggested that HIV+ CAM users were more likely than non-users to perceive conventional HIV medications as ineffective (Langewitz *et al.*, 1994). Although HAART provides substantial clinical benefits, concerns about the side-effects and long-term health consequences of HAART contribute to less favourable attitudes towards conventional medicine (Remien *et al.*, 2003; Johnson *et al.*, 2005) and such attitudes may also influence the decision to use CAM. For example, CAM use was strongly associated with more favourable attitudes towards CAM (for example the perception that CAM delays illness progression and boosts immune functioning) and less favourable attitudes towards HAART (de Visser and Grierson, 2002). In another study, patients who believe that conventional HIV medications are 'definitely not worth taking' were eight times more likely to use CAM as a substitute for conventional treatment compared to those who believe that conventional treatments are 'worth taking' (Hsiao *et al.*, 2003). Given that data collection for these studies was completed prior to the widespread use of HAART, their findings may not be representative of patients' beliefs about HAART today. Further research exploring the interplay between HAART beliefs, CAM use and adherence is needed.

Non-disclosure of CAM use to conventional care providers

Patient–provider communication about CAM use would presumably reduce the risk of adverse health outcomes that may result from drug interactions or misuse of conventional medication. CAM disclosure rates vary substantially across studies, with between 38 and 90 per cent of patients reporting that their physician is aware of their CAM use (Fairfield *et al.*, 1998; Sparber *et al.*, 2000; Standish *et al.*, 2001; Risa *et al.*, 2002; Chang *et al.*, 2003; Furler *et al.*, 2003; Hsiao *et al.*, 2003). Although no studies have investigated the link between CAM use disclosure and HIV-related health outcomes, research strongly suggests a need for routine assessment and discussion of CAM use among HIV+ patients.

Discussion

An overarching conclusion from this review is the need for research exploring the intersection between CAM use and conventional treatment for HIV. Two primary concerns have received attention: (1) the potential for CAM use to interfere with use of and adherence to conventional HIV medications; and (2) non-disclosure of CAM use to medical care providers. While there was only mixed support for an association between CAM use and HAART adherence, patients' beliefs about HAART may influence whether CAM is used as an adjunct or an alternative to conventional medications. Further investigation of patient–provider interactions regarding CAM use is needed to clarify whether non-disclosure of CAM use contributes to adverse health outcomes.

To advance this important area of study, theory-based research is required to clarify how patients' beliefs about HIV and HAART guide their decisions to use CAM. Using theory to conceptualize how patients' beliefs influence treatment decisions will help to inform the development of interventions designed to improve patient–provider communication regarding CAM, and reduce the potential for CAM use to interfere with proper use of conventional treatments. Many HIV+ patients view CAM as an important part of their care. As such, providers should strive to incorporate routine assessment of CAM use as a means of informing treatment planning and maximizing long-term health outcomes for their HIV+ patients.

Further reading

Hasan, S.S., See, C.K., Choong, C.L.K., Ahmed, S.I., Ahmadi, K. and Anwar, M. (2010) Reasons, perceived efficacy, and factors associated with complementary and alternative medicine use among Malaysian patients with HIV. *Journal of Complementary and Alternative Medicine* 16(11): 1171–6.

Thorpe, R.D. (2009) 'Doing' chronic illness? Complementary medicine use among people living with HIV/AIDS in Australia. *Sociology of Health and Illness* 31(3): 375–89.

References

Anderson, W., O'Connor, B.B., MacGregor, R.R. and Schwartz, J.S. (1993) Patient use and assessment of conventional and alternative therapies for HIV infection and AIDS. *AIDS* 7(4): 561–5.

Bica, I., Tang, A.M., Skinner, S. *et al.* (2003) Use of complementary and alternative therapies by patients with human immunodeficiency virus disease in the era of highly active antiretroviral therapy. *Journal of Alternative and Complementary Medicine* 9(1): 65–76.

Burg, M.A., Uphold, C.R., Findley, K. and Reid, K. (2005) Complementary and alternative medicine use among HIV-infected patients attending three outpatient clinics in the Southeastern United States. *International Journal of STD & AIDS* 16(2): 112–16.

Chang, B.L., van Servellen, G. and Lombardi, E. (2003) Factors associated with complementary therapy use in people living with HIV/AIDS receiving antiretroviral therapy. *Journal of Alternative and Complementary Medicine* 9(5): 695–710.

Colebunders, R., Dreezen, C., Florence, E., Pelgrom, Y. and Schrooten, W. (2003) The use of complementary and alternative medicine by persons with HIV infection in Europe. *International Journal of STD & AIDS* 14(10): 672–4.

de Visser, R. and Grierson, J. (2002) Use of alternative therapies by people living with HIV/AIDS in Australia. *AIDS Care* 14(5): 599–606.

Ernst, E. (2002) The dark side of complementary and alternative medicine. *International Journal of STD & AIDS* 13(12): 797–800.

Fairfield, K.M., Eisenberg, D.M., Davis, R.B., Libman, H. and Phillips, R.S. (1998) Patterns of use, expenditures, and perceived efficacy of complementary and alternative therapies in HIV-infected patients. *Archives of Internal Medicine* 158(20): 2257–64.

Furler, M.D., Einarson, T.R., Walmsley, S., Millson, M. and Bendayan, R. (2003) Use of complementary and alternative medicine by HIV-infected outpatients in Ontario, Canada. *AIDS Patient Care and STDs* 17(4): 155–68.

Hennessy, M., Kelleher, D., Spiers, J.P. *et al.* (2002) St Johns Wort increases expression of P-glycoprotein: Implications for drug interactions. *British Journal of Clinical Pharmacology* 53(1): 75–82.

Hsiao, A.F., Wong, M.D., Kanouse, D.E. *et al.* (2003) Complementary and alternative medicine use and substitution for conventional therapy by HIV-infected patients. *Journal of Acquired Immune Deficiency Syndrome* 33(2): 157–65.

Jernewall, N., Zea, M.C., Reisen, C.A. and Poppen, P.J. (2005) Complementary and alternative medicine and adherence to care among HIV-positive Latino gay and bisexual men. *AIDS Care* 17(5): 601–09.

Johnson, M.O., Charlebois, E., Morin, S.F. *et al.* (2005) Perceived adverse effects of antiretroviral therapy. *Journal of Pain and Symptom Management* 29(2): 193–205.

Knippels, H.M. and Weiss, J.J. (2000) Use of alternative medicine in a sample of HIV-positive gay men: An exploratory study of prevalence and user characteristics. *AIDS Care* 12(4): 435–46.

Kremer, H., Ironson, G., Schneiderman, N. and Hautzinger, M. (2006) To take or not to take: Decision-making about antiretroviral treatment in people living with HIV/AIDS. *AIDS Patient Care and STDs* 20(5): 335–49.

Langewitz, W., Ruttimann, S., Laifer, G., Maurer, P. and Kiss, A. (1994) The integration of alternative treatment modalities in HIV infection – the patient's perspective. *Journal of Psychosomatic Research* 38(7): 687–93.

Lohse, N., Hansen, A.B., Pedersen, G. *et al.* (2007) Survival of persons with and without HIV infection in Denmark, 1995–2005. *Annals of Internal Medicine* 146(2): 87–95.

London, A.S., Foote-Ardah, C.E., Fleishman, J.A. and Shapiro, M.F. (2003) Use of alternative therapists among people in care for HIV in the United States. *American Journal of Public Health* 93(6): 980–87.

Mikhail, I.S., DiClemente, R., Person, S. *et al.* (2004) Association of complementary and alternative medicines with HIV clinical disease among a cohort of women living with HIV/AIDS. *Journal of Acquired Immune Deficiency Syndrome* 37(3): 1415–22.

Ostrow, M.J., Cornelisse, P.G., Heath, K.V. *et al.* (1997) Determinants of complementary therapy use in HIV-infected individuals receiving antiretroviral or anti-opportunistic agents. *Journal of Acquired Immune Deficiency Syndromes and Human Retrovirology* 15(2): 115–20.

Owen-Smith, A., Diclemente, R. and Wingood, G. (2007) Complementary and alternative medicine use decreases adherence to HAART in HIV-positive women. *AIDS Care* 19(5): 589–93.

Remien, R.H., Hirky, A.E., Johnson, M.O., Weinhardt, L.S., Whittier, D. and Le, G.M. (2003) Adherence to medication treatment: A qualitative study of facilitators and barriers among a diverse sample of HIV+ men and women in four US cities. *AIDS & Behavior* 7(1): 61–72.

Risa, K.J., Nepon, L., Justis, J.C. *et al.* (2002) Alternative therapy use in HIV-infected patients receiving highly active antiretroviral therapy. *International Journal of STD & AIDS* 13(10): 706–13.

Smith, S.R., Boyd, E.L. and Kirking, D.M. (1999) Nonprescription and alternative medication use by individuals with HIV disease. *Annals of Pharmacotherapy* 33(3): 294–300.

Sparber, A., Wootton, J.C., Bauer, L. *et al.* (2000) Use of complementary medicine by adult patients participating in HIV/AIDS clinical trials. *Journal of Alternative and Complementary Medicine* 6(5): 415–22.

Standish, L.J., Greene, K.B., Bain, S. *et al.* (2001) Alternative medicine use in HIV-positive men and women: Demographics, utilization patterns and health status. *AIDS Care* 13(2): 197–208.

Suarez, T., Raffaelli, M. and O'Leary, A. (1996) Use of folk healing practices by HIV-infected Hispanics living in the United States. *AIDS Care* 8(6): 683–90.

Suarez, T. and Reese, F. (1997) Alternative medicine use, perceived control, coping, and adjustment in African American and Caucasian males living with HIV and AIDS. *International Journal of Rehabilitation and Health* 3(2): 107–18.

Suarez, T. and Reese, F. (2000) Coping, psychological adjustment, and complementary and alternative medicine use in persons living with HIV and AIDS. *Psychology and Health* 15(5): 635–49.

Sugimoto, N., Ichikawa, M., Siriliang, B., Nakahara, S., Jimba, M. and Wakai, S. (2005) Herbal medicine use and quality of life among people living with HIV/AIDS in northeastern Thailand. *AIDS Care* 17(2): 252–62.

Tsao, J.C., Dobalian, A., Myers, C.D. and Zeltzer, L.K. (2005) Pain and use of complementary and alternative medicine in a national sample of persons living with HIV. *Journal of Pain and Symptom Management* 30(5): 418–32.

Woolridge, E., Barton, S., Samuel, J., Osorio, J., Dougherty, A. and Holdcroft, A. (2005) Cannabis use in HIV for pain and other medical symptoms. *Journal of Pain and Symptom Management* 29(4): 358–67.

Wootton, J.C. and Sparber, A. (2001) Surveys of complementary and alternative medicine: Part III. Use of alternative and complementary therapies for HIV/AIDS. *Journal of Alternative and Complementary Medicine* 7(4): 371–7.

Wutoh, A.K., Brown, C.M., Kumoji, E.K. *et al.* (2001) 'ntiretroviral adherence and use of alternative therapies among older HIV-infected adults. *Journal of the National Medical Association* 93: 243–50.

Traditional, complementary and integrative medicine and well-being

RICHARD HARVEY

Introduction

This chapter addresses the topic of traditional, complementary and integrative medicine (TCIM) and well-being, suggesting that TCIM practices in comparison to Western allopathic medicine practices increase well-being by educating patients about self-care beyond taking care of a specific set of symptoms. The thesis of the chapter is that well-being results from patients finding meaning from their difficult circumstances, as well as the 'caring' (versus curing) that occurs with greater frequency in the context of TCIM practices. The chapter begins by examining some specific 'ways-of-knowing' related to well-being outcomes of TCIM practices. The chapter progresses by discussing types of well-being, conceptualizations of existential well-being, as well as measurements of well-being, and ends by suggesting that TCIM practices such as biofeedback enhance advice giving in support of finding meaning and increasing well-being.

Untangling TCIM intricacies and tensions using 'ways-of-knowing' perspectives

Adams *et al.* (2009) suggest that TCIM practices and resulting outcomes such as patient well-being be subject to a 'critical social science approach' that acknowledges the 'intricacies and tensions that surround the integration of different paradigms of health care practice' (Adams *et al.*, 2009: 792). Untangling the 'intricacies and tensions' that relate to well-being requires a brief discussion about 'ways-of-knowing' (Carper, 1992; Ingram, 2007).

A way-of-knowing (WOK) reflects cognitive processes that patients and practitioners use to find meaning and make sense of the world (Caseem,

2007). For example, Carper (1992) and Johns (1995) suggest that patient well-being is (1) influenced by an empirical WOK grounded in rational fact-based attitudes and beliefs, such as reflected in the hypothetical statement 'My symptoms went away and my well-being increased after being treated (by a healer who happened to be a Chinese herbalist)'; as well as (2) based on a sociopolitical WOK grounded in contextual social and political attitudes and beliefs, such as reflected in the hypothetical statement 'My symptoms went away and my well-being increased after being treated (by a healer who was an herbalist from specifically the region of China where I believe the best herbalists are trained)'.

To contrast empirical and sociopolitical WOK, an empirical WOK depends on unambiguous facts such as the fact of being treated and less sociopolitical facts such as where an herbalist was born. There are interactions between empirical and sociopolitical WOK. For example, consider a hypothetical acupuncture patient who believes in the efficacy of an acupuncture technique but faints at the sight of *any* needles; or a hypothetical acupuncturist who believes in the efficacy of needling, but lacks the needling skill of a seasoned master. In the acupuncture scenario, the patient lacks the empirical skill to receive the treatment and the practitioner lacks the empirical skill to deliver the treatment, despite a sociopolitical belief by both the patient and the practitioner that acupuncture is an effective TCIM technique. Patient well-being as a TCIM treatment outcome depends on the alignment of both the empirical knowledge and skills and the sociopolitical attitudes and beliefs of both the patient and the practitioner when delivering or receiving a treatment (Bressler, 1980).

Regarding sociopolitical WOK, Ingram (2007: 7) writes:

> Differences in WOK among people and groups often may be traced to different sources of legitimacy such as science, religion, cultural stories, symbols and artifacts. The language of a way of knowing may reflect the language of a particular scientific or professional discipline, culture, religion or method or reasoning.

Ingram (2007) argues that because people go through an inductive process when making sense of any health care practice or outcome, a sociopolitical WOK should be given primacy when understanding a health care practice or outcome such as patient well-being. Said another way, sociopolitical attitudes and beliefs about a treatment are more important to well-being than is the simple fact of being treated.

The construct of well-being in relation to TCIM practices

Facets of the well-being construct typically include describing well-being in terms of *subjective* and *psychological* well-being (Ryff, 1989), especially among patients with life-threatening illnesses such as cancer. To explore why TCIM practices lead to greater levels of well-being in contrast to western allopathic medicine practices (Barnes *et al.*, 2004), it is useful first to describe various conceptualizations of the well-being construct.

Psychological and subjective well-being

Diener (2000), Ryff (1989) and more recently Linley *et al.* (2010) describe two major domains of well-being, subjective well-being and psychological well-being, as follows:

> Subjective well-being comprises an affective component of the balance between positive and negative affect, together with a cognitive component of judgments about one's life satisfaction. Psychological well-being is conceptualized as having six components, including positive relations with others, autonomy, environmental mastery, self-acceptance, purpose in life and, personal growth. (Linley *et al.*, 2010: 878)

The label of social or psychological well-being has been used in contexts related to the measurement of 'quality of life'. For example, Ingersoll-Dayton *et al.* (2004) describe quality of life among elders facing illness in terms of intra-personal psychological well-being (for instance acceptance and enjoyment) as well as inter-personal social well-being (for instance harmony, interdependence, respect).

Whereas psychological well-being and subjective well-being are primary facets of the construct of well-being, there are other conceptualizations of well-being such as existential well-being, spiritual well-being and capital well-being.

Capital well-being

Well-being has been conceptualized in terms of acquisition or loss of capital resources. For example, Graham and Oswald (2010) suggest that when people lose material or social capital resources, they fall below their comparative well-being set point, with the likely result of entering states of 'ill-being' (Wilhelm *et al.*, 2010). Conceptualizing well-being in terms of allocating capital resources places individuals in three theoretical points of comparative well-being: above, at or below some relative well-being set point as they newly acquire or replace prior capital resources. For example, a cancer patient may experience loss of capital well-being, such as loss of mobility, loss of friends or loss of health, and have therefore fallen 'below the line' of capital well-being, which motivates them to replace their capital losses in pursuit of greater relative levels of well-being.

Spiritual well-being

Well-being has been conceptualized in terms of people having spiritual, mystical or religious/existential experiences (referred to as SMORES by Harvey,

2009) when facing a life-threatening illness of similar circumstances. For example, Edmondson *et al.* (2008) measured prayer behaviour as an operational approximation of spiritual and religious well-being among cancer patients, and found that a sense of spiritual well-being was both supported by as well as reflected in prayer behaviour. However, measuring spiritual, mystical or religious well-being using general observations of prayer behaviour may be problematic. Whittington and Scher (2010) suggest distinguishing three types of prayer associated with positive well-being – prayer giving thanks to God; prayer for being open to God; and prayer for adoration of God – from three types of prayer related to the opposite of well-being – supplicant prayer for favours; confessional prayer for forgiveness; and repetitive or mindless prayer for ritualistic adherence. Whereas spiritual, mystical or religious experiences often lead to finding meaning in life and therefore achieving a sense of well-being, unspecific measures of prayer (such as 'Do you engage in prayer?') as a sole approximation of spiritual, mystical or religious well-being are not recommended.

Existential well-being

Well-being has been conceptualized in terms of existence in relation to oneself, others, nature and a higher power, mapping on to four domains of personal, communal, environmental and transcendental existence, respectively (Ellison, 1983; Gomez and Fisher, 2003). As our existence is strengthened or threatened in any of the four domains of existence, our well-being increases or decreases accordingly. Maddi and Harvey (2006) suggest that the most important aspect of existential well-being derives from finding meaning when one or many domains of existence are threatened, such as a life-threatening illness, and people express hardy attitudes and find the 'existential courage' to persist in fighting the threat to existence. Harvey (2005: 28), quoting Maddi (1978), states that 'for hardy individuals, finding meaning, making choices and taking responsibility for those choices is the fundamental project of life' that will lead to expressions of existential courage and well-being.

Measures of well-being used in TCIM research

Scales measure reflections of a specific aspect of the construct of well-being; indexes measure the formation of a well-being construct that arises when 'subscale' facets are combined. Measuring the abstract construct of well-being in relation to TCIM practices has been attempted by a few researchers, including measures such as the single-item, Arizona Integrative Outcomes Scale (AIOS; Bell *et al.*, 2004) that uses a 0–100-millimeter visual analogue scale; the 10-item index called the CAM Health Belief Questionnaire (CBHQ; Lie and Boker, 2004); and the 29-item index called the Integrative Medicine Attitudes Questionnaire (IMAQ; Schneider *et al.*, 2003). Other recent indexes of well-being used in TCIM research have been developed by Myklebust *et al.* (2008) called the Holistic Health and Wellness Questionnaire (HHQ) and the Integrative Medicine Patient Satisfaction Tool (IMPST).

Measuring existential courage and well-being

Among the various measures of well-being, measuring existential courage and well-being facilitates the assessment of patients who express courage when they find meaning from circumstances that threaten their personal, communal, environmental and/or transcendental existence, such as having cancer. In contrast to western allopathic medicine practices that 'treat' the patient, TCIM practices engage patients in 'healing partnerships' (Frenkel and Borkan, 2003) that increase attitudes of commitment, control and challenge (Maddi and Harvey, 2006). The attitudes of commitment, control and challenge are defined as follows: challenge is a conviction that continuing to learn from experience is more fulfilling than expecting easy comfort and security; control is a conviction that the struggle to influence outcomes is more advantageous than passivity and powerlessness; and commitment is a conviction that involvement is more advantageous than detachment.

Hardiness theory (Maddi and Harvey, 2006) suggests that TCIM practices encourage engagement rather than withdrawal from dealing with illness, and therefore that engaging in TCIM treatment processes will lead to increased states of well-being. People engaging in TCIM practices increase their existential well-being because they find meaning when facing threats to their personal, communal, natural and/or transcendental existence.

Biofeedback as a TCIM technique for promoting meaning finding and well-being

Biofeedback is a TCIM treatment approach supporting 'engaged learning' that facilitates meaning finding and well-being (Stoner and Shrier, 2010). For example, biofeedback practices present patients with concrete information (empirical WOK), such as seeing or hearing feedback in direct proportion to the biological reactions. For instance, a physical therapist may place a muscle sensor on an injured limb and the patient learns how moving the injured muscles translates into sights and sounds in proportion to their muscle movement. A biofeedback session also emphasizes a (sociopolitical WOK) patient-centred 'healing partnership' (Frenkel and Borkan, 2003) that requires working with a practitioner to improve rather than merely fix a problem.

Biofeedback techniques support: (a) learning from feedback such as practising and reinforcing physiological behaviours; (b) influencing outcomes such as increasing control over physiology; and (c) engaging in pushing forward despite any difficulties.

Biofeedback techniques in particular are among the TCIM practices most frequently recommended by physicians (Blumberg *et al.*, 1995; Berman *et al.*, 2002). Biofeedback is a useful TCIM practice partly because, as Long (2009: 1) states:

> Supporting individuals to take control of their self-care requires advice-giving within a supportive treatment context and practitioner relationship, with clients who are open to change and committed to maintaining their health.

Well-being under economic pressures

Biofeedback approaches incorporate an 'improving' versus 'fixing' perspective when working with patients (Harvey and Peper, 2011). In contrast, western allopathic medicine typically treats medical problems by 'throwing pills at the problem' and is often practised with sensitivity to the economic pressures of insurance-based service providers operating in managed-care hospitals and clinics (Wolfe *et al.*, 2005). In contrast, some commentators have suggested that a common quality unifying TCIM practice is a caring attitude and necessary time spent with the client (Shuval, 2006).

Conclusion

Understanding how caring support and advice giving can lead to well-being outcomes requires understanding how patients and practitioners use various 'ways-of-knowing' (Ingram, 2007). Whereas the 'treatment' view of TCIM practices as an approach for treating or ameliorating disease, illness, pain and suffering is discussed elsewhere in this text, this chapter on well-being focuses on the 'improvement' view of TCIM as an approach for improving or enhancing growth, health and well-being. There are three recommendations for TCIM practitioners wishing to improve patient well-being:

1 *Track well-being attitudes.* Consider adding psychological measures of existential well-being, such as the hardiness measures of existential courage, with the intention of possibly tracking the extent to which patients and clients find meaning in their lives and increase their level of well-being (Maddi and Harvey, 2006).
2 *Incorporate whole-person viewpoints.* Consider giving advice that reinforces the value of optimum versus minimum levels of health (Serlin, 2007).
3 *Explore biofeedback.* Consider biofeedback theory and practice as a method for presenting objective facts that facilitate meaning finding as well as enhancing well-being (Harvey and Peper, 2011).

Further reading

Kraft, K. (2009) Complementary/alternative medicine in the context of prevention of disease and maintenance of health. *Preventive Medicine* 49(2–3): 88–92.

Sointu, E. (2006) The search for wellbeing in alternative and complementary health practices. *Sociology of Health and Illness* 28(3): 330–49.

References

Adams, J., Hollenberg, D., Lui, C. and Broom, A. (2009) Contextualizing integration: A critical social science approach to integrative health care. *Journal of Manipulative and Physiological Therapeutics* 32(9): 792–8.

Barnes, P.M., Power-Griner, E., McFann, K. and Nahin, R.L. (2004) *CDC Advance Data Report #343. Complementary and Alternative Medicine Use Among Adults: United States, 2002.* Washington, DC: US Department of Health and Human Services. Available at www.cdc.gov/nchs/data/nhsr/nhsr012.pdf, accessed 7 January 2012.

Bell, I.R., Cunningham, V., Caspi, O., Meek, P. and Ferro, L. (2004) Development and validation of a new global well-being outcomes rating scale for integrative medicine research. *BMC Complementary and Alternative Medicine* 15(4): 1–10.

Berman, B.M., Bausell, R.B. and Lee, W.L. (2002) Use and referral patterns for 22 complementary and alternative medical therapies by members of the American College of Rheumatology: Results of a national survey. *Archives of Internal Medicine* 162: 766–70.

Blumberg, D.L., Grant, W.D., Hendricks, S.R., Kamps, C.A. and Dewan, M.J. (1995) The physician and unconventional medicine. *Alternative Therapies in Health and Medicine* 1(3): 31–5.

Bressler, D. (1980) The use of guided imagery as an adjunct to medical diagnosis and treatment. *Journal of Humanistic Psychology* 20(4): 45–59.

Carper, B.A. (1992) Philosophical inquiry in nursing: An application. In J.F. Kikuchi and H. Simmons (eds) *Philosophic Inquiry in Nursing.* Newbury Park, CA: Sage.

Caseem, Q. (2007) XIV ways of knowing. *Proceedings of the Aristotelian Society* 107(3): 1–21.

Diener, E. (2000) Subjective well-being. *American Psychologist* 55(1): 34–43.

Edmondson, D., Park, C.L., Blank, T.O., Fenster, J.R. and Mills, M.A. (2008) Deconstructing spiritual well-being: Existential well-being and HRQOL in cancer survivors. *Psycho-Oncology* 17(2): 161–9.

Ellison, C. (1983) Spiritual well-being: Conceptualization and measurement. *Journal of Psychology and Theology* 11(4): 330–40.

Frenkel, M.A. and Borkan, J.M. (2003) An approach for integrating complementary–alternative medicine into primary care. *Family Practice* 20(3): 324–32.

Gomez, R. and Fisher, J.W. (2003) Domains of spiritual well-being, and development and validation of the spiritual well-being questionnaire. *Personality and Individual Differences* 35: 1975–91.

Graham, L. and Oswald, A.J. (2010) Hedonic capital, adaptation and resilience. *Journal of Economic Behavior and Organization* 76(2): 372–84.

Harvey, R.H. (2005) Hardiness at work: Psychophysiological indicators of everyday courage under stress. Dissertation, University of California, Irvine.

Harvey, R.H. (2009) *Linking Spirituality and Resilience: Implications for Whole Person Practices.* American Psychological Association Conference, Toronto, Canada.

Ingersoll-Dayton, B., Saengtienshai, C., Kespichayawattana, J. and Aungsuroch, Y. (2004) Measuring psychological well-being: Insights from Thai elders. *The Gerontologist* 44(5): 596–602.

Ingram, H. (2007) Ways of knowing: Implications for public policy. Paper presented at the annual meeting of the American Political Science Association, Chicago.

Johns, C. (1995) Framing learning through reflection within Carper's fundamental ways of knowing in nursing. *Journal of Advanced Nursing* 22(2): 226–34.

Lie, D. and Boker, J. (2004) Development and validation of the CAM Health Belief Questionnaire (CHBQ) and CAM use and attitudes amongst medical students. *BMC Medical Education* 12(4): 1–9.

Linley, A., Maltby, J., Wood, A.M., Osborne, G. and Hurling, R. (2010) Measuring happiness: The higher order factor structure of subjective and psychological well-being measures. *Personality and Individual Differences* 47: 878–84.

Long, A. (2009) The potential of complementary and alternative medicine in promoting well-being and critical health literacy: A prospective, observational study of shiatsu. *BMC Complementary and Alternative Medicine* 9(19): 1–11.

Maddi, S.R. (1978) Existential and individual psychologies. *Journal of Individual Psychology* 34(2): 182–90.

Maddi, S.R. and Harvey, R.H. (2006) Hardiness considered across cultures. In P.T.P. Wong and L.C.J. Wong (eds) *Handbook of Multicultural Perspectives on Stress and Coping.* New York: Springer.

Myklebust, M., Pradhan, E.K. and Gorenflo, D. (2008) An integrative medicine patient care model and evaluation of its outcomes: The University of Michigan experience. *Journal of Alternative and Complementary Medicine* 14(7): 821–6.

Ryff, C.D. (1989) Happiness is everything, or is it? Explorations on the meaning of psychological well-being. *Journal of Personality and Social Psychology* 57: 1069–81.

Schneider, C.D., Meek, P.M. and Bell, I.R. (2003) Development and validation of IMAQ: Integrative Medicine Attitude Questionnaire. *BMC Medical Education* 3(5): 1–7.

Serlin, I.A. (ed.) (2007) *Whole Person Healthcare.* Westport, CT: Praeger.

Shuval, J. (2006) Nurses in alternative health care: Integrating medical paradigms. *Social Science & Medicine* 63: 1784–95.

Stoner, M. and Shrier, L. (2010) Hypnosis and biofeedback as prototypes of mind–body medicine. In D.A. Monti and B.D. Beitman (eds) *Integrative Psychiatry.* New York: Oxford University Press, pp. 359–82.

Whittington, B.L. and Scher, S.J. (2010) Prayer and subjective well-being: An examination of six different types of prayer. *International Journal for the Psychology of Religion* 20(1): 59–68.

Wilhelm, K., Wedgwood, L., Parker, G., Geerligs, L. and Hadzi-Pavlovic, D. (2010) Predicting mental health and well-being in adulthood. *Journal of Nervous and Mental Disease* 198(2): 85–90.

Wolfe, S.M., Sasich, L.D., Lurie, P. *et al.* (2005) *Worst Pills, Best Pills: A Consumer's Guide to Avoiding Drug-Induced Death or Illness.* New York: Simon and Schuster.

PART B

Practice, provision and the professional interface

SECTION 4 Traditional medicine in context   105

SECTION 5 Exploring the complementary and alternative medicine–conventional medicine interface   133

SECTION 6 Integrative medicine   157

Traditional medicine in context

Introduction

Leading the reader through the contemporary history of traditional Vietnamese herbal medicine, Wahlberg (Chapter 12) provides both a critical interpretation of the highs and lows of traditional herbal medicine's popularity over this time and an insight into the progressive public health initiatives associated with more latter-day traditional herbal medicine use and policy in Vietnam. As this overview of traditional herbal medicine in Vietnam illustrates, there is much potential for TCIM to provide preventive health measures for the well-being of populations in both low-income and western countries, especially in remote areas where conventional health services may be stretched or non-existent (for parallels and discussion on this point relating more specifically to a global health agenda, see Chapter 27). In this respect, Wahlberg explains how traditional Vietnamese herbal medicine has been closely aligned with a 'drugs at home' policy directive, whereby communal clinics as well as villagers are encouraged to grow essential medicinal plants in their gardens, with a view to progressing self-sufficiency and self-care at a grass-roots level.

Drilling down from the broad-level historical and political analysis that constitutes much of Wahlberg's work, Broom and colleagues (Chapter 13) draw on empirical fieldwork to examine 'medical pluralism' within Indian cancer care, as experienced by a select group of biomedical clinicians. This research draws out the complex historical, cultural and socioeconomic conditions within which the work of Indian oncologists is embedded, highlighting how medical pluralism, while reflecting important richness in cultural knowledge and practice, is nevertheless inextricably linked to forms of social inequality and suffering. Broom and colleagues suggest that such findings exemplify the need to question a romanticized vision of plural medical cultures that often overlooks or denies the politics of human value and the restrictions placed on certain groups.

Staying with Indian culture but changing focus, Nisula (Chapter 14) advances a detailed discussion of patient health-seeking and practitioner behaviours in Mysore, South India, with specific reference to Ayurvedic medicines within the wider context of local health-care utilization. This work, based on a combination of data-collection methods, explores a number of interconnected themes that help illuminate broader issues directly related to traditional medicines in the context of models of integration, as discussed in Section 6 of this collection. More specifically, Nisula reveals the symbolic and social value of 'instruments' within Ayervedic consultations, showing how these 'props', in most cases transported from biomedical practice, can be interpreted as one (of many) manifestations of contemporary medical pluralism. As Nisula explains, one of the most debated issues among Ayurvedic practitioners concerns the advantages and disadvantages of the incorporation of biomedical instruments, techniques and concepts into Ayurvedic routines. This issue cuts to the core of a wider consideration or dilemma facing TM or CAM practitioners contemplating or involved in integrative practices: the extent to which integration may be synonymous with 'incorporation' and the many compromises that may accompany such a process (see Chapter 19 for more detailed discussion along these lines).

CHAPTER 12

Biopolitics and the promotion of traditional herbal medicine in Vietnam

AYO WAHLBERG

Introduction

The case for a traditional medicine (TM) revival can certainly be made in Vietnam, and although it is China's long-standing medical traditions that have received most attention in the region, scholars of traditional medicine in Vietnam are keen to highlight that 'far from being merely a copy of Chinese traditional medicine ... Vietnamese [TM] is made up of ancient health care practices related to the Vietnamese culture' (Hoàng et al., 1999: 1). While Chinese influence is clear, the two Vietnamese scholars Tue Tinh (fourteenth century) and Lãn Ông (eighteenth century) are considered the fathers of a form of TM that was specifically adapted 'to the physical and physiological characteristics of the Vietnamese person as well as to the particularities of Vietnamese pathology, which depends on the tropical climate of Vietnam' (Hoàng et al., 1999: 13).

Vietnam's unique history and health care system have allowed for an approach that has specifically aimed to build up a 'revolutionary movement to bring TM back to the grassroots level' (Hoàng, 2004), not only through its provision by traditional doctors but also by promoting self-sufficiency in the treatment of the most common ailments.

The role of modern medicine as a 'civilizing weapon' in colonial policy and practice throughout the nineteenth and early twentieth centuries is well documented. In Vietnam the efforts of colonial authorities to 'medicalize' French Indochina took hold at the turn of the twentieth century. Although its practice

Source: Wahlberg, A. (2006) Biopolitics and the promotion of traditional herbal medicine in Vietnam. *Health: An Interdisciplinary Journal for the Social Study of Health, Illness and Medicine* 10(2): 123–47. Abridged version reprinted with kind permission of Sage Publishing Ltd.

and use were never even close to being abolished, scholars of TM in Vietnam do suggest that colonial health care policies were responsible for 'ruthlessly dr[iving] [TM] into stagnation and decline' (Hoàng *et al.*, 1999: 25–6).

In 1954 President Ho Chi Minh set up a government of the Democratic Republic of Vietnam and it was during these times of nation building that he delivered a speech in which he echoed the words of Chairman Mao in China:

> We must build our own medicine ... Our ancestors had rich experience in the treatment of disease using local medications and those of the north [China]. To enlarge the sphere of action of medicine, it is necessary to study means of uniting the effects of oriental remedies with those of Europe. (cited in Hoàng *et al.*, 1999: 26)

Vietnamese TM was no longer to be discouraged in the name of public health. It was not so much the biopolitical goals of protecting and promoting public health in Vietnam that had changed, yet a space for Vietnamese TM in securing these was opened up. Ho Chi Minh's 1955 call led to the establishment of a network of institutions whose mandate it would be to modernize, standardize and repopularize Vietnamese TM.

Modernizing traditional herbal medicines

What has characterized the push to modernize herbal medicine in Vietnam over the past decades? As a starting point, it has required a comprehensive mapping-out exercise of botanical enlightenment, designed to put order into the rich, yet at times chaotic, unsystematic, unscientific and even unwritten records of herbs and their medicinal uses that have been around for centuries. The key challenges facing scientists were, first of all, that while the experiences of the hundreds and thousands of traditional practitioners around Vietnam were considered invaluable, they were often recorded only sporadically and, when they were, names of plants were given in their vernacular forms, which varied across region and ethnic group. Moreover, correct harvesting information (which has a significant bearing on a herb's medicinal potency) was rarely sufficiently noted. And finally, some herbal remedies were nowhere to be found in the otherwise rich archive of Vietnamese herbal records.

Parallel to this taxonomic drive to collect, collate and classify knowledge about different medicinal plants and traditional herbal formulae has been a large-scale programme to industrialize a great number of the most used and most relevant herbal remedies. It was for these reasons that the Ministry of Health, after consultations with the World Health Organization and other national health authorities in the region, approved Decision 371/BYT-QD on 12 March 1996, introducing new requirements for the safety and efficacy of herbal medicines (Ministry of Health, Vietnam, 1996). These regulations require that any new industrially produced herbal medicine applying for marketing authorization must undergo a series of tests to see whether the product meets quality, safety and efficacy standards. Product samples must be sent to the national Institute of Drug Quality Control, where one out of four quality control laboratories is specifically dedicated to herbal medicines.

The point here is not that a once 'natural' practice of preparing herbal medicines in Vietnam has now become saturated with rules and regulations, with regulators leaving no stone unturned, from the urban centres to the remotest of rural villages (if for no other reason than lack of resources); rather, it is to demonstrate how problematizations of the safety and quality of what are otherwise considered 'less aggressive and less toxic' (Bùi, 1999: 30) traditional herbal medicines in Vietnam have been dependent on the building up of bodies of expert botanical, pharmacological, phytochemical and pharmacognostic knowledge over the past 50 years or so.

While herbal medicine is widely regarded as an effective and economical means to promoting public health, especially in rural areas where access to modern pharmaceuticals can be limited, industrially augmented risks of misidentification, contamination and counterfeiting have required a range of new measures to safeguard the public from potentially dangerous 'industrially produced' herbal medicinal products.

Standardizing the practice of herbal medicine

Regulating the practice of traditional herbal medicine has also been an integral part of the Vietnamese government's programme to promote TM since 1955. As a result, Vietnam is one of the few countries in the world (together with China and Korea) that is seen as having an 'integrated approach' to health care, with TM playing a substantial role in medical education, research and practice (World Health Organization, 2002: 9). Bùi has suggested that half a century into this programme of modernization, TM practitioners can today be classed into three different groups: first, a 'dying breed' of elder practitioners who have been trained in classical traditional medical techniques with a classical theoretical and philosophical base; second, those who have received training at the TM faculties of medical colleges or secondary schools of TM; and finally, 'herb doctors' who have received no formal training but have acquired knowledge and experience through apprenticeships (Bùi, 1999: 34–6). In today's Vietnam, it is the latter two groups who provide by far the majority of herbal medicine treatment, and for this reason it is worth looking at the ways in which their (in)ability as practitioners has come to be problematized as a public health issue over the past decades.

The regulation of the practice of traditional herbal medicine in Vietnam has happened via two specific routes: first, by making both modern and traditional medicine compulsory components of medical education and practice in Vietnam; and second, by the organization of apprentice-trained 'herb doctors' into national associations, as well as the development of a licensing system for these practitioners. Students attending Vietnam's medical colleges are required to follow 16 compulsory courses in TM (covering classical theory, diagnostics, medical botany and acupuncture) in the first four years of their degrees. Those wishing to do so can then choose to specialize in TM in their final two years (see World Bank, 1993: 30). Outside of Vietnam's medical colleges, the Tue Tinh secondary colleges of TM offer three-year 'Assistant Doctor' diplomas which likewise cover both modern and traditional medicine as well as providing further education and 'refresher courses' for practising medical doctors (World Bank, 1993: 31). TM graduates from both the medical and secondary colleges are destined for work in the extensive network of health services found at national, provincial, district and commune levels in Vietnam. Further to the 40 or so specialized national and provincial hospitals of TM, the Ministry of Health stipulated by decree in 1976 that each district hospital was to have a department or section specializing in TM, which are often staffed by 'assistant doctors', although some medical doctors who have specialized in traditional medicine also work at this level. Finally, it is also governmental policy that each commune clinic strive to have at least one staff worker specialized in TM, responsible also for keeping a garden of medicinal herbs (Hoàng, 2004).

Notwithstanding this extensive state-supported health care network of hospitals and clinics to which the majority of Vietnamese people do have access through their nearest commune clinic, district hospital or provincial hospital, 'herb doctors' (apprentice-trained rather than college-educated traditional practitioners) continue to play an important role in the delivery of health care, especially in rural areas of the country. Even though these 'herb doctors' will often work in cooperation with commune clinics and district hospitals, they do constitute a separate category of traditional practitioner, subject to different practice requirements. With the passing of Vietnam's fourth constitution in 1992 according to which it became 'strictly forbidden for private organizations and individuals to dispense medical treatment, or to produce and trade in medicaments illegally, thereby damaging the people's health' (Government of Vietnam, 1992: Article 39), the qualifications of private practitioners are increasingly being examined. The constitution has since been followed up by national regulations to govern the private practice of medicine, requiring 'herb doctors' to register their practices with provincial health authorities and to apply for a practising licence, which will only be awarded after an evaluation by health authorities, often in cooperation with provincial or district associations of TM practitioners. As noted in a report for the World Bank, 'a strong thrust of [this] legislation is to ensure that practitioners are properly qualified' (World Bank, 1993: 41). This process is for the most part still in its beginnings, as by 2003 the Ministry of Health had 'only' licensed 3715 private practices of TM (Huu and Borton, 2003: 89), which is in sharp contrast to the estimated 20,000 members of the national Association of Traditional Practitioners.

Yet, whatever the gaps between regulatory intentions and outcomes, it is clearly this group of apprentice-trained traditional practitioners or 'herb doctors' who have come under increasing scrutiny in the past decade or so, especially as regards their training and qualifications. For, although they are often highlighted for the important role that they can and should play in the provision of primary health care especially, a number of public health concerns about their abilities have been raised. For example, the World Health Organization in Vietnam lists as key obstacles that their explanations can appear 'mysterious'; some practitioners are not sufficiently qualified while others overstate their abilities; their lack of knowledge of modern medicine can be harmful to patients; and they tend to keep their 'know-how' secret (World Health Organization, 2004b).

Again, the point to be made is not that an ancient master–apprentice tradition is now becoming saturated by licensing rules and regulations. Rather, what is evident is that the art or skill of practising traditional herbal medicine in Vietnam is also in the process of becoming the object of an expert knowledge that is being called on to determine safety, competency and quality criteria as a means to prevent the 'damaging of the people's health'. Vietnam has embarked on a normative process, which is only just in its beginnings, to identify what is meant by the terms 'proper' and 'safe' in the practice of traditional herbal medicine.

'Re-educating the people'

What of the users of herbal medicine in Vietnam, the great majority of which continue to live in rural areas, often far away from the ministries, associations, departments and institutions of traditional medicine that issue decrees, guidelines or training manuals? These are the people who are often self-medicating with herbs, not necessarily as a matter of some kind of personal choice but sometimes because access to other medical services is all but non-existent. Nevertheless, while one would perhaps assume that since Vietnam has had such a long history of herbal medicine use its promotion has never been a problem, this is far from being the case, and the popularity and use of traditional herbal medicines have had their peaks and troughs since the battle of Dien Bien Phu in May 1954 (see Hoàng *et al.*, 1999; Hoàng, 2004). The period might be roughly divided into three parts, with the first three decades up to 1985 characterized by a chronic shortage of modern medicinal supplies as a direct result of trade embargos against Vietnam. As a way to overcome this shortage, the Vietnamese government launched a 'revolutionary movement to bring traditional medicine back to the grassroots level' (Hoàng, 2004), especially since colonial policies had done so much to discourage the use of traditional medicine. Starting in the early 1960s and inspired by China's 'barefoot doctors' programme, the National Institute of TM organized a number of training courses aimed at mobilizing and training some 2000 activists who were to return to their districts as focal persons for the promotion of TM, initially in North Vietnam. The Institute also nominated groups of three to four people who were then sent out to a number of villages to work with medical staff in the area on ways to promote TM. Following the reunification of Vietnam in 1976, these efforts were expanded to the rest of the country, with the Ministry of Health issuing a decree requiring every district to have a department or institute that provided traditional medical treatment. It is estimated that 40–50 per cent of all medical treatment being provided at the time was based on TM, herbal medicine and acupuncture being the most popular therapies (see Huu and Borton, 2003; Hoàng, 2004).

However, when the Vietnamese government embarked on a series of economic reforms starting in 1986, it had a marked impact on the provision and practice of traditional medicine, with 'many herbal pharmacists and acupuncturists abandon[ing] their practices' (Huu and Borton, 2003: 87), mainly because the subsidies they had been receiving from health authorities were rescinded. At the same time, modern drugs were becoming more freely available, since trade embargos were gradually being lifted. As a result, TM experienced a period of decline that lasted until about 1992. Since then, the Ministry of Health has led an active campaign to 'revitalize' or 'revive' TM once again. Important components of this 'revival' campaign have been the 'Drugs at Home' and 'Doctor at Home' programmes of the Ministry of Health (see World Bank, 1993) and a 'national policy for traditional medicine through 2010' launched in 2003.

The 'Drugs at Home' programme was designed to encourage communal clinics as well as villagers to grow 35 species of essential medicinal plants in their gardens that are known for their anti-influenza, anti-inflammatory, anti-dysenteric, anti-rheumatic, anti-tussive, anti-diarrhoeic and emmenagogic properties. Each commune is encouraged to reserve more than half a hectare for such cultivation and the goal is to have about 40 per cent of patients treated with herbal remedies at communal clinics (Bùi, 1999: 30–31). As part of the 'Doctor at Home' programme, a book entitled *Herbal Medicines for Families* has been published, providing users with instructions on how to prepare remedies for some of their most common ailments, including diarrhoea, whooping cough, allergies, hormonal imbalance and colitis (see World Bank, 1993; Bùi, 1999). The national policy on TM through 2010 has set TM usage targets of 10 per cent at the central level, 20 per cent at the provincial level, 25 per cent at the district level and 40 per cent at the communal level, while also suggesting that sales of traditional medicinal products could be pushed up to 30 per cent of the domestic pharmaceutical market (Ministry of Health, Vietnam, 2003).

This revitalization effort, spearheaded by the Ministry of Health but involving traditional practitioners, rural hospitals, a number of trained activists as well as the rural populations themselves, has been described as a programme to 're-educate the local people on the use of herbal remedies and [to] encourage them to grow and use medicinal plants' (Huu and Borton, 2003: 67).

While colonial programmes definitely tended to objectify Vietnamese individuals as 'inferior' or 'backward', contemporary programmes view individuals as fully capable partners and resources in the quest to improve public health. 'Re-education' is required to the extent that colonial policies were successful in discouraging the use of traditional herbal medicines. At the same time, in Vietnam, as in many other countries, consumers of herbal medicines have become the target of very practical health programmes (such as the 'Doctor at Home' programme) that, in the words of the WHO, 'promote the *proper* use of TM/CAM through consumer education/training' (World Health Organization, 2004a: x, emphasis added).

Conclusion: Quackery transformed

Vietnam has experienced a tangible TM 'revival' over the past 50 years. The strategy of scientific modernization that has played out in Vietnam also bears a number of similarities to what has been happening in many other countries, such as Malaysia and Ghana. But what has made the Vietnamese case relatively unique is the extent to which the practice and use of traditional herbal medicine have been integrated into the national public health delivery system. More specifically, there is a strong case for arguing that the efforts to encourage especially those people in more rural areas to become self-sufficient in the traditional herbal treatment of their most common ailments continue to be among the most comprehensive in the world, which, as noted, can be directly linked to a proud history of TM use dating back many centuries, a prolonged period of postcolonial isolation (due to conflict and embargos) and an impressively far-reaching health delivery network. Indeed, it must surely stand as one of the great ironies of Vietnam's tragic history that just as modern medicine had been used as a 'civilizing weapon' against what were considered 'backward' natives by Vietnam's colonizers, modernizing and repopularizing TM in Vietnam became a concrete element of their own grass-roots-based efforts to drive these very colonizers out.

Vietnam has experienced a palpable shift in public health strategies from the colonial marginalization of 'quackery' and 'sorcery' to the postcolonial promotion of a new, responsibilized – that is, 'safe', 'proper', 'appropriate' – form of Vietnamese TM. For this reason, there are perhaps some who would make the case that what I have described is but a continuation of the bio-medical hegemony of the colonial days in a different guise, that herbal medicine in Vietnam has been 'scientifically colonized' or co-opted, stripped of its original value as a 'natural', 'eastern' or epistemologically distinct form of medicine (notwithstanding that in Vietnam this process has been cast in terms of 'building our own medicine'). While I have clearly shown that Vietnamese TM is currently being bio-politicized – appropriated by expert bodies of knowledge that make authoritative and often contested claims as to what constitute the most 'appropriate', 'effective', 'safe' and 'responsible' ways of practising and utilizing it in the service of public health – I would not argue that this bio-politicization has come at the cost of a lost 'authenticity' or 'legitimacy'. As it always has been, traditional herbal medicine is under constant revision in Vietnam and it is currently being recast into a form that fits the biopolitical aims of safeguarding and promoting public health in Vietnam, which importantly is by no means limited to the maintenance of biological norms of vitality, but equally embraces notions of 'quality of life', 'balance' and 'harmony'.

Further reading

Eisenberg, D., Harris, E., Littlefield, B. *et al.* (2010) Developing a library of authenticated Traditional Chinese Medicinal (TCM) plants for systematic biological evaluation – rationale, methods and preliminary results from a Sino-American collaboration. *Fitoterapia* 82(1): 17–33.

Hsu, E. (2009) Chinese propriety medicines: An 'alternative modernity'? The case of the anti-malarial substance Antemisinin in East Africa. *Medical Anthropology* 28(2): 111–40.

Timmermans, K. (2003) Intellectual property rights and traditional medicine: Policy dilemmas at the interface. *Social Science and Medicine* 57: 745–56.

References

Bùi, C.H. (1999) Integration of traditional medicine into the health care system. In B.C. Hoàng, T. Phó and N. Huu (eds) *Vietnamese Traditional Medicine*. Hanoi: Gioi, pp. 29–36.

Government of Vietnam (1992) *Constitution*. Hanoi: Government of Vietnam.

Hoàng, B.C. (2004) Promotion of herbal medicine in the rural areas of Vietnam. Personal communication from former Director of Institute of Traditional Medicine (1975–95), Hanoi, 4 November 2004.

Hoàng, B.C., Phó, T. and Huu, N. (1999) *Vietnamese Traditional Medicine*. Hanoi: Gioi .

Huu, N. and Borton, L. (2003) *Traditional Medicine: Vietnamese Culture*. Hanoi: Gioi.

Ministry of Health, Vietnam (1996) Decision on the safety and efficacy of herbal medicines, Decision 371/BYT-QD. Hanoi: Ministry of Health.

Ministry of Health, Vietnam (2003) *National Policy on Traditional Medicine 2010*. Hanoi: Ministry of Health.

Nguyen, V. (1999) Traditional pharmaceutical activities in Vietnam and their possible development. In B.C. Hoàng, T. Phó and N. Huu (eds) *Vietnamese Traditional Medicine*, Hanoi: Gioi, pp. 37–49.

World Bank (1993) *Traditional Medicine in Vietnam*. Consultant's report prepared by Gerard C. Bodeker. Washington, DC: World Bank.

World Health Organization (2002) *Traditional Medicine Strategy 2002–2005*. Geneva: World Health Organization.

World Health Organization (2004a) *Guidelines on Developing Consumer Information on Proper Use of Traditional, Complementary and Alternative Medicine*. Geneva: World Health Organization.

World Health Organization (2004b) *Traditional Medicine: Challenges and Opportunities*. Hanoi: World Health Organization, Vietnam.

CHAPTER 13

The inequalities of medical pluralism: Hierarchies of health, the politics of tradition and the economies of care in Indian oncology

ALEX BROOM, ASSA DORON AND PHILIP TOVEY

Introduction

As is the case in other South Asian nations, medicine is intimately interwoven with religiosity and ethnic identities in India (Tovey and Broom, 2007). Common therapeutic modalities like Ayurveda and Unani are deeply embedded in local cultural sensibilities and religious ideologies, producing a complex interplay of medicine, culture and identity (Alavi, 2005).

The context of cancer in India is in many ways quite peculiar to the Indian subcontinent, although it has some parallels with issues facing other developing countries. Increased wealth (although stratified) has in turn increased life expectancy through better standards of living and reduced communicable diseases in certain populations (Hammer *et al.*, 2007). Cancer has thus shifted from being of limited importance, in health policy terms, to being a considerable issue with an ageing population (Pal and Mittal, 2004). Yet the majority of the Indian population do not have access to biomedical cancer facilities (Pal and Mittal, 2004), and those who do have access bring with them a complex history of engagement with a multiplicity of therapeutic modalities and paradigms of care (Naraindas, 2006).

Source: Broom, A., Doron, A. and Tovey, P. (2009) The inequalities of medical pluralism: Hierarchies of health, the politics of tradition and the economies of care in Indian oncology. *Social Science and Medicine* 69: 698–706. Abridged version reprinted with kind permission of Elsevier Ltd.

In order to begin to explore these complex and multilayered issues, the current study takes as its point of departure the experiences of oncology clinicians, whose everyday work is embedded in these complex historical, cultural and socioeconomic conditions. In this chapter we explore 'pluralism' (Indian cancer patients' use of both traditional medicines and biomedical oncology treatments) as perceived and experienced by a select group of biomedical clinicians.

Background

Out of the million people diagnosed with cancer in India each year, 50 per cent will die within 12 months, and less than 10 per cent of those in need will receive biomedical palliative care (Pal and Mittal, 2004). Deaths from cancer in India are predicted to rise significantly by 2030, to nearly 1.5 million annually (World Health Organization, 2005a).

The plethora of therapeutic practices used in India makes a comprehensive overview impossible, but some reflection on the most common practices is useful. Ayurveda (Hindu), Unani (Muslim) and Siddha (Hindu) are the most common traditional practices; – homeopathy is widespread and virtually considered 'indigenous' by Indians despite being introduced from Germany in the nineteenth century. Likewise, practices such as yoga, acupuncture and meditation are normalized forms of everyday life and health practice (Alter, 2004).

Theoretical context: Postcolonialism, tradition and the modern Indian state

A critical concept in many developing countries, and in Indian society in particular, is the complex interplay of identity, culture and medicine. In the context of colonial and contemporary postcolonial India, medicine and its use are intimately and explicitly interwoven in caste, class, gender and religious dynamics (Khan, 2006). As such, therapeutic decision making can be informed as much by notions of 'effectiveness' as by conceptions of place, community and identity (see Chapter 14 for an example). Thus, priorities in and around therapeutic decision making can be quite different to those in western contexts: medicine-as-culture is more pronounced in India due to the plurality of modalities operating, many of which existed long before the presence of biomedicine. Biomedicine is often not the sole paradigm through which other practices are measured in India (cf. Naraindas, 2006). Its centrality is limited by the fact that it is not the only state-legitimated medicine (Ayurveda, Unani, homeopathy and other practices are also supported), thus creating a more diversified and open therapeutic environment. Finally, in a postcolonial India, localized and indigenous practices are held up by some as integral to contemporary Indian identity politics (Khan, 2006).

This intermingling of identity, culture and medicine necessarily shapes hierarchies and dynamics between professional groups and systems of medicine (Naraindas, 2006). Biomedicine is relatively new to India and the dynamics between TCAM (Traditional, Complementary and Alternative Medicine) and biomedical practitioners are constantly evolving and are differentiated according to the region examined. It is evident that TCAM practitioners hold certain forms of cultural capital and local knowledge that are acknowledged, if not supported, by many practising biomedical clinicians (see Chapter 14). While efficacy in a biomedical sense may be disputed, there is widespread acceptance of the fundamental assumptions underlying many practices that would receive little recognition from the biomedical community in western contexts (Frank and Ecks, 2004). As such, biomedical clinicians' approaches to TCAM are embedded as a set of cultural sensibilities that tend to embrace traditional and other non-biomedical treatments. Forms of therapeutic engagement also denote notions of class, faith and sociocultural status. Consumption of medicine can thus interplay with the (re)production of class and urban/rural distinctions (Khan, 2006). For the individual, therefore, medical pluralism may be transformed into 'hierarchies of health', mediated by existing social inequalities, including those of class, gender, age and place.

Understanding the role of the state is critical for situating medical pluralism in India and, in particular, the politics of tradition and regulatory devices of modernity (Cant and Sharma, 1999; Benner, 2005; Attewell, 2007). In India, 'tradition' has also been politicized and strategically deployed; it has been reshaped and appropriated to suit contemporary sentiments and ideological trajectories (Alter, 2000).

The modern state in India has witnessed the relegation of many traditional practices to the margins (Cant and Sharma, 1999, p. 177), imposing controls and supervising its usage in unsanctioned spaces (Pinto, 2004). The state in India has been instrumental in the shaping of what should be protected and what should be discouraged in terms of medical knowledge and practice.

By drawing on these conceptual issues, we explore 'pluralism' as seen in the everyday experiences of cancer clinicians in India. How is medical pluralism perceived in the everyday working lives of cancer clinicians, and how would they make sense of their patients' therapeutic decisions and their engagement with TCAM?

Methods

The methodology for this project draws on the interpretive traditions within the social sciences, focusing on establishing an in-depth understanding of the practices, views and experiences of respondents. We selected three hospitals and one palliative care service that provide cancer and end-of-life services for Delhi and the surrounding areas. In total, 22 clinicians participated in a 30–60-minute in-depth interview. We interviewed 16 medical specialists (medical oncologists, radiation oncologists, palliative care specialists, surgeons, haematological oncologists, paediatric haematologists), 5 oncology nurses and one oncology clinical psychologist. The interviews explored perceptions of patient decision making and therapeutic trajectories; cultural/structural processes in and around TCAM and biomedicine usage; distinctions/similarities between biomedicine and TCAM; and the broader implications of therapeutic diversity for their everyday clinical work. From our position as qualitative researchers, we do not seek to validate or contest these clinicians' perspectives, but we present their accounts as situated interpretations of pluralism in Indian cancer care.

Results

Tradition and modernity in contemporary India

We asked the clinicians to reflect on the relationship between different health care practices in Indian culture. A key theme that emerged was the 'everyday' nature of the use of TCAM and its integral role in Indian sensibilities and the home environment:

> CLINICIAN 5: Because you are born [in India] with so many things in place, even the spices that you use for, in food for example. Steadily I learned that each of them also has some kind of medicinal use. I mean, turmeric and cumin, yeah, that's what we've been hearing about [in the literature]. The traditional medicines are our way of life without our even knowing it. [Consultant, medical oncologist]

For such clinicians, 'being Indian' necessarily involved use of traditional practices, at least in the context of 'everyday' ailments. Traditional medicine comprised part of their habitus, deeply internalized through various structures of community membership. Not surprisingly, therefore, each of the clinicians interviewed had personally used TCAM for minor issues (such as colds or cuts and bruises) and the response 'of course I use them' was typical. Yet there was consistent reflection on being rather precariously placed between support for the 'traditional' versus the pre-eminence of modern science. This ambivalence seemed to centre on being implicated in 'community' structures as part of their everyday life, while concurrently serving as strong advocates for the validity of modern values and scientific rationality. A way of making sense of this disjunction seemed to be the placing of traditional medicine firmly within the domestic sphere – the home (cf. Das, 1999). As one consultant stated, 'we tell our cancer patients not to use them and then we go home and use them ourselves'. These parallel lives, on the part of the clinicians, reflected a wider trend whereby structures and knowledge systems of the modern India coexist, albeit with tensions. Yet while traditional practices were broadly accepted as 'normal' and 'Indian', a high value was placed on scientific rationality and these clinicians deployed such notions discursively as a means of ascribing and reinforcing their professional legitimacy.

Practices of distinction and distinction in practice: Evidence, faith and the politics of care

In distinguishing between TCAM and biomedical practice, scientific rationality and its various manifestations (global-defined efficacy, objectivity, quantification and trial evidence) were articulated as central. Those who practised traditional medicine were marked by mystification and even false consciousness; they were represented by the consultants as actors who were yet to achieve the degree of self-reflexivity that characterizes modern social order (Beck, 1994). Despite this binary conception of TCAM and biomedicine, there was an underlying ambivalence regarding the grass-roots separation of 'rational' biomedical science and the 'metaphysical' referencing ascribed to traditional medicine. For example, while initially suggesting an incompatibility of TCAM and biomedicine, as the interviews continued these distinctions were problematized and deconstructed, with important reflections around the incompleteness (and even fallacies) of claims to rationality and objectivity in the grass-roots biomedical treatment of cancer patients in India:

> CLINICIAN 14: ... when it comes to religion and politics versus science, religion and politics will always win. I mean, we consultants. I have always been amazed, that the doctors [in this hospital] are so intense about their treatment, their way of treating, that it has become religion and politics, more or less. So whenever we [try to] form a single protocol, we cannot sit down and agree on a single protocol. So when it comes to religion and politics, whether allopathic or alternative, science will always lose. [Consultant, paediatric haematologist]

As shown in the above excerpt and in the accounts of other interviewees, as the discussion continued, bias, politics and the subjective, intuitive elements of biomedical work were consistently emphasized. While maintaining a theoretical distinction of rationality/accountability as delineating biomedical cancer care from TCAM, the influences of politics (whether departmental, organizational or societal) on biomedical cancer care were viewed as ultimately blurring the distinctions between 'us' and 'them'. Despite this blurring of inter-professional boundaries, there was overwhelming concern regarding TCAM and its role in Indian cancer care.

Treatment trajectories and traditional practices

A key issue for each of the clinicians interviewed was what their patients were using before presenting to hospital. Use of TCAM was viewed as a critical factor in explaining why patients presented late to hospital.

CLINICIAN 8: I would say that fifty percent of them [patients] would have already used alternative therapies. They want to try for two, three months, all those [alternative] methods of treatment. Then they come up at stage four disease, stage three disease. Then we say, 'we cannot operate', we cannot offer them curative treatment, it is going to [be] palliative, that is an unfortunate situation. [Consultant, head and neck surgeon]

Furthermore, the interviews revealed consistent anger at the so-called tendency of TCAM practitioners to treat in contexts 'out of their depth' and delay biomedical treatment. However, as the interviews continued, the picture emerged as far more complex than the 'lure of alternatives' and 'erroneous claims to efficacy'. Rather, complex sociocultural understandings of cancer and structural inequalities emerged as intertwined in people's engagement with TCAM. The initial blame ascribed to TCAM was transformed into discussion around the intersectionality of biography, disease type, social structures and treatment trajectories.

Socioeconomics and the economies of care

While ascribing some blame to TCAM practitioners, these clinicians emphasized the centrality of 'cost of care' in shaping their patients' therapeutic trajectories, stressing the hugely expensive private sector and the costly public system. Furthermore, economics were articulated as interplaying with notions of the 'hopelessness of cancer' in shaping decisions regarding whether or not to pursue biomedical versus TCAM treatments. The issue of cost came up in subsequent interviews as inter-playing with the cultural stigmas in and around cancer, with the clinicians describing how perceptions of 'terminality' mediate use of biomedical treatment, rather than distinctly 'modern' beliefs or understandings of effectiveness:

CLINICIAN 5: ... in India, [people think] cancer is equal to death. So, then all the assessments start from that point for many patients. It's a serious diagnosis, it affects my [long pause] it's a question of my life and my death, now let me take stock of things. And then finances become a major, major issue, so if there is [traditional medicine] which take care of my pain, and it doesn't cost me much, I would rather go for that. [Consultant, medical oncologist]

A self-perpetuating process is recounted by these clinicians whereby perceptions of cancer as a death sentence promote a view of costly biomedical treatment as 'not worth it'. Friends and family members were represented as in some ways complicit in preventing individuals from accessing the domain of biomedical and rational knowledge. While these accounts reflect clinician perspectives, their explanations also shed light on potentially important sociocultural processes in and around treatment selection and access. Specifically, treatment selection may be more than simply patients not understanding best treatment or supporting TCAM. Rather, it may be a decision informed by cultural stigmas and understandings of cancer and a broader sense of hopelessness around chances of success. This process of strategic selection of treatment, based on notions of cost, value and benefit, was viewed by these clinicians as further complicated by the gendered landscapes of Indian culture and complex notions of human value.

Gender, social value and treatment trajectories

Indian society is considerably patriarchal in character and men retain a position of significant power and authority in the family and wider society. A consistent theme in the interviews was the value placed on males within the family structure and its relationship to whether the family could 'afford' treatment or not. The interviews revealed major concerns regarding community and family decisions not to treat women based on financial constraint, and, furthermore, the (related) perceived tendency of some Indian women to conceal their symptoms until they would be 'untreatable' from a biomedical perspective. The patriarchal structures of Indian society were viewed as complicit in the paucity of women accessing biomedical cancer care; the view of female family members as of less 'value' to the family was a common theme in the accounts of these clinicians. In certain cases, TCAM was perceived as being used for family members of a 'lower priority'. However, this notion of social value also crossed gender lines, impacting on older men:

> CLINICIAN 21: … males they get treatment faster, because he is the bread earner for the family, so family is very concerned, so they quickly come to us. But children I feel, especially girl child, they are not that, not keen. I feel males, young males get very fast, middle aged men also get fast, but old age, not so much. [Consultant, radiation oncologist]

While younger men may be viewed as 'benefiting' from quicker access to biomedical cancer care, the broader valuing of human life and health is highly differentiated between groups of Indian men. As such, these hierarchies of health should be viewed as impacting on men and women, albeit differentially depending on their class and age, among other factors.

Discussion

The key finding from this study was the embeddedness of patient disease and therapeutic trajectories in vast social inequalities and, indeed, the intermingling of pluralism and the politics of social value. Medical pluralism, while reflecting important richness in cultural knowledge and practice, emerged as inextricably linked to forms of social inequality and suffering. The use of Indian practices (including Ayurveda, Unani and Siddha) reflects a complex combination of religion, identity and belief, but also severe economic constraint and restrictive notions of human value. In turn, patriarchal relations and the politics of ageing seemed strongly linked to engagement with TCAM, with women and older people viewed as less of a priority than younger or male members of their family.

Given these results, we argue that presenting 'medical pluralism' as a desirable development trajectory creates an illusion of linearity and evades forms of structural constraint. Such illusions of linearity and agency/choice in plural contexts have previously been identified by others who also question pluralism as deployed by some medical anthropologists (for example Connor, 2001 [see Chapter 2 in this collection]; Cant and Sharma, 1999). These romantic visions of plural medical cultures conceal social–cultural cleavages, overlooking (or even denying) the politics of human value and the restrictions placed on certain groups.

It is vital that the 'hierarchies of health' evident in the accounts presented here be situated within an understanding of the role of the state. The modern Indian state has drawn on and utilized nostalgia and the 'rediscovery' of tradition, while concurrently (and differentially) pursuing the values of modernity and progress. Indeed, notions of pluralism fit comfortably with this tradition/progress political trajectory, with nostalgia for tradition placed carefully beside the desire for progress in the pursuit of what is distinctly Indian. Yet the state in postcolonial India has not achieved this balance in many areas of health service delivery. Rather, as shown here, in grass-roots contexts medical pluralism is often transformed into forms of marginalization and polarization (cf. Farmer, 1996) and the deployment of pluralism may actually act to conceal forms of suffering and structural problems in and around health care delivery (Das, 1999, 2003).

Further reading

Tovey, P., Chatwin, J. and Broom, A. (2007) *Traditional, Complementary and Alternative Medicine and Cancer Care: An International Analysis of Grassroots Integration.* London: Routledge.

References

Alavi, S. (2005) The Unani public sphere: Urdu medical texts and the Oudh Akhbar in 19th Century India. *Indian Economic and Social History Review* 42: 101–29.

Alter, J. (1996) Gandhi's body, Gandhi's truth: Nonviolence and the biomoral imperative of public health. *Journal of Asian Studies* 55: 301–22.

Alter, J. (2000) *Gandhi's Body: Sex, Diet and the Politics of Nationalism.* Philadelphia: University of Pennsylvania Press.

Alter, J. (2004) *Yoga in Modern India: The Body between Science and Philosophy.* New Jersey: Princeton University Press.

Attewell, G. (2007) *Refiguring Unani Tibb: Plural Healing in Late Colonial India*. New Delhi: Longman.

Beck, U. (1994) The reinvention of politics: Towards a theory of reflexive modernization. In U. Beck, A. Giddens and S. Lash (eds) *A Reflexive Modernization*. Cambridge: Polity Press.

Benner, D. (2005) The medical ethics of professionalised Ayurveda. *Asian Medicine* 1: 185–203.

Cant, S. and Sharma, U. (1999) *A New Medical Pluralism?* London: Routledge.

Connor, L. (2001) Healing powers in contemporary Asia. In L.H. Connor and G. Samuel (eds) *Healing Powers and Modernity*. Westport, CT: Bergin and Garvey, pp. 3–21.

Das, V. (1999) Tradition, pluralism, identity: Framing the issues. In V. Das (ed.) *Tradition, Pluralism, Identity*. New Delhi: Sage, pp. 9–21.

Das, V. (2003) Technologies of the self: Poverty and health in an urban setting. In *Sarai Reader*. Delhi: Sarai.

Farmer, P. (1996) On suffering and structural violence: A view from below. *Daedalus* 25: 261–83.

Frank, R. and Ecks, S. (2004) Towards an ethnography of Indian homeopathy. *Anthropology & Medicine* 11: 307–26.

Hammer, J., Aiyar, Y. and Samji, S. (2007) Understanding government failure in public health services. *Economic and Political Weekly* 42: 4049–57.

Khan, S. (2006) Systems of medicine and nationalistic discourse in India. *Social Science and Medicine* 62: 2786–97.

Khare, R. (1996) Dava, daktar and dua: Anthropology of practiced medicine in India. *Social Science and Medicine* 43: 837–48.

Naraindas, H. (2006) Of spineless babies and folic acid: Evidence and efficacy in biomedicine and Ayurvedic medicine. *Social Science & Medicine* 62: 2658–69.

Pal, S. and Mittal, B. (2004) Improving cancer care in India. *Asian Pacific Journal of Cancer Prevention* 5: 226–8.

Pinto, S. (2004) Development without institutions: Ersatz medicine and the politics of everyday life in rural North India. *Cultural Anthropology* 19: 337–63.

Tovey, P. and Broom, A. (2007) Cancer patients' negotiation of therapeutic options in Pakistan. *Qualitative Health Research* 17: 652–62.

World Health Organization (2005a) *India: Core Health Indicators*. Geneva: World Health Organization.

World Health Organization (2005b) *WHO Global Atlas of TCAM*. Kobe: World Health Organization Centre for Health Development.

CHAPTER 14

In the presence of biomedicine: Ayurveda, medical integration and health seeking in Mysore, South India

TAPIO NISULA

This chapter is based on research (conducted via interviews, participant observation and survey material) examining medical integration and health seeking in Mysore, South India. It explores the use of Ayurvedic services, the impact of biomedicine on Ayurvedic practices and the meaning of instruments with respect to the expectations of patients and healers.

Ayurvedic medicine serves as a health reserve in urban Mysore. For the majority of informants biomedical treatment was an obvious choice, a form of therapy that was taken for granted, if compared with the preference for Ayurvedic services, which were usually utilized because of the failure of biomedicine. Regarding the position of Ayurveda, three issues are vital: the lack of experience and first-hand knowledge of Ayurveda on the part of health seekers; the significance of instruments, tools and technology as regards the expectations of proper consultation; and the impact of medical integration, which seems to be critical in order for modern Ayurveda to thrive in the health market. In short, in order to gain popularity in an urban context, Ayurvedic practitioners favour institutional integration and the adoption of items and practices particular to biomedicine.

Although there are people who are familiar with Ayurvedic treatment, knowing that it is a long process based on various dietary instructions and advice for personal conduct, many patients are first and foremost preoccupied with the instructions concerning the daily regimen of medicines produced by

Source: Nisula, T. (2006) In the presence of biomedicine: Ayurveda, medical integration and health seeking in Mysore, South India. *Anthropology and Medicine* 13(3): 207–24. Abridged version reprinted with permission of Routledge (Taylor and Francis Ltd).

the ever-growing Ayurveda industry and bolstered by the accelerating commercialization. Interestingly, if the association of biomedicine with pharmaceuticals and hospital technology characterizes a Southern Indian medical context, so does the association of Ayurveda with manufactured drugs. The most common answer one receives in Mysore city after asking about the benefits of Ayurvedic treatment is that it does not have side-effects. Apparently, the medical, cosmological and philosophical basis of Ayurveda is obscure and imprecise for most laypeople. In short, whether allopathy or Ayurveda, the medicine is frequently reduced to the icons of efficacy: if one offers quick fixes, the other has no side-effects.

This connection between Ayurveda and biomedicine – or English medicine, as it is often referred to in everyday life in South India – leads us to issues that are relevant for the arguments set out in this chapter. Generally speaking, the issues under discussion are related to the popularity of biomedical treatment in relation to Ayurveda and the use of biomedical instruments and technology in the context of Ayurvedic services. It is significant that according to many Ayurvedic practitioners in Mysore city, they have to fall back on the display of instruments designed for biomedical check-ups and treatment – although they might not use them – because of their patients' expectations concerning the effectiveness of therapy. Successful treatment is often associated with a practitioner's familiarity with technical devices, as stated by Ayurvedic practitioners themselves. It is worth mentioning that while patients seem to expect to find these instruments from Ayurvedic clinics, most of them tend to consult Ayurvedic practitioners only as a secondary resort.

The conceptual approach to Ayurveda that has been chosen here represents the standpoint of an officially qualified Ayurvedic practitioner, a college-trained doctor who is recognized by the government of India and registered with government bodies. These doctors represent the majority of *vaidyas*, Ayurvedic practitioners, in Mysore city. It should be added, however, that Ayurvedic medicine as it is practised today in South India could not be regarded as an expression of orthodox medicine. It has various local manifestations, which are not often consistent with the canonical textual sources. Moreover, it is well known that there are various kinds of Ayurvedic practitioners whose medical knowledge is based on diverse sources, and who are not necessarily trained in colleges, nor skilled in Sanskrit, the language of classical texts, and whose awareness of these texts might be rather rudimentary. Consequently, the border between Ayurvedic and non-Ayurvedic treatment is often relative.

Ayurveda and the question of medical integration

One of the most debated issues among Ayurvedic practitioners concerns the advantages and disadvantages of the incorporation of biomedical instruments, technology and concepts into Ayurvedic routines. This process has often been referred to as 'medical syncretism' or 'integration' (Leslie, 1992).

The contrast between pure (suddha) and impure Ayurveda has been an important element in the discourse of health and healing in India. Several practitioners referred to the split between the purists and integrationists. Although these characterizations are probably ideal types, they have relevance to a discussion about Ayurveda and its future, and certainly there are practitioners who could be seen to represent one or the other type.

According to the purist, Ayurveda is a self-sufficient medicine, a science with a divine history, capable of dealing with any affliction; according to the integrationist, in turn, only by accepting the use of modern technology and integrating it into Ayurvedic methods and education will the existence of Ayurveda and its popularity and utilization in a clinical setting be secured. It could be argued, however, that whatever the benefits or detriments of medical integration, the point is that in the face of the emergence of commercial forms of Ayurveda, the question of integration in relation to purity appears to be of secondary importance. Clearly, the aim of this chapter is not to defend medical orthodoxy, to advocate pure Ayurveda or to stress harmful influences of other medical approaches, which could be seen, from the point of view of a purist, to deteriorate the classical foundation of Ayurveda.

The crux of the problem is that as a result of omnipresent health markets, the differentiation of care has also had an impact on Ayurvedic treatment. And, as far as the Ayurvedic industry is concerned, it has even been remarked that the 'encounter with the modern market is successful only to the extent that Ayurvedic pharmaceuticals accept the ground rule; the industry responds and caters only to those who could afford its products' (Banerjee, 2002: 464). Hence, despite the importance of the question of purity, a more crucial issue seems to be the relationship between integration and increasing inequality in the non-biomedical sector.

So, if in order to be successful in domestic and global markets, 'Ayurvedic medicine had to be cast in the mould of modern medicine and disconnected from its relationship to the knowledge system' (Banerjee, 2002: 438), it follows that the growing inequality in the field of Ayurveda goes hand in hand with market-oriented Indian medicine, which, in turn, fosters the integration between Ayurveda and biomedicine. Whether opposed or not, medical integration between therapeutic approaches in India will, obviously, become more intense, irrespective of repercussions. And since it is a multidimensional phenomenon, it has implications that have ramifications throughout the health care system. However, in order to understand these implications as far as Mysorean health culture is concerned, we must turn first to health-seeking behaviour, and second to healing objects.

Health seeking in Mysore

Like most cities in India, Mysore is packed with clinics, pharmacies and hospitals. In terms of quantity, people have easy access to health services, mainly allopathic, Ayurvedic and homeopathic. This does not mean that every Mysorean can afford these services or choose between different alternatives; they have to consult the practitioner they can afford or who is available to them.

Despite these options, the choice of therapies follows a specific path. It is also interesting that clients' ignorance of the details of specific medical approach(es) does not necessarily contribute to the decline of medical pluralism or a lessening of integration, at least in Mysore. The ignorance of one approach, however, does contribute to the popularity of other approach(es).

It could be argued that there is a general pattern behind health-seeking behaviour in Mysore city. Regarding the patients interviewed, the first choice of treatment, for the majority, was biomedical treatment. Certainly many people, before consulting a doctor, rely on self-medication, consisting of various methods, medicines and articles, such as allopathic and Ayurvedic drugs, herbs, liquids and food items, which form the basis of medical knowledge in a local popular sector. Needless to say, however, not everyone has specific knowledge of herbs and spices.

This finding does not come as a complete surprise. The incompleteness of laypeople's medical knowledge, whether in the biomedical context, Ayurveda or grandmother's medicine, is the rule rather than the exception. Familiarity with healing techniques directs the choices of health seekers by giving preference usually to those who are known over those who are not. However, in a plural medical culture the knowledge or lack of knowledge of therapeutic options and techniques has specific outcomes when it comes to choosing among therapies. Clearly, the disinterest in or lack of first-hand knowledge of other approaches does not necessarily threaten the existence of plural culture, but patterns it.

Ignorance of Ayurvedic practices is shaping health seeking in Mysore. Biomedical treatment was an obvious choice, a form of therapy that was taken for granted, if compared with the preference for Ayurvedic practitioners who were consulted usually because of the failure of biomedical interventions. Consistent with these findings is that biomedicine, in terms of hospitals, clinics and pharmacies, dominates the medical scene in the city. The difference in quantity between allopathic and Ayurvedic services is considerable. Everyone who was interviewed was familiar with biomedical fixes, and had used either pharmaceuticals or injections. Everyone had consulted a practitioner who identified himself/herself with biomedicine. And whatever the outcome of biomedical treatment, the experiences of consultations followed in most cases the expectations of consultations. This is not to say that when searching for treatment, patients, because of the setbacks and disappointments involved, would not have visited several allopathic doctors, but to emphasize the commonplace nature of consultations in a biomedical context. Furthermore, even though some of the informants were familiar with their doctors prior to the initial visit, one could not assume that the reason to consult a practitioner who was trained or assumed to be trained in biomedicine would follow, mechanically, from one's prior acquaintance with him or her.

Conversely, consultation of an Ayurvedic practitioner was based, in most cases, on recommendations and suggestions that were obtained from friends and relatives after unsuccessful biomedical treatment. The impact of social relations is evident whenever people choose among the therapies. However, with regard to information about Ayurvedic treatment it appears to be extremely important, as most of the informants had no previous experiences of Ayurvedic treatment. People tend to consult allopathic practitioner, and only if the treatment and medicines are not able to improve their condition do they turn to Ayurvedic practitioners, usually after they have consulted several practitioners practising English medicine. Clearly, Ayurveda was an obvious choice for only a small proportion of Mysoreans interviewed and, moreover, most of them had only rudimentary knowledge of Ayurveda, if any.

This is an extremely interesting finding. One would have expected that because of the energetic marketing of mass-produced Ayurvedic medicines and their advertising through pharmacies and the media, information about Ayurveda would have been more widespread (cf. Banerjee, 2002). But possibly because of the advertising, informants were usually able to name one or two Ayurvedic products manufactured by the leading companies, such as Himalaya or Dabur, mentioning that Ayurvedic drugs are not supposed to have side-effects. This was, however, often all they knew about Ayurveda.

If there is a need to improve knowledge of the conceptual foundation of Ayurveda among practitioners, surely this holds good in the case of patients. Evidently, there is nothing like a shared Ayurvedic knowledge in Mysore city. Although there exists an Indian medicine, which is available to most Mysoreans, there are so many people 'who don't know anything about it', as many Ayurvedic practitioners mentioned.

An obvious argument is that in the Mysorean plural medical culture Ayurvedic services work as a secondary health resort, and as such they offer a health exit for dissatisfied patients. They are known to exist, but it is not usually known what is included in them.

In modern urban Mysore the users of Ayurvedic services are in the minority among health seekers, and Ayurvedic services have an auxiliary role to play. This is not to argue, however, that Ayurvedic medicine is of no value. Despite its position as a secondary resort in health care, it makes up a considerable health resource. Patients who were interviewed were usually satisfied with the treatment they had obtained from Ayurvedic practitioners.

Furthermore, the position of Ayurveda is anything but static. First, because of the promotion of Indian systems of medicine and their integration into the state health care system, the status of Ayurvedic medicine, in proximity to biomedicine, is increasing, at least with reference to health policy, if not in the minds of health seekers. Secondly, because of the booming Ayurvedic industry and medicine marketing, the relationship between Ayurveda and biomedicine is intensifying. Manufacturers and entrepreneurs from both fields, with homogenized strategies to reach the consumer, are equally active players in the health market. The border between Ayurveda and biomedicine is becoming more indefinable as regards the marketing of medicines and services. And finally, when searching for treatment and consulting various practitioners, possibly to a growing extent due to the former reasons, health seekers are creating bonds between various approaches and at the same time blurring their boundaries. All these reasons bolster integrated health care and increase the awareness of Ayurveda. However, there is nothing indicating that Ayurvedic services in Mysore city will not continue as a secondary health resort in the years ahead, or that the health-seeking pattern in the city will change radically. This view is supported by the issue discussed below.

The appeal of instruments

If the health-seeking pattern in Mysore city has a specific nature, one could assume that it might also have specific implications that are related to the expectations with regard to consultations and treatment. If instruments designed for biomedical check-ups and treatment are widely used in the context of Ayurveda, one could argue that this is an additional example of medical integration, as has been suggested above. Clearly, the same tools, the same professional etiquette, the same attitude to medicines and the same figures – gods and gurus, divinities and teachers – are embodied in the routines taking place in various forms of health services. If so, patients' familiarity with medical instruments, pharmaceuticals and technology within the framework of biomedical treatment possibly has something to do with the expectations occurring in other fields of therapy.

According to the interviews, many clients were expecting to see instruments in Ayurvedic clinics. A very popular clinic that is run by Doctor R, who is qualified in both allopathy and Ayurveda, offers a good example. Some of the patients preferred Doctor R over other doctors because of his knowledge of both approaches and because he is well equipped for diagnosing patients. Doctor R's clinic was not exceptional. Many informants in other clinics with whom the issue was discussed regarded the presence of tools as important. And moreover, all of the informants who had experiences of consultations with Ayurvedic practitioners had visited one who possessed instruments.

Secondly, it is paradoxical that even the most eager defenders of pure Ayurveda were forced to rely on the symbolic power of instruments and were dependent on the technological solutions characterizing biomedical services and practices, such as X-rays. Only one Ayurvedic practitioner, out of 25 interviewed, did not have a stethoscope or other instruments associated with biomedical check-ups and treatment in his consulting room. Furthermore, clients often ask, in order to estimate a doctor's ability, whether he or she has distinct instruments, such as a stethoscope or a sphygmomanometer. Three Ayurvedic practitioners claimed that they never use their 'allopathic' equipment and that their role was purely to offer 'mental' images to their patients. So, however apparent is the therapeutic relevance of articles utilized by various healers, as apparent, it seems, is their symbolic and social relevance. These findings are in accordance with previous studies. It has been stated that 'most registered practitioners [of Ayurveda], and particularly those trained in colleges, are convinced that for the good of their patients, and to support themselves in practice, they cannot give up vitamin and antibiotic injections, or symbols of medical expertise such as the stethoscope' (Leslie, 1992: 185).

These examples inform us about the commodification of health. In Mysore city a well-known Ayurvedic practitioner mentioned that earlier in his career he used to fill empty capsules with powdered Ayurvedic drugs to attract suspicious patients with a form of medicine they were expecting to be given. Nowadays he is prescribing only the powders to his patients, rather than in capsules, but, as he stressed, in order to do that he had to familiarize his patients with Ayurvedic medication.

It follows that in spite of differences in the treatment process (biomedical substances and methods versus Ayurvedic substances and methods) and theoretical sources (biomedical theory versus Ayurvedic theory), there are no significant differences between biomedicine and Ayurveda as regards the significance of the presence of instruments. What is at issue here is that most Ayurvedic colleges in South India follow a policy of integration. Because courses in biomedicine are included in the curriculum, college-trained Ayurvedic practitioners have usually learned the principles of biomedicine and are familiar with biomedical concepts and instruments. And, as a result, the ancient categories of nosology and physiology are often replaced by biomedical ones in a clinical reality where the difference between Ayurvedic and allopathic practitioners disappears.

Apparently, in order to gain popularity and succeed in a Southern Indian medical setting, Ayurvedic practitioners are favouring institutional integration and exploitation of items and practices that are peculiar to biomedicine. Furthermore, it has been underscored that the educational policy related to Ayurveda 'has been implemented by people who feel that they have to prove the value of Ayurveda by using the language of modern science' (Leslie, 1992: 184–5). The discursive change in Ayurveda and the establishment of integrated colleges during the last five decades has, however, had an additional consequence; namely, the professionalization of Ayurveda, which is an ongoing process. Present-day Ayurvedic practitioners form a profession that has as its foundation a standardized and formal education obtained from medical colleges. Due to professionalization, conceptual change and familiarity with instruments and technology, most Ayurvedic hospitals have adopted a culture particular to biomedical institutions. Plainly, in an urban context, like in Mysore city, there are no significant differences between biomedicine and Ayurveda as regards the professional and intellectual context of health and healing.

But how should we interpret these findings? It seems that besides the official status of Ayurvedic treatment – acknowledged by the government of India as a significant sector of health care – and the formal promotion of medical integration, which strengthens the integration of Ayurveda into the state health care system, the integration has other dimensions, as noted, such as the exploitation of instruments and technology in Ayurvedic clinics and hospitals. This particular aspect seems to advance the relevance of tools and things. Health seekers' expectations of consultations as well as practitioners' expectations concerning those of their patients are both related, at least partly, to the significance of instruments. In this specific sense the impact of biomedicine on Ayurvedic practices is explicit.

In general, the role of instruments and technology should be considered in relation to the omnipresent medical integration, dominance of biomedicine and a specific health-seeking pattern, in which Ayurvedic services operate as a secondary health resort. All of these aspects seem to strengthen the positive meaning of things and tools that have their origin in biomedicine, and by doing so they are fortifying biomedical therapy against other therapies, which in turn is sustaining the existing health-seeking pattern.

Further reading

Schensul, S., Mekki-Berrada, A., Nastasi, B., Saggurti, N. and Verma, R. (2006) Healing traditions and men's sexual health in Mumbai, India. The realities of practiced medicine in urban poor communities. *Social Science and Medicine* 62: 2774–85.

References

Banerjee, M. (2002) Power, culture and medicine: Ayurvedic pharmaceuticals in the modern market. *Contributions to Indian Sociology* 36: 435–67.
Leslie, C. (1992) Interpretations of illness: Syncretism in modern Ayurveda. In C. Leslie and A. Young (eds) *Paths to Asian Medical Knowledge*. Berkeley: University of California Press, pp. 177–208.

Exploring the complementary and alternative medicine–conventional medicine interface

Introduction

As health-care utilization studies have repeatedly shown, the vast majority of people who utilize CAM products, technologies, practices and practitioners also continue to seek conventional health care. In tandem with this patient-led demand for CAM (as an accompaniment or supplement as opposed to an alternative to biomedical care), conventional providers have also developed closer relationships with these other medicines. Some have introduced direct integrative practices adopting CAM therapies, techniques or products often without consultation or input from complementary health providers; others have introduced both formal and informal collaborations and referral networks with complementary practitioners (often working outside the practice settings of public health-care systems); and others still have at minimum acknowledged what they perceive as their responsibility to inform and education themselves (and their patients) about CAM in the interests of consumer choice and safety. While it is important to note that such mainstreaming practices and behaviours often remain ad hoc pockets of activity that do not always receive official approval or support (from professional associations or practice-setting management), it would appear that a climate increasingly sympathetic to health-care pluralism and integration is emerging across many conventional practice fields.

One area of conventional practice that has attracted much research attention and commentary with regard to CAM is primary health care. Indeed, general practice/family medicine has traditionally been the focus of choice for gauging interest, attitudes and prospects of future fortunes or limitations to collaboration and/or integration across the conventional/CAM divide. In line with this focus, the first chapter in this section (Chapter 15) explores the dynamics driving and inhibiting communication between primary health-care clinicians and their patients about traditional medicine/CAM. Interpreting data from a qualitative study with both clinicians and patients, Shelley and colleagues compare the perspectives of both groups with regard to traditional

133

medicine/CAM communication, as well as identifying strategies for enhancing this important aspect of the primary health-care consultation.

Alongside general practice/family medicine, another important professional group providing first-line patient care is community-based pharmacy. As Boon and colleagues (Chapter 16) explain, pharmacists are an integral part of the conventional health-care team currently providing an important interface for patients with regard to the use of and information about dietary supplements and natural health products. However, following a systematic assessment of the pharmacy literature, Boon and colleagues highlight what they interpret as a predominantly deterministic and circular message and call for consultation with practising pharmacists, educators and policymakers to foster open debate and ensure that proactive decision making characterizes the future of pharmacy practice in relation to dietary supplements and natural health products.

The last chapter in this section (Chapter 17) also presents a narrative analysis of professional documentation regarding CAM. However, attention is redirected to the portrayal of CAM (in this case mostly techniques and therapies as opposed to products) within nursing circles. Analysing journal articles via the conceptual framework of social worlds theory, Tovey and Adams illustrate the use of nostalgic and nostophobic referencing as ways in which nursing authors advocate, legitimize and/or defend CAM integration to others in their professional world. Identifying and understanding such dynamics not only provides a window to the ever-evolving debates regarding professional identity and territory and the position and role of CAM therein (in nursing and all other professional worlds), but also alerts us to the importance of critically examining such topics that have until recently remained largely the terrain of advocacy.

CHAPTER 15

'They don't ask me so I don't tell them': Patient–clinician communication about traditional, complementary and alternative medicine

BRIAN SHELLEY, ANDREW SUSSMAN, ROBERT WILLIAMS, ALISSA SEGAL AND BENJAMIN CRABTREE ON BEHALF OF THE RIOS NET CLINICIANS

Introduction

Most users of traditional medicine and complementary and alternative medicine (TM/CAM) also use allopathic care. There are numerous studies, however, documenting a lack of communication in the conventional care setting between patients and their primary care clinicians about patients' use of TM/CAM (Adler 1999; Sleath *et al.*, 2001; Herman *et al.*, 2004).

Patient-centred communication is an evolving construct, defined by Epstein *et al.* (2005) as a set of strategies (or a 'way of being') designed to enhance a sense of partnership in the patient–clinician relationship. Applied to TM/CAM use, patient-centred communication can be important because it may result in closer agreement between the clinician and the patient about treatment plans; reduce misunderstandings between patients and clinicians; uncover potential herb–drug interactions; strengthen the quality of the patient–clinician relationship; and provide an opportunity to discuss specific

Source: Shelley, B., Sussman, A., Williams, R., Segal, A. and Crabtree, B. (2009) 'They don't ask me so I don't tell them': Patient–clinician communication about traditional, complementary, and alternative medicine. *Annals of Family Medicine* 7(2): 139–47. Abridged version reprinted with permission of American Academy of Family Physicians.

TM/CAM modalities with high-quality evaluative evidence (Corbin Winslow and Shapiro, 2002; Flannery 2006).

A first step towards improving communication between patients and their primary care clinicians about TM/CAM use is to better understand the factors influencing that communication. We conducted a qualitative study to explore the dynamics driving and inhibiting communication between clinicians and their patients about TM/CAM. Our specific aims were to compare perspectives of patients and primary care clinicians on communication about TM/CAM, and to identify strategies for enhancing patient–clinician communication about TM/CAM.

Methods

We conducted this study in southwestern Hispanic and Native American communities in New Mexico, where TM/CAM use is common (Cherrington *et al.*, 2003; Zeilmann *et al.*, 2003; Shelley, 2006). We carried out a multistage qualitative study using focus groups, in-depth interviews and a video vignette to investigate processes of communication about TM/CAM. In total, 41 staff participated in the 8 clinic staff focus groups, 93 patients were interviewed, 14 clinicians were interviewed, 5 clinicians participated in the clinician focus group, and 6 community advisory board members and 21 patients participated in the reflective patient interviews (for more details about design, see the original paper).

Findings

Acceptance and non-judgement

Patients' perceptions of how their clinicians would react to their use of TM/CAM were generally the most important factor in their openness to discussions with the clinician about this topic. An accepting and non-judgemental attitude by the clinician contributed to willingness by the patient to reveal use of TM/CAM. Many patients told stories about previous experiences during which they felt rebuked by a clinician for using TM/CAM; others avoided the discussion out of fear that the clinician would respond negatively.

> [PATIENT] When my little boy was born, I used to give him herbs for his stomach aches. And I used to come in for his well-child check-up and I wouldn't tell [the doctor] because ... I'd be like, 'she'll get madder.' So I don't tell them that I use herbs on the kids.
> [INTERVIEWER] And what makes you think the doctor would get mad?
> [PATIENT] Well, when I had my first little girl they did get mad at me. They told me that I'm not supposed to give them anything for the colic.

Importantly, patients did not expect clinicians to be experts on TM/CAM, beyond having broad awareness of local types of TM/CAM. This attitude appeared to reflect an understanding that TM/CAM is outside the realm of the training and expertise of most conventional care clinicians.

Clinicians, for their part, varied in their approach to communicating acceptance or non-acceptance of TM/CAM use. For some clinicians, discussions about TM/CAM were viewed as important in communicating respect for patient autonomy and culture and as a mechanism to enhance the patient–clinician relationship. Although these clinicians often still maintained a degree of caution towards the efficacy, cost and safety of TM/CAM, it appeared that communicating encouragement of the patient's efforts towards self-care was of equal importance and was linked to the clinician's value in a more comprehensive definition of patient health and wellness.

> If they're getting a benefit out of having their aura stroked or something, I don't believe in auras, but I'm not going to even betray with a facial muscle that I don't believe in auras. I'm just going to say, 'Great, I think that's great.' Because I think anything that somebody does for themselves to try to take care of themselves is a positive.

These clinicians pointed out that the language used to introduce and discuss TM/CAM was critical; they emphasized an open and non-judgemental approach. While rejecting the idea of themselves as content experts in TM/CAM, they emphasized the importance of not dismissing the patient's use of TM/CAM as a way to support a positive therapeutic relationship with potentially greater benefits than those that might come from criticizing the TM/CAM practice.

Other clinicians considered their role as scientific experts advising their patients and their commitment to 'do no harm' as compelling them to warn the patient about concerns they had about TM/CAM practices. These clinicians also mentioned a value in being open and honest with their patients about their clinical views.

> There's a lot of shyster kind of stuff out there. A couple years ago there was a diabetic thing that actually had glyburide ground up in it. So I had these people taking this herbal thing. What they were taking, however, was pulverized glyburide and people were having hypoglycemia with it. I have no problem with [patients using TM/CAM]. I just want to make sure that there's no contraindication.

Initiation of communication

The differing perspectives between patients and clinicians with regard to the initiation and timing of discussion about TM/CAM influenced communication about this topic. Many patients reported either no or low levels of communication about their TM/CAM use with their primary care clinicians. Patients were generally receptive to, if hesitant about, increasing discussion about TM/CAM, but they consistently expressed a preference for the clinician to initiate the TM/CAM discussion: 'In my situation, I don't see myself ever just giving him information or just pouring it out. I think he needs to start the dialogue.'

In contrast, clinicians often did not perceive high levels of TM/CAM use among their patients, and therefore would not initiate the conversation.

> [INTERVIEWER] So, where does TM/CAM fit in your hierarchy of things?
> [CLINICIAN] I think if I heard more of it coming from my patients, I would feel more stimulated to go out there and get myself informed. But if they're not bringing it up, then I'm not.

At the same time, we found that many clinicians believed that their own understanding of the TM/CAM practices their patients were using was insufficient to be able to discuss the practices intelligently or to provide scientifically based medical advice to their patients should the topic come up. This perceived lack of understanding appeared to act as a barrier to the clinician in initiating discussions about TM/CAM.

> If you're interested in Pap smears or mammograms, I would be more than happy to help you with that, but on the other stuff, trying St John's Wort or whatever for your depression, don't come to me. I mean, that's the depth of my herbal depression knowledge. I don't know how many times a day, I don't know what brand, I don't know what dosage.

If the clinician did initiate a discussion about TM/ CAM, the phrasing of questions appeared to be important. Patients seemed not to understand that a question about what else he or she is taking is a question about TM/CAM use, assuming instead that the clinician is asking about allopathic care treatments, such as prescription or over-the-counter medications. Multiple competing demands for time within the brief clinical encounter limited when and how clinicians discussed TM/CAM with patients. For example, several clinicians indicated that if they ask patients about the use of these practices, they do so typically only as part of an initial medical history.

Safety and efficacy concerns

Views about the safety and efficacy of the TM/CAM practices also appeared to influence communication. Clinicians, trained to base their therapeutic decision making on the best available scientific evidence, expressed scepticism where evidence of the effectiveness and safety of TM/CAM is lacking.

Some clinicians, driven by their concerns about the safety and efficacy of TM/CAM, reported an assertive approach aimed at dissuading patients from using TM/CAM by calling on their medical authority and expertise.

[INTERVIEWER] If the use of [TM/CAM] does come up in the context of a patient whose diabetes isn't well controlled, we're wondering what you're trying to know about that use.

[CLINICIAN] I want to know what it is they're taking and the rationale for taking it. It's not always taking medicine, sometimes it's not taking medicine, because I've had people come and say, 'Well I'm not taking my Lipitor because my neighbor told me it does this and it does that.' Usually I can answer that with, 'Well, where did they go to medical school?' and I think they get the idea right away that they shouldn't be listening to the neighbor and they should be listening to the doctor.

Discussion

We found three main themes that largely determine whether and how communication about TM/CAM takes place between patients and their primary care clinicians: acceptance/non-judgement, initiation of communication and safety/efficacy concerns. Patients' perspectives about TM/CAM communication were clear and consistent. Most patients who are using TM/CAM for health or illness expect the clinician to initiate the discussion on this topic if communication is to occur. Patient data suggested that clinician initiation, when carried out in a non-judgemental fashion, would demonstrate openness to TM/CAM and would help patients overcome anticipated or previous negative interactions in discussions about TM/CAM. Patients usually did not expect their clinicians to be experts on the TM/CAM they were using.

Paradoxically, some clinicians interpreted the low levels of communication about TM/CAM as a sign of low use in their clinical practices. This assumption, together with the clinician's lack of understanding about TM/CAM, appeared to limit discussion of TM/CAM in the brief clinical encounter. Many clinicians expressed scepticism about TM/CAM safety and effectiveness out of genuine concern for their patients, and some believed that their duty is to protect patients from the potential adverse effects of certain practices or possible delay of effective conventional care resulting from TM/CAM use. Other clinicians, while still sceptical, see non-judgemental discussions with their patients about TM/CAM to be a way to improve their understanding of and relationships with their patients. Many clinicians, however, mention limited time as a restricting factor.

This project aimed to better understand the dynamics of communication about TM/CAM between primary care clinicians and their patients, and to identify strategies for enhancing that communication. One study has reported that patient anticipation of a negative response to their TM/CAM use by clinicians is high (Adler, 1999), whereas two other studies suggest that clinicians are open to discussing this topic, perhaps more than patients realize (Crock *et al.*, 1999; Frenkel and Borkan, 2003). In contrast, we found variability among the clinicians interviewed in their openness to this discussion.

Traditionally, strategies to increase communication with patients about

TM/CAM have recommended that clinicians acquire wider knowledge about specific TM/CAM therapies. We suggest investigating a different approach. We believe that clinicians must initiate this discussion, yet in so doing they do not have to be experts in TM/CAM therapies; they simply need to show non-judgemental interest and candour regarding limited knowledge. Such an approach was preliminarily confirmed during our video vignette process, but this model will require rigorous investigation with actual patients and clinicians (Barrett *et al.*, 2007). Open and non-judgemental questioning is consistent with patient-centredness theory (Epstein *et al.*, 2005), which is intended to facilitate eliciting the patient's perspective, understanding the patient, acting in a manner consistent with patients' values and involving patients in medical decision making. In addition, patient disclosure of TM/CAM is correlated with having a physician with a participatory decision-making style (Sleath *et al.*, 2001).

Our research took place in Hispanic and Native American communities where TM/CAM use is an important component of personal health care, which could limit the generalizability of our findings. We believe, however, that the themes we identified as influencing TM/CAM communication share a common basis with concepts about patient-centred communication in general. Our findings have implications for TM/CAM communication skills training that could be integrated into clinical curricula and continuing medical education. It may be easier to educate clinicians with brief training in targeted communication skills, which have been shown to increase clinicians' discussion of challenging topics (Ryan *et al.*, 2001; Stewart *et al.*, 2007). Future investigation should also explore factors contributing to why patients and clinicians are or are not comfortable with discussing TM/CAM. Such information would help gain further understanding of what motivates patients to discuss TM/CAM and what motivates clinicians' willingness to listen.

Further reading

Adams, J. (2004) Demarcating the medical/non-medical border: Occupational boundary-work within GPs' accounts of their integrative practice. In P. Tovey, G. Easthope and J. Adams (eds) *The Mainstreaming of Complementary and Alternative Medicine: Studies in Social Context.* London: Routledge.

Robinson, A. and McGrail, M. (2004) Disclosure of complementary and alternative medicine use to medical practitioners: A review of qualitative and quantitative studies. *Complementary Therapies in Medicine* 12(203): 90–98.

Sussman, A., Williams, R.L.W. and Shelley, B.M. (2010) Can we rapidly identify traditional, complementary and alternative medicine users in the primary care encounter? A RIOS Net study. *Ethnicity and Disease* (20)1: 64–70.

References

Adler, S.R. (1999) Disclosing complementary and alternative medicine use in the medical encounter: A qualitative study in women with breast cancer. *Journal of Family Practice* 13(2): 214–22.

Barrett, B., Rakel, D., Chewning, B. *et al.* (2007) Rationale and methods for a trial assessing placebo, echinacea, and doctor–patient interaction in the common cold. *Explore (NY)* 3(6): 561–72.

Cherrington, A., Lewis, C.E., McCreath, H.E., Herman, C.J., Richter, D.L. and Byrd, T. (2003) Association of complementary and alternative medicine use, demographic factors, and perimenopausal symptoms in a multiethnic sample of women: The ENDOW study. *Family and Community Health* 26(1): 74–83.

Corbin Winslow, L. and Shapiro, H. (2002) Physicians want education about complementary and alternative medicine to enhance communication with their patients. *Archives of Internal Medicine* 162(10): 1176–81.

Crock, R.D., Jarjoura, D., Polen, A. and Rutecki, G.W. (1999) Confronting the communication gap between conventional and alternative medicine: A survey of physicians' attitudes. *Alternative Therapies in Health and Medicine* 5(2): 61–6.

Epstein, R.M., Franks, P., Fiscella, K. *et al.* (2005) Measuring patient-centered communication in patient-physician consultations: Theoretical and practical issues. *Social Science and Medicine* 61(7): 1516–28.

Flannery, M. (2006) Communication about complementary and alternative medicine: Perspectives of primary care clinicians. *Alternative Therapies in Health and Medicine* 12(1): 56–63.

Frenkel, M.A. and Borkan, J.M. (2003) An approach for integrating complementary–alternative medicine into primary care. *Family Practice* 20(3): 324–32.

Herman, C.J., Allen, P., Hunt, W.C., Prasad, A. and Brady, T.J. (2004) Use of complementary therapies among primary care clinic patients with arthritis. *Preventing Chronic Disease* 1(4): A12.

Ryan, G.L., Skinner, C.S., Farrell, D. and Champion, V.L. (2001) Examining the boundaries of tailoring: The utility of tailoring versus targeting mammography interventions for two distinct populations. *Health Education Research* 16(5): 555–66.

Shelley, B.M. (2006) Integrative medicine research in New Mexico: Lessons from the published literature. *Complementary Health Practice Review* 11(2): 107–19.

Sleath, B., Rubin, R.H., Campbell, W., Gwyther, L. and Clark, T. (2001) Ethnicity and physician–older patient communication about alternative therapies. *Journal of Alternative and Complementary Medicine* 7(4): 329–35.

Stewart, M., Brown, J.B., Hammerton, J. *et al.* (2007) Improving communication between doctors and breast cancer patients. *Annals of Family Medicine* 5(5): 387–94.

Zeilmann, C.A., Dole, E.J., Skipper, B.J., McCabe, M., Dog, T.L. and Rhyne, R.L. (2003) Use of herbal medicine by elderly Hispanic and non-Hispanic white patients. *Pharmacotherapy* 23(4): 526–32.

CHAPTER 16

The ethics of dietary supplements and natural health products in pharmacy practice: A systematic documentary analysis

HEATHER BOON, KRISTINE HIRSCHKORN, GLENN GRIENER AND MICHELLE CALI

Introduction

Pharmacists are an integral part of the conventional health care team within the context of the North American health care system. The introduction of new categories of products such as natural health products (NHPs) in Canada and dietary supplements (DSs) in the United States has created new challenges for pharmacists striving to provide comprehensive patient-centred pharmaceutical care for patients.

Although NHPs and DSs are widely available in pharmacies across North America, there has been relatively little discussion among members of the profession about what professional responsibilities pharmacists have with respect to these products. Pharmacists' responsibilities to detect and prevent interactions between NHPs/DSs and conventional medications has consistently been identified in the literature as important (Cardinale, 2000; Levy, 2000; Chavis, 2001; Jurgens, 2001) and a recent study suggested that use of prescription drugs in conjunction with NHPs/DSs is high enough (16 per cent) to raise concerns about unintended interactions (Kaufman, 2002).

Source: Boon, H., Hirschkorn, K., Greener, G. and Cali, M. (2010) The ethics of dietary supplements and natural health products in pharmacy practice: A systematic documentary analysis. *International Journal of Pharmacy Practice* 17(1): 31–8. Abridged version reprinted with permission of John Wiley & Sons Ltd and Royal Pharmacy Society.

Several information papers suggest that pharmacists should provide objective information to help patients make informed choices about NHP/DS use (NAPRA, 1999; Boon, 2001). These reports seem to imply that there is relative agreement within the profession of pharmacy, not only that pharmacists have professional responsibilities with respect to NHPs/DSs, but also with respect to key aspects of what those responsibilities are (or should be). However, there is evidence that this is not an accurate portrayal of the opinions and practices within the profession (Bouldin *et al.*, 1999). Pharmacists' practices also lag behind at least some of the expectations outlined in the information papers, since most pharmacists do not routinely document, monitor, or inquire about patients' use of NHPs or DSs (Bouldin, 1999).

The purpose of this study was to complete a comprehensive, systematic assessment of the pharmacy literature to identify how the pharmacist's role with respect to NHPs and DSs is portrayed.

Methods

A systematic search was conducted in a variety of health databases to identify all literature that pertained to both pharmacy and natural health products and dietary supplements. Of the 786 articles identified, 665 were broad-coded and 259 were subjected to in-depth qualitative content analysis for emergent themes (for more details of methods, see the original paper).

Results

Here we review the themes of whether pharmacists have a role with respect to NHPs/DSs and whether pharmacists should be selling NHPs/DSs. Following these themes, we explore the ethics of the message that emerges in this literature.

Do pharmacists have a role with respect to NHPs/DSs?

Most of the literature either explicitly or implicitly identified that pharmacists have a key role to play with respect to NHPs/DSs. Support for counselling about NHPs/DSs as a key role for pharmacists was extremely widespread and general. Indeed, the vast majority of content reviewed contained reference to pharmacists' counselling role, implying that most authors assumed that pharmacists should be involved in this area.

> Although pharmacists may be reluctant to discuss the use of herbal therapies with patients for fear that such discussion may imply endorsement or approval, it is nonetheless the pharmacist's professional responsibility to advise patients about potentially harmful aspects of herbal remedies, including possible interactions or contraindications

with synthetic medications and/or current disease states. To do otherwise could leave patients at risk for major problems and jeopardize the public trust accorded pharmacists. (Bennett and Brown, 2000)

A very common subtheme was that pharmacists' role(s) arose from consumer demand for NHPs/DSs. The general argument was that since so many patients are using these products, pharmacists need to have some knowledge in this area.

However, it seems inevitable that patients' increasing demand for and use of alternative therapies will continue to increase the need for information and advice from pharmacists, particularly regarding alternative therapies that are medicinal in nature. In fact, the current findings, along with other research, indicate that pharmacists are already experiencing an increased demand for such information, especially in pharmacies that stock herbal medicines. (Brown, 1998)

Another variation on this theme was that pharmacists are one of the most accessible health care practitioners and they are available at the point of sale.

The availability of these products in many pharmacy settings and the rapidly growing body of knowledge regarding the potential for significant interactions between drugs and natural products have led to the emergence of pharmacists as a 'front line' for provision of information regarding the safety and efficacy of natural products. (Clauson *et al.*, 2003)

Several authors made the point that NHPs/DSs were the future of pharmacy.

In the future pharmacists will need to be the information providers for more than just conventional pharmaceuticals and medical devices. Those pharmacists that do not continue to move forward and keep up, particularly in herbal medicine and especially in combination with conventional medications, could put their patients in danger and the reputation of their profession at risk. (Rowell and Kroll, 1998)

However, not everyone agreed that NHPs/DSs should be part of pharmacists' scope of practice. 'As the columns of *The Pharmaceutical Journal* have shown in recent years, some pharmacists would ban from pharmacies all herbal and homoeopathic products that have not been validated by clinical trials' (Sturgess, 2002). '[S]keptics declare that pharmacists have no business selling and promoting products whose medical worth is still in question' (Johne *et al.*, 1999).

Others simply questioned what role pharmacists can have when there is evidence that patients are not asking pharmacists for advice. 'One study showed that 72 per cent of respondents who used alternative medicine (including herbals) did not inform any health care professional of their use [in reference to Eisenberg *et al.*, 1993]' (Bouldin *et al.*, 1999). Overwhelmingly, however, the message that emerges in these documents is that pharmacists do indeed have a role to play with respect to NHPs/DSs, particularly with respect to counselling.

Should pharmacists sell NHPs?

Most documents made the point that the NHP/DS (and especially the herbal) market is growing overall and within pharmacies. There was almost unanimous support that NHPs/DSs should be sold in pharmacies (the only disagreement was over the sale of homeopathy). Some of the documents were clearly intended to encourage pharmacists to sell NHPs, extolling the good profit margins of these products. A large proportion of documents on this topic made the point that NHPs/DSs are profitable for pharmacies, highlighting the age-old challenge that pharmacists face because they are both health care professionals and also business people expected to generate a profit. 'Good health care outcomes mean satisfied customers/patients who gladly keep their business where their good health lies. This leads to increased sales, in both natural medicine as well as prescriptions' (Grauds, 2001). 'The outlook for this market niche is optimistic and by incorporating alternative medicine in these services, pharmacists can be assured that their profit margin will increase' (Kattis, 1999).

The profit motivation for selling NHPs/DSs was further highlighted in articles that described niche pharmacists/pharmacies that specialized in these products. This is not to suggest that profit was the only motivation for NHP/DS sales in pharmacies. The following author, for example, highlights that patient-centred care is the justification for carrying these products:

> [F]inancial gain is not the main reason pharmacists get involved. As in any profession, there are, no doubt, some pharmacists who see the alternative medicine movement as a 'cash cow.' Most pharmacists, however, focus more on their patients and what they are using, particularly if it has the potential for disrupting the benefits of their medication regimens. Thinking that any pharmacist who has an interest in learning more about alternative therapies is doing so just to make money is an unfair and, most likely, erroneous assumption. (Montagne, 1999)

It was also clear from the documents that NHP/DS sales are already a core part of pharmacy business and that this decision may be made by corporate headquarters rather than by an individual pharmacist working at store level:

> In the real world, many pharmacists don't have the option of remaining aloof from the issue. If they are employees, they will have to deal with the reality that herbal products will very likely be sold in their store. And if they own their own pharmacy, they have to decide whether they should refuse to sell herbals on principle – and thereby lose profits while leaving their patients to the mercies of possibly unskilled health food store staff. (Johne *et al.*, 1999)

Consequently, many pharmacists do not make decisions about the products carried in their workplaces, and are simply left to make the best of this situation that we would characterize as an ethical conflict, as described below.

The ethics of the message: An emerging ethical conflict?

Although there is widespread support that pharmacists should be selling NHPs/DSs and that patient counselling about these products is an important and growing part of the pharmacists' role, some authors pointed to the emergence of ethical issues. There were two main ethical conflicts identified in the documents. The first is the issues raised by the sale of products for which there is no scientific evidence of effectiveness or safety. This issue is generally described in terms of consumers' enhanced choice being in conflict with the pharmacists' duty to help and protect the patient. The following quotations sum up this first ethical issue:

> Is it unethical for pharmacies to carry and promote herbal remedies? Is it unethical for traditional pharmaceutical companies to lend their trusted names to these dietary products? Is it unethical for pharmaceutical laboratories to support these products by certifying standardization of constituents while knowing that efficacy studies are lacking? These are just a few questions that pharmacy must address in the years to come. The immediate dilemma that today's pharmacist faces with alternative medicine lies in determining what really works and what does not. And how does one determine the truth about the medical safety and efficacy of any herbal product in today's market? (Williamson and Wyandt, 1999)

> A pharmacist may not recommend a product whose safety or quality is in doubt, but there is nothing, apparently, to prevent him or her selling dubious remedies. (Sturgess, 2002)

Homeopathy was a special case of this first ethical issue that was highlighted in several articles because of the theoretical incompatibility of homeopathic principles with conventional pharmacology.

> [T]he incompatibility of homeopathic paradigms with all of basic science must be appreciated. Although some pharmacists may wish to keep an 'open mind' about the use of such dubious products, they should be reminded that the 1996 revision of The Ontario College of Pharmacists Code of Ethics clearly states that, 'pharmacists never knowingly condone the dispensing, promoting or distributing of drugs ... which are not of good quality'. (Harrison et al., 1999)

The second issue identified here is whether it is ethical for pharmacists to sell NHPs/DSs if they do not have the knowledge to counsel patients about them (including knowledge about evidence that is in existence). 'Pharmacists have an ethical responsibility for currency of knowledge about any medicines that they offer for sale or supply to the public' (Blenkinsopp, 2005).

Even where ethics was not identified explicitly with respect to lack of knowledge or evidence, there are numerous passages that highlight this gap in pharmacy practice and education:

> Pharmacists know that our patients are using these products, yet we have little understanding of them. Lack of knowledge about interactions and dosage and administration is a major concern and will continue to be if we do not develop a scientific body of knowledge to address these issues. (Beal, 1998)

> Health care providers should be concerned about the lack of scientific evidence present to make a solid decision about supplements. (Semaan, 2000)

What becomes apparent in the passages quoted here is that an information or knowledge gap is either the source of an ethical conflict, or compounds an already existing ethical conflict between patient care and profit. Whereas a lack of information focuses on the lack of research and evidence, the knowledge gap refers to pharmacists' lack of knowledge even about what information and evidence do currently exist. Despite the identification of these information/knowledge gaps and the raising of related ethical concerns by some commentators, the overwhelming message in these documents has still been that pharmacists should have a role and should be selling NHPs/DSs.

Conclusion

The notable message that emerges in these documents, with the exception of a small number of detractors, is that pharmacists do have a role to play with respect to NHPs/DSs and that they should be selling NHPs/DSs. What is problematic about this message – beyond the concerns raised about the information and knowledge gap confounding existing issues – is that it is largely deterministic and circular: patient demand for NHPs/DSs exists, therefore pharmacies should be selling NHPs/DSs, and since pharmacies are already selling NHPs/DSs, pharmacists should have a role with respect to NHPs/DSs (for instance they should counsel about these products). However, none of these conclusions necessarily or logically follows from the ones before, leading us to argue that open debate and discussion about the merits of pharmacists undertaking a role have largely been precluded by this line of thinking. While the message in these documents might be clear-cut (if presumptuous), it by no means represents the profession of pharmacy at large or even the views of most practising pharmacists. It is simply what we called it, a message, granted a powerful and one-sided message that charts a particular future course for pharmacy, but a future course that is not wholly determined. This message strongly underscores the need to consult with practising pharmacists, pharmacy educators and policymakers to foster debate about the issues raised here and ensure that proactive decision making, rather than abandonment to the determinism suggested by the status quo, characterizes the future of pharmacy practice.

Further reading

Barnes, J. (2003) Pharmacovigilance of herbal medicines: A UK perspective. *Drug Safety* 26(12): 829–51.

Cramer, H., Shaw, A., Wye, L. and Weiss, M. (2010) Over-the-counter advice seeking about complementary and alternative medicine (CAM) in community pharmacies and health shops: An ethnographic study. *Health and Social Care in the Community* 18(1): 41–50.

References

Beal, F.C. (1998) Herbals and homeopathic remedies as formulary items?' *American Journal of Health-System Pharmacy* 55: 1266–7.

Bennett, J. and Brown, C.M. (2000) Use of herbal remedies by patients in a health maintenance organization. *Journal of the American Pharmacists Association* 40: 353–8.

Blenkinsopp, A. (2005) St John's wort – an ethical dilemma? *Pharmaceutical Journal* 274(7340): 296.

Boon, H. for the CSHP Alternative Medicine Task Force (2001) *Information Paper: The Role of the Pharmacist with Respect to Complementary/Alternative Medicine* (CSHP Official Publication 1999). Ottawa: Canadian Society of Hospital Pharmacists, pp. 181–6. Available at www.cshp.ca/productsServices/official Publications/index_e.asp (accessed 28 October 2008).

Bouldin, A.S., Smith, M.C., Garner, D.D. *et al.* (1999) Pharmacy and herbal medicine in the US. *Social Science and Medicine* 49: 279–89.

Brown, C.M. (1998) Use of alternative therapies and their impact on compliance: Perceptions of community. *Journal of the American Pharmacists Association* 38(5): 603–08.

Cardinale, V. (2000) How you and your patients can stay out of botanical trouble. *Drug Topics* 144(3): 70–72.

Chavis, L.M. (2001) Pharmacy-based consulting on dietary supplements. *Journal of the American Pharmacists Association* 41(2): 181–91.

Clauson, K., McQueen, C.E., Shields, K.M. and Bryant, P.J. (2003) Knowledge and attitudes of pharmacists in Missouri regarding natural products. *American Journal of Pharmaceutical Education* 67(2): 1–9.

Grauds, C. (2001) Clinical pharmacist talks to plants, too. *Alternative Therapies in Health and Medicine* 7(4): 19–20.

Harrison, A., Pablo, A. and Verhoef, M. (1999) The consumer's role in co-ordination: Making sense of transitions in health care. In A. Mark and S. Dopson (eds) *Organizational Behaviour in Health Care – the Research Agenda*. London: Macmillan, pp. 47–62.

Johne, A., Brockmöller, J., Bauer, S., Maurer, A., Langheinrich, M. and Roots, I. (1999) Pharmacokinetic interaction of digoxin with an herbal extract from St

John's wort (Hypericum perforatum). *Clinical Pharmacology and Therapeutics* 66(4): 338–45.

Jurgens, T. (2001) Who should be providing information to patients about herbal medicine? *Canadian Journal of Clinical Pharmacology* 8(4): 186–7.

Kattis, T. (1999) Alternative medicine and its impact on the pharmacy profession. *Canadian Pharmacists Journal/Revue des Pharmaciens du Canada* 132(3): 11, 7.

Kaufman, D.W. (2002) Recent patterns of medication use in the ambulatory adult population of the United States. The Slone Survey. *Journal of the American Medical Association* 287(3): 337–44.

Levy, S. (2000) What they're asking about herbs – and what you can tell them. *Drug Topics* 144(2): 42–4.

NAPRA Inter-Provincial Pharmacy Regulatory Committees (1999) *NAPRA Position Statements. Pharmacist's Responsibility in Providing Advice About or Selling Alternative Health Products.* www.napra.org/practic/information/response.html (accessed 21 February 2002).

Rowell, D.M. and Kroll, D.J. (1998) Complementary and alternative medicine education in United States pharmacy schools. *American Journal of Pharmaceutical Education* 62(4): 412–19.

Semaan, N. (2000) Integration of complementary disciplines into the oncology clinic. Part III. Herbal medicine. *Current Problems in Cancer* 24(4): 213–22.

Sturgess, R. (2002) Is it possible to move towards a consensus on homeopathy? *Pharmaceutical Journal* 269: 138.

Williamson, J.S. and Wyandt, C.M. (1999) The herbal generation: Trends, products, and pharmacy's role. *Drug Topics* 143(7): 69–78.

CHAPTER 17

Nostalgic and nostophobic referencing and the authentication of nurses' use of complementary therapies

PHILIP TOVEY AND JON ADAMS

Introduction

The recent expansion of interest in CAM within nursing should not be conflated with consensus and there is a clear line of thinking that is critical of CAM nursing integration (Giuffe, 1997). As a consequence, one important aspect of the current CAM nursing context is the pressure to advocate, legitimize or at least defend integration.

One issue of immediate interest is whether those centrally involved in CAM nursing are engaging in strategies to underpin and encourage mainstreaming, and, if they are, what form these strategies are taking. Any attempt to address this issue will necessitate awareness of the quite distinct historical, cultural and structural characteristics of nursing, and its occupation of a quite different space from medicine within orthodox provision (Allen, 2000).

Conceptual background

Nostalgia and nostophobia
Our work draws on the notion of nostalgic and nostophobic referencing. Nostalgic referencing can be defined as allusion to the past, grounded in a partial, contentious, arguably romanticized and necessarily constructed

Source: Tovey, P. and Adams, J. (2003) Nostalgic and nostophobic referencing and the authentication of nurses' use of complementary therapies. *Social Science and Medicine* 56(7): 1469–80. Abridged version reprinted with permission of Elsevier Ltd.

view of events; one that aims to legitimize current thoughts or actions of individuals and their world and includes the rediscovery or redeployment of all or some of a cited historical event or period. We can conceptualize nostophobic referencing as the mirror of this: a negative interpretation of past events or periods, applied to underpin its rejection or removal from future action in favour of an identified alternative that is in keeping with specific objectives.

Social worlds and rhetorics

The theory we employ here to interpret and frame the texts under analysis is based on a conceptualization of society as being made up of multiple social worlds, each of which is essentially inter-connected. Of importance here is the theoretical assertion of the inevitability of the fragmentation of these worlds into subworlds, and that such subworlds will be actively engaged in processes that are geared towards establishing worth and validity.

Crucial to such attempts to gain validity and worth are the rhetorics of worlds and their subworlds. Indeed, worlds are themselves constituted and reconstituted by rhetorical practices and have been conceptualized as 'universes of discourse' by earlier theorists (Shibutani, 1955). Examining the different worlds of health care draws attention to 'representational practices' and also highlights the inherently political dimension to these practices as groups attempt to gain epistemic authority, raise their market profile and attract or maintain financial resources for their world.

CAM nursing can appropriately be seen in these terms (Tovey and Adams, 2002), and rhetorics employed in such public presentations as the journal texts analysed here can be seen as constituting attempts by those within the subworld of CAM nursing to accrue validity and authentication for their 'new-found' practices and technologies.

Method

We conducted a text analysis of papers published in four nursing journals: *Complementary Therapies in Nursing and Midwifery, Journal of Advanced Nursing, Nursing Standard* and *Nursing Times* between 1995 and 2000 (for more details of method, see the original publication).

Results

The following data illustrate how a particular view of the past is called on by authors in their presentations of CAM nursing. This is evident both in relation to an interpretation of the 'true' meaning of nursing in a broad historical context, and in more precise references to defining moments and a 'golden age', specifically in relation to the pivotal figure of Florence Nightingale.

CAM and the historical 'reality' of nursing

The attempt to establish both that there is a general, deeply ingrained affinity between nursing (principles and practice) and CAM practice, and that an examination of the history of nursing practice lends support to this, are pivotal themes running through the papers analysed.

Caring in an increasingly rationalized world

Underpinning much of the discussion in the texts is a conceptualization of nursing as above all else an essentially human activity, concerned to promote those values that have become increasingly marginalized in an ever more rationalized environment of health care; one in which medicalized treatment regimes have dominated at the expense of human contact. The historical task of nursing is seen, within the texts, as something very different from this technical fix. There is a dual approach to historical referencing: a nostalgia for care-oriented, human-level practice, and a nostophobia about more recent institutional arrangements.

Many of the developments of recent history are an anathema to the presentations of appropriate practice offered in the texts. There are many references to the desirability of 'getting back' to a style of practice associated with an earlier period in nursing:

> For nurses in particular, incorporating a complementary therapy into their practice has allowed many to get back to what they see as real nursing, that is hands-on, individualised care.

Elsewhere, 'traditional' nursing practice is contrasted with that of CAM. Nostophobic referencing of an era dominated by restrictive hierarchical structures and professional relations is introduced to underline the practice-level impediments to integration within a 'traditional' structure.

> Nursing as a profession is nothing if not bound by hierarchy, and it may be difficult where a nurse is expected to be subservient to her supervisors or medical colleagues with her traditional nursing hat on, but wishes to take full responsibility as a holistic CAM practitioner with her CAM hat on.

Innovation and flexibility

Beyond these broad, essentially conceptual discussions of the place of CAM in the historical evolution of nursing, authors of texts drew out rather more practical dimensions of professional character and action, to support the authenticity of CAM in nursing. One example of this is the presentation of nursing as intrinsically innovative and flexible. The basis of the argument is that throughout history nursing has repeatedly incorporated techniques to extend the profession's boundaries. Given that change – be that the rediscovery of lost arts, the appropriation of new skills or whatever – is essential to the CAM nursing agenda, a partial or romanticized image of nursing on this issue clearly offers potential strategic benefit.

The presentations of nursing as flexible and innovative are also directly contrasted with interpretations of medicine as historically restrictive on, and controlling, nursing practice. Nurses' introduction of CAM is seen to provide a point of demarcation from medicine (Adams and Tovey, 2001). Thus, what is taken to be an essential element of nursing through the ages (innovation) facilitates the appropriation of CAM; this in turn provides the potential for success in 'the long struggle to establish epistemological demarcation from medicine' (Allen, 2000: 387) that has been the characteristic of nursing over recent years. In the following quotation, attention centres on the unequal power relations between the two professions that are seen to underlie the historical conflict between them:

> It is difficult for nurses to introduce complementary therapies into their practice without the permission of medical colleagues. This sort of dynamic is well documented in the literature and has frequently been the rock on which nursing innovations falter.

Once again, the nostophobic allusion to an era of medical dominance is grounded in a belief that such structures are not just contrary to the principles of CAM nursing, but are actively engaged in preventing its development. This dynamic – set within the historical relations between the two professions – is presented as an impediment not only to the utilization of CAM, but to the full expression of nursing innovation more broadly.

> Nurses, a largely female workforce, have been constrained by an imposed traditional view of healers as men that are, typically, medics or clerics. Any challenges will inevitably be met with a degree of scepticism, and on some cases, distrust.

Professional selflessness and the patient interest

Another feature of the image of nursing presented in the texts is of a profession historically shaped by a fundamental selflessness: a depiction of the profession's behaviour as being ultimately guided by client interests. The appropriation of the core rhetoric of client-centredness serves to reinforce the authentic character of the affinity between CAM and nursing.

> A fundamental tenet of nursing practice ... has always been to put the needs of the patient [first] ... the profession owes patients and their families the opportunity to utilise every resource available in order to accelerate the healing process.

CAM nursing as historical reality

In certain texts nurses themselves were presented as early pioneers of CAM. Here the suggestion is of nursing returning to a mode of holistic practice that has existed previously – at least within a section of the profession. In these terms CAM and nursing are historically bound as well as conceptually linked.

It is interesting that early moves towards the integration of certain healing therapies within healthcare was initiated by nurses ... perhaps we share more in common with our ancestors than we thought.

The use of massage by nurses is not a new phenomenon. In 1895 a small group of nurses employed as 'medical rubbers' in London hospitals formed the Society of Trained Masseurs.

CAM and Florence Nightingale: Appropriating the defining icon

Perhaps the single most interesting historical theme to be drawn from the texts is the use of Florence Nightingale both to underpin the conceptual affinity between nursing and CAM, and to provide a legitimacy to the case for ongoing incorporation. While the specific content of presentations varies, in each case a level of consistency is evident. We see constant reference to how CAMs' reliance on the 'natural' is matched by a similar emphasis by Nightingale. Now the potential for authentication is enhanced by being able to draw on the defining icon of nursing for evidence.

Certainly Nightingale's [definition of nursing], 'to put the patient in the best condition for nature to act upon him (sic)' is indication for the inclusion of complementary therapies into nursing care.

Many complementary therapies are based on the principle that disease is caused by an imbalance in a person's energy ... and that re-establishing a balance will help people heal themselves. Nightingale believed that the goal of nursing was to 'put the patient into the best condition for nature to act upon him (sic)', so nursing could be said to share many of the same values and beliefs as the complementary therapies that could be incorporated into nursing care.

In the reclaiming of Nightingale, CAM-oriented writers are providing a new take on a strategy previously employed by other nursing subgroups in professional debates surrounding nursing's role and identity (Duff, 1998; McDonald, 1998; Wheeler *et al.*, 1999). However, it is worth highlighting something of a contradiction (or at least a point of potential contestation) in the use of Nightingale. This use is occurring at a time when some within the profession are distancing themselves from her image in an attempt to assemble a culturally dynamic base to modern nursing (Hallam, 2000). Thus, while often presenting themselves as the forerunners of an innovative and daring expansion of nursing boundaries, on this dimension at least, CAM nursing may be seen to be operationalizing an inherent conservatism in its attempt to authenticate therapies.

Discussion

Our analysis illustrates the use of nostalgic and nostophobic references across a range of issues and in each case the interpretation of history fed a wider agenda: CAM integration. Now, if we acknowledge that nurses are using nostalgic and nostophobic referencing as strategies to authenticate the use of CAM, we are led on to the inevitable question of why.

To begin to make sense of this we need to acknowledge, and return to, two important features of context. The first is that the future character of nursing remains contested. Both externally, and crucially within nursing, there is debate about the nature of nursing, its responsibilities, its roles and, of course, the place of CAM within it. The second point relates closely to this. It is that the authors of the texts presented here should not be seen to represent nursing. In so far as they can be taken to represent any unified grouping, they can be combined as advocates of CAM/nursing integration. These CAM advocates occupy a subworld of nursing and in order for that subworld to be successful they need to engage in processes of persuasion. The nostalgic and nostophobic referencing examined here constitutes one crucial component of such attempts to persuade others within the nursing profession of the worth of CAM integration.

Further reading

Adams, J., Lui, C., Sibbritt, D., Broom, A., Wardle, J. and Homer, C. (2011) Attitudes and referral practices of maternity care professionals with regard to complementary and alternative medicine: An integrative review. *Journal of Advanced Nursing* 67(3): 472–83.

Adams, J. and Tovey, P. (eds) (2007) *Complementary and Alternative Medicine in Nursing and Midwifery: Towards a Critical Social Science*. London: Routledge.

References

Adams, J. and Tovey, P. (2001) Nurses' use of professional distancing in the appropriation of CAM. *Complementary Therapies in Medicine* 9(3): 136–40.

Allen, D. (2000) Doing occupational demarcation: The 'boundary-work' of nurse managers in a district general hospital. *Journal of Contemporary Ethnography* 29(3): 326–56.

Duff, E. (1998) Florence Nightingale: Basing care on evidence. *RCM Midwives Journal* 1(6): 192–3.

Giuffe, M. (1997) Science, bad science and pseudoscience. *Journal of Perianesthesia Nursing* 12(6): 434–8.

Hallam, J. (2000) *Nursing the Image: Media, Image and Professional Identity*. London: Routledge.

McDonald, L. (1998) Florence Nightingale: Passionate statistician. *Journal of Holistic Nursing* 16(2): 267–77.

Shibutani, T. (1955) Reference groups as perspectives. *American Journal of Sociology* 60: 562–8.

Tovey, P. and Adams, J. (2002) Towards a sociology of CAM and nursing. *Complementary Therapies in Nursing and Midwifery* 8: 12–16.

Wheeler, W., Spinks, M. and Attewell, A. (1999) Florence: Death of an icon? *Nursing Times* 95(19): 24–6.

Section 6

Integrative Medicine

Introduction

As Hsiao and colleagues outline (Chapter 18), integrative medicine can occur at a number of levels, ranging from the patient (whereby the integration of complementary and conventional medical paradigms does not necessarily require a collaboration or even meeting of different providers; for examples see Chapters 1 and 2) through to integration established and supported at a health policy or system level (as seen via the integration outlined in Chapters 12–14, for example). Furthermore, as Coulter (Chapter 30) and others have illuminated, the very definition of integrative medicine has been difficult to establish, with some preferring to refer to integrative health care, a term that does appear to accommodate more comfortably the full extent of integrative models as outlined by Hsiao and colleagues (Chapter 18), among others.

Much debate, commentary and research has evolved around the combination of conventional medicine and health care with elements of TCIM. Yet until recently, little investigation had explored the meaning and understanding of 'integrative medicine' from the perspective of providers themselves engaged in such combined practice. Hsiao and colleagues help address this important research gap in their empirical work presented in Chapter 18, showing that integrative medicine is a multidimensional construct on the 'shop floor' of practice and highlighting how clinicians' orientation towards integrative medicine may be an important factor to measure in evaluating crucial aspects of integrative medical care.

Any attempt to combine and integrate practices, techniques, practitioners and systems of knowledge from across the conventional/non-conventional border must inevitably face issues around power relations and the like. In Chapter 19, Fan and Holliday critically explore such issues and, with reference to a number of different forms of medical integration attempted in modern Chinese history, question the often implicit assumption that conventional medicine (modern scientific medicine, as they refer to it) should retain its principal dominant status in terms of deciding which medicine (conventional or traditional/complementary and alternative) should be emphasized and whose medical standard should be adopted.

As the attitudes and practice behaviours of conventional providers increasingly reflect an interest in and engagement with CAM (see Chapters 15–17), so the general education and teaching of these subjects become ever more central to debates regarding the content and philosophy of conventional medical education (and the education of other conventional provider groups such as pharmacy, as outlined in Chapter 16). Rakel and colleagues (Chapter 20) explore the inclusion of CAM education within conventional medical schools and how this allows a salutogenic focus to care. This focus on healing and prevention, as the authors argue, has pertinence to the wider task of addressing the epidemic rates of chronic disease related to poor lifestyle choices and, of equal significance, also constitutes an opportunity to train healthier and happier health care practitioners through encouraging self-care and reflection.

CHAPTER 18

Variations in provider conceptions of integrative medicine

AN-FU HSIAO, GERY RYAN, RONALD HAYS, IAN COULTER,
RONALD ANDERSEN AND NEIL WENGER

Introduction

Consumer demand and political pressure have contributed to recent interest in combining CAM and conventional medical paradigms, termed integrative medicine (Trachtman, 1994; Pelletier *et al.*, 1999). Integrative medicine can occur at six levels: consumer, health care provider, clinic, institution, professional/regulatory and health policy or system (Tataryn and Verhoef, 2001). We focus on integration at the provider level because providers play a pivotal role in the clinical encounter.

Patients commonly combine CAM modalities with conventional medical treatments outside the purview of their physicians and CAM providers, yet the clinical effect of such patient-initiated 'integrative medicine' may be hampered by the lack of provider supervision, may be unsafe (Fugh-Berman, 2000) and may result in poor quality of care due to poor coordination between clinician-initiated and patient-initiated therapies (Weeks, 1996). Therapeutic benefits may be most likely to emanate from skilled providers of divergent clinical paradigms treating an interested patient according to a shared, coherent conceptual framework (Bell *et al.*, 2002).

Yet it is unclear what 'integrative medicine' means to providers and to different provider groups. Different commentators have forwarded different views of integrative medicine: as replacing the biomedical paradigm (Weil, 2000); as constituting conventional medicine's 'co-optation' of CAM

Source: Hsiao, A., Ryan, G., Hays, R., Coulter, I., Andersen, R. and Wenger, N. (2006) Variations in provider conceptions of integrative medicine. *Social Science and Medicine* 62(12): 2973-87. Abridged version reprinted with permission of Elsevier Ltd.

(Coulter, 2004); or as a component of the patient-centred care movement. As such, the development of a conceptual framework of integrative medicine at the provider level is necessary to understand the practice, structure and quality of integrative medical care.

Methods

We employed a qualitative design, using the grounded theory approach (Glaser and Strauss, 1967) and conducted in-depth interviews with conventional and CAM practitioners. We chose acupuncturists, physicians, chiropractors and physician acupuncturists because they reflect the main types of providers who practise integrative medicine. We conducted interviews with 50 health care practitioners: 13 physicians, 13 physician acupuncturists (physicians who have also completed acupuncture training), 12 chiropractors and 12 acupuncturists (for more details of project design, see the original paper).

Results

Four key domains of integrative medicine emerged from our interviews: provider attitudes towards integrative medicine, knowledge of integrative medicine, referral to other practitioners and the practice of integrative medicine. These key dimensions and their respective subdomains represent how providers think about and practise CAM and conventional medicine and the merging of these two paradigms.

Provider attitude towards integrative medicine

Some practitioners expressed blanket faith in the value of conventional medicine and CAM, while others expressed blanket disbelief in these modalities. They also made statements approving or disapproving of integrative medicine as well as practitioner groups and broad types of treatment modalities. Respondents described four types of attitudes towards integrative medicine: practitioners' openness, philosophical scope, confidence in CAM and conventional medicine, and faith in integrative medicine. Each subdomain represents a spectrum with two opposing views: open-mindedness/close-mindedness, holism/reductionism, effectiveness/ineffectiveness, and faith/scepticism towards the integrative medicine paradigm. Although respondents within each provider group spanned the full range from approval to disapproval of integrative medicine, physician acupuncturist, chiropractor and acupuncturist provider groups were more likely to be open-minded, holistic and have faith in integrative medicine compared with the physician provider group.

Practitioners' openness

Openness refers to practitioners' ability to see the advantages of both CAM and conventional medicine from their own medical paradigms and the potential benefits of combining them. In contrast, some close-minded practitioners believed that medicine ought to be practised 'their way or no way at all.' They tended to stereotype practitioners who were outside their own medical paradigms.

Many respondents, however, felt that openness to both conventional and CAM paradigms was the key to successful integration. One physician described an ideal integrative practice setting as caring for patients as a series of 'case reports', where both physicians and CAM practitioners jointly discussed the 'strengths and weaknesses of the different healing modalities' in order to arrive at 'shared treatment plans and goals'.'

Philosophical scope

The interviews revealed holism as a central concept in integrative medicine. Traditional Chinese medicine and chiropractic both embrace the notion of holism. In the words of one chiropractor, who had practised for 20 years in the community:

> One key concept of integrative medicine is the understanding that a human being is more than his physical body … the whole human being contained physical, emotional, as well as spiritual dimensions.

Although some physicians also believed in the bio-psycho-social model of health, other physicians often dismissed the spiritual aspects of health as 'lacking scientific merits' and 'New Age hocus pocus'. One physician recalled her experience during gross anatomy class as follows:

> When you come to medical school, the first thing they give you is a dead body to dissect. So right off the bat, in medical school, they are telling you that the only thing that matters is the body and that the emotional or spiritual aspects are not important.

However, many physicians also consider their patient's emotional and social states when developing a treatment plan. Acupuncturists, chiropractors and physician acupuncturists in general were more likely to embrace holism than were physicians, and practitioners who were holistic were more likely to refer patients to CAM practitioners.

Confidence in CAM and conventional medicine

Confidence refers to practitioners' state of feeling certain about the effectiveness and safety of their own medical paradigm. Physicians tended to believe that practice should be based on scientific evidence. Some physicians believed that most CAM modalities failed the evidence-based standard and were 'no more effective than placebos', thereby undermining their confidence in integrative medicine.

Many physicians and physician-acupuncturists were reluctant to prescribe herbs and supplements because of concerns about their safety and quality. As one physician explained, 'I am reluctant to advise my patients to use herbs or supplements because I don't know what kind of stuff is in the bottles.'

On the other hand, many CAM practitioners strongly believed that their healing modalities and traditions are effective and safe because they have stood 'the test of time'; acupuncturist and chiropractor provider groups often lacked confidence in conventional medicine because of its 'high-tech' approach and severe side-effects. One acupuncturist explained:

> Most of my patients prefer to be treated with acupuncture, manipulation, or herbs because they believe that these treatments are natural and safer than Western drugs. These treatments are safe and effective because they have stood the test of time. Western medicine, on the other hand, has only been around about 50 years, since WWII.

Practitioners who held strong beliefs about their own medical traditions but acknowledged the limitations of these paradigms were more likely to endorse integrative medicine.

Faith in integrative medicine

Faith refers to the strength of a provider's convictions about integrative medicine. Since CAM and conventional treatments are based on different, contradictory theories and paradigms, some practitioners expressed scepticism about whether it would be possible to merge the two paradigms into a single, unified care plan. A physician acupuncturist explained why he predominantly chose traditional Chinese medicine over western medicine:

> I think integrative medicine can create quite a schism within the personality or practice style of the person if they're trying to practice Western medicine and Oriental medicine at the same time. For me, the way to deal with the schism was to practice what I believed in most.

On the other hand, some practitioners strongly believed that it was possible to 'harmonize' the biomedical and CAM paradigms into a single, unified paradigm. An example of such integration was found in a physician acupuncturist who believed that traditional Chinese medicine could be integrated successfully with western medicine. He viewed western medicine and traditional Chinese medicine as two different languages and himself as a 'bilingual' provider. He felt that integrative medicine was superior to conventional medicine or traditional Chinese medicine because he was able to 'take the best of both worlds and fuse them into a more powerful kind of medicine'.

Many physicians cited lack of knowledge and exposure as the reasons they were sceptical towards integrative medicine. Some chiropractors and acupuncturists also distrusted integrative medicine because they were afraid that CAM might be 'co-opted' by conventional medicine. This scepticism contributed to the lack of a shared understanding of the meaning of integrative medicine across provider groups.

Knowledge of integrative medicine: Knowledge proficiency
Practitioners and provider groups varied in their expectations of how much integrative medicine providers should know in order to blend conventional medicine successfully with CAM. Many practitioners believed that a 'fully integrative' practitioner ought to have 'complete knowledge of both conventional medicine and CAM'. In the words of one physician, a highly integrative provider ought to be 'a master' of both paradigms and 'be as good in either realm as the next best guy'. In contrast, a 'less integrative' practitioner was perceived as a 'dabbler', someone who did not practise integrative medicine on a regular basis and had a lower skill level compared with a fully integrative practitioner. Most practitioners agreed that someone who was unwilling to dedicate effort to learn about alternate medical paradigms would be less integrative.

Referral to other practitioners

Respondents viewed referral to other practitioners as a key component of integrative medicine. Referral behaviour was divided into two key elements: location and timeliness of referral.

Referrals to consultants in the same practice setting were classified as 'on-site' referrals, in contrast to referrals to consultants at other practice sites, classified as 'off-site' referrals. A key issue was whether providers referred outside their own medical paradigm, and if so, whether this was early or late in a patient's course. Referral outside one's own medical paradigm is defined as referrals from CAM practitioners to conventional practitioners and vice versa.

Referral location: On-site and off-site

For some providers, 'on-site' referral marked one end of the integrative/non-integrative conti- nuum. When asked the question 'What is an ideal setting for integrative medicine?', one physician replied that 'physicians and alternative practitioners would work together under one roof ... they would have ongoing back and forth knowledge about the different medical traditions. They would be constantly referring patients to each other.' Another advantage of making on-site referrals was sharing one common patient chart with other practitioners, which may 'open lines of communication' and 'promote collaboration' between CAM and conventional practitioners.

Nevertheless, few respondents worked in an 'integrative medicine' setting, where conventional and CAM practitioners share the same office and most respondents made off-site referrals. This was largely because few shared the same practice setting with practitioners of another paradigm.

Readiness to refer outside one's own medical paradigm

Practitioners consistently mentioned the importance of referring outside their own medical paradigm. Some practitioners 'had no qualms' and were 'faster' to refer out to other practitioners when patients were not getting better. Other practitioners would refer to outside practitioners only after exhausting all options within their own medical paradigm; there were still other practitioners who wanted to treat all their patients 'in-house' and refused to refer patients to practitioners outside their medical paradigm.

Chiropractors, in general, felt that they were better prepared to refer patients to practitioners outside their own medical paradigm compared with acupuncturists and physicians. This could be attributed to their education and training during chiropractic school, which emphasized the need for multidisciplinary care and the importance of teamwork. In contrast, many physicians would consider referring to acupuncturists and chiropractors only after exhausting all options within conventional medicine. They were described as 'stuck in one model of care' and were close-minded about other medical traditions. To enhance practitioners' readiness to refer, conventional and CAM practitioners agreed that they needed to develop 'strong working relationships' or 'connections' with each other. However, 'turf wars' and 'big egos' often limited referral and communication between CAM and conventional practitioners, which might drive patients to 'mix conventional and CAM treatments' outside the purview of their providers.

Practice of integrative medicine

The final aspect of integrative medicine was the ability to practise. Practice was defined as what practitioners could do or use to treat patients, including the following: prescriptions, ordering laboratory tests, surgery, manipulation, acupuncture, preventive services, co-management and treatment recommendation. Treatment using CAM and conventional healing modalities and co-management with practitioners outside one's own medical paradigm were critical parts of practice. Co-management often required the cooperation of both conventional and CAM practitioners to develop a unified treatment plan. Co-management differed from referral because practitioners communicated with each other to devise a coordinated care plan, whereas referral usually lacked the coordination component.

Treatment with both CAM and conventional healing modalities

Dual-trained practitioners were able to treat their patients with at least two healing modalities: one from conventional medicine and the other from CAM. Practitioners viewed someone who was able to provide both CAM and conventional treatments as more integrative than a practitioner who could provide only one type of treatment.

Practice setting appeared to play a role in determining whether a dual-trained practitioner used conventional or CAM treatment. One physician acupuncturist who worked in an academic medical centre explained, 'I frequently used Chinese herbs in my private practice. I don't use Chinese herbs in the inpatient setting because of my fear of being sued.' Practitioners were more likely to use conventional medicine when they were in a hospital setting, whereas they were more likely to use CAM or integrative medicine when they were in an outpatient setting.

Co-management with practitioners outside one's own medical paradigm

Practitioners who communicated and coordinated their patients' care with practitioners outside their medical paradigm defined their actions as co-management. Since many patients seek care from both physicians and CAM practitioners, co-management among practitioners was considered to be an important aspect of the practice of integrative medicine. One physician explained:

> I think an excellent integrative medicine practitioner would be a physician who actually had a working relationship with different types of practitioners outside of conventional medicine and who coordinated care between his patients and those practitioners. He would get letters back and forth about what was going on with his patients.

When asked to describe a 'fully integrative medicine model', many respondents emphasized the importance of physicians and CAM practitioners working together as a 'team' in order to develop a coordinated treatment plan for patients.

Many chiropractors and acupuncturists expressed willingness to co-manage patients with physicians, but found obstacles to this type of multidisciplinary care because physicians did not treat them as 'equal'. Many physicians pointed out the lack of a working relationship with acupuncturists and chiropractors as a barrier to co-management. They also felt that there were inadequate 'scientific data' to support the effectiveness and safety of integrative medicine treatments. Interestingly, one CAM practitioner noted that a large number of medical treatments in biomedical practice are also not based on randomized controlled trials.

Discussion

Our study shows that integrative medicine is a multidimensional construct, including provider attitudes, knowledge, referral and practice. The conceptual model explains the linkage between provider characteristics and provider behaviours, as mediated by provider attitudes and knowledge.

Variations of provider behaviours were linked to provider knowledge of alternate paradigms, which were strongly influenced by their education and postgraduate training. Most physician acupuncturists also viewed traditional Chinese medicine as 'complementary' to biomedicine, whereas most physicians viewed traditional Chinese medicine as 'alternative' to biomedicine.

The 'faith in integrative medicine' subdomain described the range of provider faith in developing a unifying paradigm of integrative medicine, spanning from disbelief to fully embracing integrative medicine. This debate over the feasibility of merging the biomedical and CAM paradigms is consistent with Kuhn's theory of scientific revolution, which postulated that two paradigms were 'incommensurable' if they are based on contradictory principles or dogma (Kuhn, 1962; Coulter, 1999). However, Boon and colleagues recognize this dilemma, and have proposed a conceptual framework of integrative health care at the system level, which represents one possible way to resolve the incompatibility between the biomedical and CAM paradigms (Boon *et al.*, 2004).

A limitation of our study pertains to the sampling frame. Participants represented a purposive sample recruited from a particular geographical region, thereby limiting the external validity of our results. Another limitation is the exclusion of other practitioners of integrative medicine, such as naturopaths and massage therapists, and of medical specialists, such as anaesthesiologists. Additional interviews with these providers may uncover new domains of integrative medicine at the provider level. Future studies should evaluate how well our conceptual model fits these provider groups.

We believe that this is the first attempt to develop a conceptual model of integrative medicine at the provider level. We used a qualitative, grounded approach to uncover key domains of integrative medicine, thereby elucidating how different providers view and practise integrative medicine. Since provider groups varied in their conceptualizations of integrative medicine, clinicians' orientation towards integrative medicine may be an important factor to measure in evaluating the effectiveness, safety and quality of integrative medical care.

Further reading

Hollenberg, D. (2006) Uncharted ground: Patterns of professional interaction among complementary/alternative and biomedical practitioners in integrative health care settings. *Social Science and Medicine* 62(3): 731–44.

References

Bell, I.R., Caspi, O., Schwartz, G.E. (2002) Integrative medicine and systemic outcomes research. *Archives of Internal Medicine* 162: 133–40.

Boon, H., Verhoef, M., O'Hara, D. and Findlay, B. (2004) From parallel practice to integrative health care: A conceptual framework. *BMC Health Services Research* 4: 15–19.

Coulter, A. (1999) The new Cedars-Sinai alternative medicine clinic. Expansion of health care for the community. *Journal of Alternative & Complementary Medicine* 5(2): 93–8.

Coulter, I. (2004) Integration and paradigm clash. In P. Tovey, G. Easthope and J. Adams (eds) *The Mainstreaming of Complementary and Alternative Medicine: Studies in Social Context.* London: Routledge, pp. 103–22.

Fugh-Berman, A. (2000) Herb–drug interactions. *Lancet* 355: 134–8.

Glaser, B. and Strauss, A. (1967) *The Discovery of Grounded Theory: Strategies for Qualitative Research.* Chicago: Aldine.

Kuhn, T. (1962) *The Structure of Scientific Revolutions.* Chicago: University of Chicago Press.

Pelletier, K., Astin, J. and Haskell, W. (1999) Current trends in the integration and reimbursement of CAM by managed care organizations and insurance providers: 1998 update and cohort analysis. *American Journal of Health Promotion* 14(2): 125–33.

Tataryn, D. and Verhoef, M. (2001) Combining conventional and complementary and alternative health care. *Perspectives on Complementary and Alternative Health Care.* Toronto: Health Canada.

Trachtman, P. (1994) NIH looks at the implausible and the inexplicable. *Smithsonian* 25: 110–23.

Weeks, J. (1996) Operational issues in incorporating complementary and alternative therapies and providers in benefits plans and managed care organizations. *Complementary and Alternative Medicine: Issues Impacting Coverage Decisions.* Tucson, AZ: US NIH Office of Alternative Medicine, US Agency for Health Care Policy and Research, Arizona Prevention Center.

Weil, A. (2000) The significance of integrative medicine for the future of medical education. *American Journal of Medicine* 108: 441–3.

CHAPTER 19

Which medicine? Whose standard? Critical reflections on medical integration in China

RUIPING FAN AND IAN HOLLIDAY

Introduction

There is a prevailing conviction that if traditional medicine (TM) or complementary and alternative medicine (CAM) are integrated into health care systems, modern scientific medicine (MSM) should retain its principal status. In this chapter, we contend that this position is misguided in medical contexts where TM is established and remains vibrant. Attention is not here directed to TM as it has developed among the Han people of China. This form of TM roughly constitutes what most in the West identify as 'Chinese medicine', which has been explored elsewhere (Fan, 2003; Holliday 2003).

Against those who take the dominance of MSM for granted, we argue that in order to develop an appropriate integrative system for MSM and TM, it is first necessary to explore two fundamental questions. Which medicine should be emphasized? Whose medical standard should be adopted?

These fundamental questions have not been seriously addressed. The dominant position is implicit in World Health Organization (WHO) documents that promote the claims of TM within an integrative system. WHO states that '[i]n an integrative system, TM/CAM is officially recognised and incorporated into all areas of healthcare provision' (WHO, 2002). However, 'officially recognised and incorporated' is a vague requirement, implying an open-ended spectrum. At one extreme, there is presumably considerable state support for research and education in TM practices, and TM therapies are widely available from hospitals and clinics. At the other extreme, TM may have no more than

Source: Fan, R. and Holliday, I. (2007) Whose medicine? Whose standard? Critical reflections on medical integration in China. *Journal of Medical Ethics* 33: 454-61. Abridged version reprinted with permission of BMJ Publishing Group.

a limited presence, even though it is indeed present in 'all areas': research, education, clinical practice and pharmacy. In such a case, incorporation of TM into a so-called integrative system is no more than token, which is clearly problematic.

The question of 'whose standard' is even more fundamental. Every medicine embodies a medical standard in the form of a set of professionally and popularly approved norms, rules and mechanisms by which specific diagnostic, therapeutic and pharmaceutical practices are validated for use in health care settings. Evidently, there are as many different and incommensurable medical standards as there are various and incommensurable medical traditions. In order to set up an integrative system, such as for TM and MSM, government therefore needs to formulate a policy regarding the medical standard that is to be adopted for selecting, operating and regulating integrative practice. In principle, there are several possibilities: TM standard based, MSM standard based, dual standard based (whereby TM and MSM operate independently according to their own standards) and new standard based (whereby a new standard is framed out of mixed TM and MSM standards). Which of these possible standards should inform the integration of TM and MSM?

This chapter explores these issues by reflecting on the special case of China. In particular, it focuses on three formally autonomous regions in the north and west: Inner Mongolia, Tibet and Xinjiang. The chapter concludes that the proper integrative system for TRM and MSM is a dual-standard-based form in which both TM and MSM are free to operate according to their own medical standards.

From marginalization to fusion

It is clear that MSM is now stressed in the integrative systems of Inner Mongolia, Xinjiang and Tibet, although TM is active in the ordinary medical practice undertaken in clinics or by individual practitioners in villages and small towns. In all areas, MSM has been given priority over TM, and TM has been pushed virtually to the margins of the health care system. Moreover, in addition to its small size, TM faces an identity crisis in each region: TM is evaluated in the Weberian sense as 'disenchanted' and reformed according to the MSM standard. It is therefore increasingly difficult for each TM to stand independently, free from the intervention and amendments of MSM designed to change its substance. These tendencies are driving not only the marginalization of TM, but also a fusion of TM into MSM.

In education, TM colleges have invested greater amounts of time and resources into teaching MSM and related modern scientific theories and technologies, rather than focusing on TM classics and techniques. Traditional practitioners are now required to know a great deal of modern medicine, although the reverse is not the case. In research, TM researchers tend to choose more 'scientific' topics for their research projects, and graduate students prefer more 'scientific' scholars as their supervisors. In the pharmaceutical sector, for instance, research projects are designed and conducted under the direction of modern scientific theories to discover effective chemical ingredients from traditional drugs and prescriptions. In clinical practice, reforming TM has been the dominant attitude of health care administrators, who implicitly or often explicitly value MSM over TM. TM hospitals have equipped themselves with advanced modern western diagnostic and therapeutic facilities in order to 'scientificize' themselves and compete with MSM hospitals.

TM physicians in such TM hospitals usually administer 'double diagnosis' and 'double therapy' in their practice. For every patient they make two diagnoses: one according to TM explanations and another according to MSM theories. As a result, although MSM physicians only conduct MSM therapy, TM physicians take double therapy for granted. This practice has strengthened the popular impression that, for most medical problems, MSM should do the main work, although TM may offer some minor, complementary assistance.

In evaluation and regulation, the scientific standard of MSM is used to evaluate every aspect of TM. In addressing TM, the government has emphaszsed 'scientificization' (*kexuehua*), created through 'scientific' research, 'scientific' explanations and the 'scientific' reorganization of TM. Such policies have caused enormous difficulties for TM physicians, especially young physicians applying for promotion, in practising TM in official medical institutions. They often find themselves facing a review committee consisting mainly of MSM experts. These experts are either unable or unwilling to evaluate TM physicians solely according to TM standards. Moreover, TM physicians are afraid that if they are subject to a malpractice lawsuit, the assessment norms will primarily be drawn from MSM. This has induced them to adopt more MSM than TM in their practice.

The ideology of science

What has caused the asymmetry between the popularity of folk TM practices and the institutional marginalization (or fusion into MSM) of TM? The answer lies primarily in the ideology of science that has been adopted by the Chinese authorities to evaluate all forms of medicine. This ideology can be condensed into the following argument: the more scientific, the more effective (premise 1); MSM is more scientific than TM (premise 2); therefore, (a) MSM is more effective than TM; and (b) in the integrative system of TM and MSM, TM should be improved according to the MSM standard so as to become more scientific and therefore more effective.

Logically, we could block the two conclusions by rejecting premise 2. For instance, some Chinese have tried through coining a special understanding of science to contend that TM is as scientific as MSM, or even more scientific than MSM. However, this strategy is nothing more than quarrelling about the conventional modern understanding of science. Like it or not, the modern sense of science is now solidly established, with a series of arranged empirical knowledge and rules regarding observation, evidence and inference. They have been widely adopted and manifested in the core disciplines of modern science, such as physics, chemistry and biology. Because this sense of science has been broadly accepted in modern China, challenging premise 2 is equivalent to offering a new definition of science, which is at best missing the point of the issue being debated.

Alternatively, we could block the two conclusions by rejecting premise 1, which is indeed what this chapter intends to do. We believe that premise 1 cannot stand. Moreover, because it is the crux of the scientific ideology that has directed the shaping of inappropriate integrative systems in the three regions, it must be rejected in order to return the major indigenous medicines to their proper places. Before explaining how and why we refute premise 1, a particular issue generated by conclusion (b) will be addressed in the next section.

Improving traditional medicine: Whose standard?

Conclusion (b) states that TM should be improved according to the MSM standard so as to become more scientific and thereby more effective. The issue is, is it possible to improve TM according to the MSM standard without changing the nature of TM? We hold that the answer depends on which of two different types of improvement is made to TM.

The first type is an MSM standard that inspires or suggests a reform or revision of a particular TM measure or practice, while allowing the reform or revision to be accredited by the TM standard. One example is the use of modern technologies and facilities to manufacture TM drugs in more efficient ways. In this sense, a medical system does learn and can benefit from the methods of a different medical system, and can gain improvement according to its own standard, even though distinct medical systems operate on parallel lines defined by their unique theoretical underpinnings. This reveals the complexity of mutual medical learning. In theory, it is difficult, indeed largely impossible. In practice, however, it can be helpful for physicians to draw insights and borrow measures from more than one tradition. The crucial point is that the newly learnt measure should be incorporated into its own system of medical standard.

The second type occurs when MSM therapies and strategies are forced on TM, but cannot be accredited by the TM standard. A typical example is attempting to find and abstract effective chemical ingredients from TM prescriptions in order to make MSM medications. Because such an activity is also incommensurable with basic TM theories and principles regarding prescriptions and medications, it cannot be accredited by the TM standard.

Although it is legitimate for MSM to conduct such activities in order to develop its pharmaceutical industry, the medications thus produced are indeed

MSM drugs, not TM drugs. Hence, instead of seeing such activities as successful 'improvements' of TM, they should be seen as MSM activities in nature.

Comparing effectiveness: Whose standard?

If premise 1 holds, the dominant position of MSM in the integrative systems of the three regions is warranted. Unless it can be challenged, the fate of TM in these regions will inevitably be doomed.

Is it true that the more scientific a medical measure, the more effective it is? In particular, is it true that MSM is more effective than TM? In order to disclose an end hidden behind a medical judgement that a particular treatment is effective, it is necessary to ask the question 'effective for what?' Although distinct medical traditions share the same formal goals of preserving health, preventing disease and treating illness, this formal goal is useless in comparing the effectiveness of different medical traditions. Different medical traditions have developed different substantive goals expressed in their various, incompatible understandings of health, disease and illness. That is, they do not understand health, illness and disease in similar (mutually commensurable) ways.

Distinct medical traditions have set up different goals and expectations based on their unique, underpinning religions and philosophies. Their different conceptual frameworks lead to different empirical systems, expressed in particular values and goals and in distinct rules of evidence and inference, which may overlap but never coincide with one another. To demonstrate this point in a concrete manner, we turn to Tibetan medicine, which holds different and incommensurable substantive goals (manifested in its views of prevention, treatment and pharmacy) from those of MSM.

Incompatible goals

The substantive goals of Tibetan medicine contrast sharply with those sought by MSM. Tibetan medicine holds that the Tantric Buddhist principle of the essence aspect is involved in all creatures and operated and identified through the 'Wisdom Mind'. This belief significantly directs and shapes the specific Tibetan medical goals. In prevention, the goal includes avoiding karma (negative actions), discharging physical desires smoothly, and seeking the proper union of man and woman in sexual ways. In treatment, the goal involves fulfilling complete therapy by pursuing fundamental rather than mere mundane treatment. In pharmacy, the goal covers enhancing the effect of medication through Tantric rituals. Seeking these specific goals leads to a comprehensive positive ideal of health in the Tibetan Buddhist way of life. As a result, Tibetan medicine contains a system of end–means structures that is entirely alien to and incommensurable with that of MSM. Accordingly, when

MSM physicians see some Tibetan medical interventions as ineffective, they may simply make the judgement in terms of the substantive ends of MSM, while being ignorant of the particular goals that Tibetan medicine pursues.

For instance, if one claims that the Tibetan medical attempt to improve the humour disturbance of a terminally ill patient by examining his family member's 'family pulse' is less effective than MSM palliative care, one must overlook the fact that a goal of Tibetan medicine is to offer fundamental treatment regarding the patient's essence aspect, which is closely related to the essence aspect of his family members. This is to say, given that Tibetan medicine does not hold the same set of substantive medical ends or goals as MSM, it is not possible to state that MSM is more effective than Tibetan medicine, or vice versa. As substantive medical goals indicate concrete values that a medicine is pursuing through certain mechanisms and means, then unless we can judge that the substantive goals of MSM are more appropriate than those of TM in promoting health, preventing disease and curing illness in the formal sense, we cannot claim that MSM is more effective than TM. Comparing TM and MSM is ultimately comparing their incompatible substantive medical goals.

Can we tease out a set of 'neutral' substantive goals for evaluating MSM and TM? Some may want to argue that indices such as life expectancy, morbidity and mortality rates in general, and infant and maternity mortality rates in particular, plus emergency rescue success rates and other indices, can be used as neutral standards to compare the effectiveness of MSM and TM. That is, they may contend that both MSM and TM should accept these indices as fair criteria to evaluate their respective medical practices, even if they hold incompatible substantive medical goals. However, the difficulties with such a 'neutral' standard strategy are multiple. First, many factors other than medicine contribute to the variation of these indices. An effective medicine is at best a necessary, but not sufficient, condition for good scores on these indices. Second, there is the issue of discrepancy between theory and practice. Supposing that medicine P is in theory more effective than medicine Q means that, all other things being equal, a set number of doctors using P will generate better indices than the same number of doctors using Q. However, the reality may well be that doctors using Q do more effective work than doctors using P because the latter have not received such good training and proper regulation as the former, even though their medicine is theoretically superior (indeed, this was the complaint of many TM physicians in the three regions during our investigation). Third, the values manifested in these indices may not be evenly promoted by each medicine. Today, many people believe that TM is better than MSM in promoting long-term health and thereby increasing average life expectancy, whereas MSM is better than TM in critical care, especially for the very elderly. Supposing that this belief is true, judging which medicine is more effective will depend on which index is taken to be more important: average life expectancy or critical care.

The values manifested in these indices cannot always be pursued consistently with other human values involved in medical practice. For instance, all three TM systems have developed useful knowledge and skills in aiding birth at home, fitting well into the local religious beliefs in favour of home delivery. It may be the case that no matter how perfect such home delivery techniques become, home delivery will still involve slightly higher rates of infant and maternity morbidity and mortality than delivery at a well-resourced MSM hospital. However, in this case, the effectiveness of a medicine can no longer be judged only in terms of the 'neutral' values of the indices. If people take it to be fundamentally important to deliver at home (for they may want to hold a religious ritual that can only proceed at home, in addition to cherishing the mother's psychological comfort in the company of her family members in a familiar environment), the most effective medicine will be the one that can offer most assistance at home rather than in hospital.

Conclusion

Different forms of medical integration have been attempted in modern Chinese history: TM standard based, MSM standard based and new standard based. The Chinese have broadly recognized the failure of the TM standard-based integration (primarily in the nineteenth century) and the defect of the new standard-based integration (primarily in the mid-twentieth century). If this chapter's argument is sound, then the currently dominant MSM standard-based integration is also indefensible. Regions with vibrant established TM systems (such as Tibet, Inner Mongolia and Xinjiang) should change to a dual-standard-based system whereby TM and MSM operate independently according to their own standards (Fan, 2003).

To be fair, the Chinese authorities have made efforts to preserve the indigenous medical sectors in the medical institutions of all three regions. They are staffed by highly skilled practitioners, and overseen by deeply committed and able officials in the State Administration of Traditional Chinese Medicine and its regional and local offices. However, the ideology of science is all pervasive and thus disenchants practitioners of TM. MSM is simply too dominant and TM is in retreat. In order to reframe proper integrative systems in these regions, greater attention needs to be paid to ensuring that modern and traditional medicines are able to function on different but equal bases. As each is founded on unique conceptual underpinnings carrying particular values and goals and distinct empirical rules, it becomes difficult to hold that a single measure could ever be found to evaluate competing traditions. In this domain, as in so many others, there is no universal standard, and a positivistic search for the 'evidence-based high ground' is likely to be counterproductive (Richardson, 2002). The choice, then, is either to arrange medical traditions in a hierarchy and distribute status privileges among them, or to set them on equal bases. We know of no good argument for building a hierarchy, and can think of many valid reasons why setting medical traditions on an equal footing should be the approach taken (Holliday, 2003).

Further reading

Adams, J., Hollenberg, D., Lui, C. and Broom, A. (2009) Contextualising integration: A critical social science approach to integrative health care. *Journal of Manipulative and Physiological Therapeutics* 32(9): 792–8.

References

Fan, R. (2003) Modern western science as a standard for traditional chinese medicine: A critical appraisal. *Journal of Law, Medicine and Ethics* 31: 213–21.

Holliday, I. (2003) Traditional medicines in modern societies: An exploration of integrationist options through East Asian experience. *Journal of Medicine and Philosophy* 28: 373–89.

Richardson, J. (2002) Evidence-based complementary medicine: Rigor, relevance, and the swampy lowlands. *Journal of Alternative and Complementary Medicine* 8: 221–3.

World Health Organization (2002) *WHO Traditional Medicine Strategy 2002–2005*. Geneva: World Health Organization.

CHAPTER 20

Complementary and alternative medicine education: Promoting a salutogenic focus in health care

DAVID RAKEL, MARY GUERRERA, BRIAN BAYLES, GAUTAM DESAI AND EMILY FERRARA

Introduction

Complementary and alternative medicine: The evolution of medical education

Complementary and alternative medicine (CAM) education in conventional medical schools has evolved since the US National Institutes of Health (NIH) began awarding R-25 CAM education Project Grants in 2000 to encourage curriculum development in this field. The momentum of change continues to define the field as we realize the importance of bringing a stronger emphasis on healing into our health care delivery system. Complementary and alternative medical education has led to a better understanding of the importance of teaching students about the dynamic, multidimensional process of how the body heals (Snyderman and Weil, 2002).

Many of the areas taught in a CAM curriculum address fundamental ingredients of health and healing such as nutrition, mind–body influences and spiritual connection (Kligler *et al.*, 2004). The curriculum recognizes the importance of both physical and non-physical, internal and external influences. Education in CAM has triggered a deeper understanding of what is needed to shift our health

Source: Rakel, D., Guerrera, M., Bayles, B., Desai, G. and Ferrara, E. (2008) Complementary and alternative medicine education: Promoting a salutogenic focus in health care. *Journal of Alternative and Complementary Medicine* 14(1): 87–93. Abridged version reprinted with kind permission of Mary Ann Liebert, Inc.

care delivery model towards a better balance of facilitating health and treating disease. Investing in health and healing-oriented education will enhance health care delivery by reducing health care costs (Sarnat and Winterstein, 2004); creating insight into the process of healing; and improving satisfaction and well-being in the next generation of health care practitioners (Ball and Bax, 2002).

Education focused on salutogenesis

The term salutogenesis (*salud* [Spanish], *salute* [Italian]: health, genesis: creation of) is making a resurgence in health literature. It emphasizes training health professionals in healing-oriented care in order to improve quality, particularly in a primary health care system. If we are to prepare students to provide health-oriented care in a culture with epidemic rates of chronic disease related to poor lifestyle choices, it is imperative that health education include a core understanding of healing and prevention.

Balancing salutogenesis and pathogenesis

Pathogenesis (pathos: suffer, genesis: creation of) has been at the forefront of medical education. Students learn about how and why the body develops disease, its causes and how to treat them. CAM education is helping to develop a better understanding of how the body develops health, its influences and how to reproduce them. This salutogenic process requires an investment in educating health care professionals to be as skilled in facilitating health as in treating disease. The purpose of healing-oriented education is to improve health care by developing competencies that transcend the dichotomies between CAM and conventional medicine.

Methods

A survey of CAM educational leaders at institutions awarded grants for incorporating CAM education into medical curricula was performed to address how CAM education can improve health care delivery in America (for details of methods, see the original publication).

Results and discussion

Themes to support salutogenic education and improved health care delivery

Five core themes were noted to be successful in achieving this goal. These included education on the importance of relationship-centred care; understanding holism; the promotion of self-reflection and self-care; collaboration with CAM providers to enhance communication; and the need for faculty development in CAM.

Investing in relationship-centred care

Our survey highlights the importance of relationship in the facilitation of health. Educating health care professionals about CAM is an essential component towards a broader movement that will enhance patient-centred and relationship-centred models of care, which will improve health outcomes, adherence and efficiency (Stewart *et al.*, 2000). Relationship-centred care can reduce the need for medical tests and referrals (Stewart *et al.*, 2000) and nurture a patient's comfort at expressing emotions, resulting in increased optimism and positive therapeutic expectations (Branch *et al.*, 2001). The ability of a clinician to develop rapport and trust with a patient appears to be a vital characteristic of an effective healer regardless of the therapeutic tool (Moerman and Jonas, 2002).

People seek health care relationships that will provide a 'participatory experience of empowerment and authenticity when illness threatens their sense of intactness' (Kaptchuk and Eisenberg, 1998). Our present health care system, with long waiting times, brief impersonal visits and lack of continuity, is not meeting this need. Many CAM practitioners are more effective in this regard, and the conventional US health care system can improve by engaging in active dialogue and collaboration with them.

Human relationships give the clinician insight and understanding into an individual's unique interaction with her/his environment that may have multiple biopsychosocial and spiritual influences. Investing in education to stress the importance of this holistic influence has the potential to improve diagnostic accuracy, efficiency and cost of care (Starfield, 1991; Epstein *et al.*, 2005).

Understanding holism

Engel described the importance of the biopsychosocial model in the 1970s (Novack, 2003) and its importance in medical education is well established (Benbasset *et al.*, 2003). This concept, however, has been overshadowed by the massive explosion of technology and the success of disease-focused care. Public interest in CAM has been attributed to the field's attention to the unique aspects of individuals within their biopsychosocial environment (Astin *et al.*, 2006). The public sees CAM as more individualized compared to allopathic medicine (Barrett *et al.*, 2003). Ten people with low-back pain who live in the same neighbourhood and go to the same church will have ten different belief systems, emotions and definitions of what gives their lives meaning and purpose. Developing an understanding of 'what type of person has the disease compared to what disease a person has' will better prepare for teaching healing-oriented medicine (Bryan, 1997). Holism validates the power that non-physical influences have on disease. It also engenders respect and enables practitioners to care competently for patients from widely different cultural backgrounds and belief systems than their own, because they will learn the unique ways in which each patient defines health and thus what healing practices may be personally acceptable.

Only focusing on the physical causes of a symptom rewards interventions that are often very costly and still may not work. Teaching students the importance of recognizing how emotions can influence a physical process (such as pain) will improve the efficiency and cost of health care delivery (Price *et al.*, 2005). This can only be completely understood by considering the patient's entire biopsychosocial and spiritual environment.

Promotion of self-reflection and self-care

Self-reflection leads to a greater sense of self-awareness defined as the ability to attend, in a non-judgemental way, to one's own physical and mental processes during ordinary everyday tasks in order to act with clarity and insight (Epstein, 1999). This allows the individual to see things as they truly are so that beliefs are not inappropriately projected. These are key ingredients in facilitating health and developing cultural competency. In order to do this for patients, students have to start by understanding how to do this for themselves.

A study of nine US medical schools showed that 47 per cent of 1964 students interviewed had at least one mental health or substance-related health issue. The majority linked their subjective distress and physical health needs to training and school-related stress (Roberts *et al.*, 2001). Many NCCAM education programmes have used various CAM modalities to encourage self-care. These include reflective diary keeping, mindfulness stress reduction, defining healing through the humanities, guided imagery and encouraging the student to define their own sense of spirituality. Physicians who are most likely to practise healthy lifestyle habits are also more likely to encourage their patients to do the same (Frank *et al.*, 2000).

Collaborating with CAM practitioners to enhance communication

Once the student is taught the importance of developing accurate insight into what the patient may require to facilitate health, there is often a need to collaborate with other health care practitioners. The health care team that is utilized to stimulate healing may be very different from the one used to diagnose and treat disease. A salutogenic approach requires the services of those skilled in areas such as counselling, manipulation, energetics, nutrition and spiritual connection.

Our survey of the NCCAM educational programmes stressed the importance of not only learning about CAM therapies but also collaborating with CAM practitioners. As students become familiar with CAM therapies, they will understand how relationship-centred care may direct them towards understanding the most appropriate therapy. If students are not aware of CAM therapies, they will not enquire about or recommend them (Wynia *et al.*, 1999).

A team-based approach may decrease adverse events when compared to a fragmented approach. In fact, fragmentation of care is reduced as patients and CAM practitioners share information regarding CAM therapies with conventional practitioners (Astin, 1998).

Faculty development

A major challenge in CAM education in medical schools is the limited number of faculty who have knowledge, understanding and awareness of these therapeutic concepts. If curricula during the first two years of medical school are not actualized by faculty mentors during clinical rotations, it is seen as unimportant and irrelevant to standard care. NCCAM educational programmes found it necessary to invest in faculty development for sustainable change for their educational endeavours. Success involves attracting interested faculty and providing education that influences future medical practice while maintaining involvement through programmes that promote faculty leadership (Rakel and Rindfleisch, 2004).

One way of incorporating faculty development in CAM is to weave it into existing courses that value and allot time to such activities. For example, many schools have clinical medicine courses in the first and second years where behaviour change and lifestyle modifications are emphasized. Some schools involved in NCCAM grants successfully conducted mind–body–medicine faculty development sessions by linking both didactic and experiential components to these course objectives.

Conclusions: Potential benefits of salutogenic education

Providing more efficient health care with reduced cost

In a disease-focused health care model, the economy benefits when more therapies are prescribed. The majority of costs in health care are a result of hospital care, physician services and prescription drugs. Since the 1980s, prescription drug costs have doubled, reflecting an increasing reliance on pharmaceutical technology (NCHS, 2005). More attention is given to treating or suppressing symptoms than to exploring their root cause.

Having a primary medical infrastructure based on continuity and relationship-centred care has been found to improve quality of health care (Starfield, 1991), reduce hospital admissions (Gill and Mainous, 1998), reduce expenditure on diagnostic testing (Epstein *et al.*, 2005) and lower total health care costs (De Maeseneer *et al.*, 2003). This cost saving comes, in part, from the attention given to the internal, non-physical influences on health that are often addressed in CAM. These include helping patients feel understood by exploring their needs and expectations, addressing psychosocial issues and expanding the patient's involvement and understanding in their health (empowerment) (Mead and Bower, 2000; Epstein *et al.*, 2005). If the importance of healing-oriented education is not stressed, medical costs will continue to escalate as dependence on the most expensive aspects of care, pharmaceuticals, physician visits and diagnostic tests continues to rise.

Training healthier and happier health care practitioners

In a medical culture that is often filled with belittlement associated with poor mental health and career satisfaction (Frank *et al.*, 2006), there is a tremendous opportunity to combine scientific competence and student health successfully. The key is through the process of self-care and reflection. The result will be professionals who are more empathetic and caring while simultaneously nurturing a reconnection to the values that attracted them to the field. This self-reflective process is the least developed in medical education and also offers the most potential for training happier and healthier professionals. CAM education has pointed to exploring ways in which innovative curricula may address this need.

Further reading

Perlman, A. and Stagnaro-Green, A. (2010) Developing a complementary, alternative, and integrative medicine course: One medical school's experience. *Journal of Alternative and Complementary Medicine* 16(5): 601–05.

Weil, A. (2000) The significance of integrative medicine for the future of medical education. *American Journal of Medicine* 108: 441–3.

References

Astin, J.A. (1998) Why patients use alternative medicine: Results of a national study. *Journal of the American Medical Association* 279: 1548–53.

Astin, J.A., Soeken, K., Sierpina, V.S. and Clarridge, B.R. (2006) Barriers to the integration of psychosocial factors in medicine: Results of a national survey of physicians. *Journal of the American Board of Family Medicine* 19: 557–65.

Ball, S. and Bax, A. (2002) Self-care in medical education: Effectiveness of health-habits interventions for first-year medical students. *Academic Medicine* 77: 911–17.

Barrett, B., Marchand, L., Scheder, J., *et al.* (2003) Themes of holism, empowerment, access, and legitimacy define complementary, alternative, and integrative medicine in relation to conventional biomedicine. *Journal of Alternative and Complementary Medicine* 9: 937–47.

Benbassat, J., Baumal, R., Borkan, J.M. and Ber, R. (2003) Overcoming barriers to teaching the behavioral and social sciences to medical students. *Academic Medicine* 78: 372–80.

Branch, W.T., Jr, Kern, D., Haidet, P. *et al.* (2001) The patient–physician relationship: Teaching the human dimensions of care in clinical settings. *Journal of the American Medical Association* 286: 1067–74.

Bryan, C.S. (1997) *Osler: Inspirations from a Great Physician.* New York: Oxford University Press.

De Maeseneer, J.M., De Prins, L., Gosset, C. and Heyerick, J. (2003) Provider continuity in family medicine: Does it make a difference for total health care costs? *Annals of Family Medicine* 1: 144–8.

Epstein, R.M. (1999) Mindful practice. *Journal of the American Medcial Assoication* 282: 833–9.

Epstein, R.M., Franks, P., Shields, C.G. *et al.* (2005) Patient-centered communication and diagnostic testing. *Annals of Family Medicine* 3: 415–421.

Frank, E., Carrera, J.S., Stratton, T. *et al.* (2006) Experiences of belittlement and harassment and their correlates among medical students in the United States: Longitudinal survey. *British Medical Journal* 333: 682.

Frank, E., Rothenberg, R., Lewis, C. and Belodoff, B.F. (2000) Correlates of physicians' prevention-related practices: Findings from the women physicians' health study. *Archives of Family Medicine* 9: 359–67.

Gill, J.M. and Mainous, A.G. (1998) The role of provider continuity in preventing hospitalizations. *Archives of Family Medicine* 7: 352–7.

Kaptchuk, T.J. and Eisenberg, D.M. (1998) The persuasive appeal of alternative medicine. *Annals of Internal Medicine* 129: 1061–5.

Kligler, B., Maizes, V., Schachter, S. *et al.* (2004) Core competencies in integrative medicine for medical school curricula: A proposal. *Academic Medicine* 79: 521–31.

Mead, N. and Bower, P. (2000) Patient-centredness: A conceptual framework and review of the empirical literature. *Social Science and Medicine* 51: 1087–110.

Moerman, D.E. and Jonas, W.B. (2002) Deconstructing the placebo effect and finding the meaning response. *Annals of Internal Medicine* 136(6): 471–6.

National Center for Health Statistics (2005) *Health, United States, 2005: With Chartbook on Trends in the Health of Americans.* Hyattsville, MD: Centers for Disease Control and Prevention. Available at www.cdc.govJnchsJhus.htm (accessed November 26, 2006).

Novack, D.H. (2003) Realizing Engel's vision: Psychosomatic medicine and the education of physician-healers. *Psychosomatic Medicine* 65: 925–30.

Price, C., Arden, N., Coglan, L. and Rogers, P. (2005) Cost-effectiveness and safety of epidural steroids in the management of sciatica. *Health Technology Assessment* 9: 1–58.

Rakel, D. and Rindfleisch, A. (2004) Optimal healers: Igniting the spark and fanning the flame. Training academic medical faculty in optimal healing. *Journal of Alternative and Complementary Medicine* 10(1): S113–S120.

Roberts, L.W., Warner, T.D., Lyketsos, C. *et al.* (2001) Perceptions of academic vulnerability associated with personal illness: A study of 1,027 students at nine medical schools. Collaborative research group on medical student health. *Comprehensive Psychiatry* 42:1–15.

Sarnat, R.L. and Winterstein, J. (2004) Clinical and cost outcomes of an integrative medicine IPA. *Journal of Manipulative Physiology and Therapeutics* 27: 336–47.

Snyderman, R. and Weil, A.T. (2002) Integrative medicine: Bringing medicine back to its roots. *Archives of Internal Medicine* 162: 395–7.

Starfield, B. (1991) Primary care and health. A cross-national comparison. *Journal of the American Medical Association* 266: 2268–71.

Stewart, M., Brown, J.B., Donner, A. *et al.* (2000) The impact of patient-centered care on outcomes. *Journal of Family Practice* 49: 796–804.

Wynia, M.K., Eisenberg, D.M. and Wilson, I.B. (1999) Physician–patient communication about complementary and alternative medical therapies: A survey of physicians caring for patients with human immunodeficiency virus infection. *Journal of Alternative and Complementary Medicine* 5: 447–56.

PART C

Knowledge production, research design and perspectives

SECTION 7 Evidence, safety and regulation   185

SECTION 8 Traditional, complementary and integrative
          medicine in perspective   229

SECTION 9 Future agendas: Key debates and themes   255

Evidence, safety and regulation

Introduction

The field of TCIM research and practice has long been subject to demands from others located outside its perimeters (and also from some within its borders) to produce an evidence base and it is no surprise that many commentators and researchers have examined the role, relevance and relationship between evidence-based medicine [EBM] (as a movement within modern health care and evaluation) and TCIM. In Chapter 21 Barry rehearses this examination, but does so in a somewhat thought-provoking fashion, providing a contrast between the biomedical and anthropological approaches to the role of evidence in CAM. Barry attempts to raise questions about the suitability of the EBM approach (and the gold standard randomized controlled trial therein) for gathering evidence on CAM. She suggests a role for social scientists in contributing to raising consciousness of this issue and in offering alternative models of evidence such as anthropological evidence, which she argues is much more closely aligned to the knowledge system of non-biomedically trained CAM practitioners.

Starting from a similar premise to Barry in as much as they also acknowledge that there is an apparent 'gap' between the results of randomized controlled trials showing little or no effect and the widespread use and reports of beneficial outcomes of CAM treatments, Fonnebo and colleagues nevertheless embark on a different scholarly journey in response to this dilemma (Chapter 22). Exploring the strengths and weaknesses of conventional biomedical research strategies and methods as applied to CAM, the authors suggest a new research framework for assessing and building a rigorous evidence base for these treatment modalities – one that does not contain new methodological elements but instead reorganizes existing elements in a way tailored to pragmatic clinical practice and ultimately challenges the conventional research paradigm in this area and beyond. Returning briefly to the more direct relationship between the EBM movement (and evidence-based practice [EBP]) and CAM, Coulter (Chapter 23) draws on his insider experience and perspective of doing research in an evidence-based CAM centre to reflect on some of the methodological challenges involved in establishing such a project.

Often accompanying calls for evidence of CAM effectiveness are references to the potential risks of traditional and complementary medicine practice, especially with regard to integrated patient use alongside conventional treatments and the subsequent possible dangers of polypharmacy. These are issues made ever more significant given the challenges facing patient–clinician communication (and specifically the issue of non-disclosure) relating to CAM use (see Chapter 15 for more details). However, the consideration and discussion of safety and risk around CAM have remained limited to issues of direct risk, including adverse events and the monitoring of these events. In response, Wardle and Adams (Chapter 24) outline a novel approach focusing on the inherent indirect risks associated with these medicines, fitting within the development of a mature public health agenda for CAM and broadening the debate in this area of study.

Addressing the challenges of the indirect risks associated with CAM requires policy and research attention in the area that is commensurate with the contemporary use of CAM, including among other things a need to develop minimum standards of training and appropriate levels of regulation in relation to these medicines. Taking up this lead and providing context of a related but different nature, Weir closes this section by outlining a detailed examination of the liberalization of the regulatory structure of CAM and exploring the implications for consumers and relevant professions, both conventional and otherwise.

CHAPTER 21

The role of evidence in alternative medicine: Contrasting biomedical and anthropological approaches

CHRISTINE BARRY

Introduction

Concurrent with the rise in alternative and integrated medicine, there has been a movement towards increasing reliance on science-based research to judge the effectiveness of treatments, otherwise known as evidence-based medicine (EBM). In this chapter, I focus on the UK context in discussing debates connecting the EBM movement with alternative medicine. I then go on to investigate the different notions of evidence produced in anthropological research on alternative medicine.

I wish to problematize the call from within biomedicine for more evidence of alternative medicine's effectiveness via the medium of the randomized clinical trial (RCT). This call originates in part from the motive of ensuring that alternative medicine 'works' before providing it in a publicly funded service. However, this call is also, in part, political and relates to the agenda of controlling the threat posed by alternative medicine to the long-standing hegemony of biomedicine in the West. I highlight possible omissions and biases inherent in the RCT method, not always visible to its supporters. RCTs usually omit the measurement of important elements of 'what works' in alternative medicine, which often acts in a different way to biomedical drugs. By presenting ethnographic evidence, I show how evidence, when seen from the perspectives

Source: Barry, C. (2006) The role of evidence in alternative medicine: Contrasting biomedical and anthropological approaches. *Social Science and Medicine* 62: 2646–57. Abridged version reprinted with kind permission of Elsevier Ltd.

of the users and practitioners of alternative medicine, hinges on a very different notion of therapeutic efficacy.

Integrating alternatives into the NHS: The role of the RCT

In Britain the CAM integration debates have been most vocal from within the medical establishment, albeit at the fringes. In a medical system currently dominated by discourses of EBM, the integration debate has centred on the pivotal issues of regulating CAM professions and producing evidence to prove that such therapies merit inclusion in the NHS. Evidence in this CAM context is conceived of as therapeutic efficacy for biomedically diagnosed disorders, within the individual body (or body part), and as measurable utilizing science-based research strategies, most notably the randomized controlled trial. These assumptions reflect a biomedical orientation towards 'health care technologies' (such terminology itself denotes a separation of treatments from the people they treat, the people providing them and the settings in which they are provided).

RCTs carried out on alternative therapies necessarily entail reducing the complexity of the intervention to fit the reductionist nature of the RCT method. As a result, the therapeutic intervention as tested in RCTs is in most cases quite different to the interventions used by alternative practitioners in everyday clinic situations.

Evidence-based epistemology can in itself have transformative effects on alternative therapies. Villanueva-Russell's (2004) sociological case study shows how the development of clinical guidelines has influenced some practices within chiropractic. She suggests that such guidelines are at odds with the approach and work of purist chiropractors, whom she calls 'straights', who follow a vision of vitalism, seeing their work as aiming to ensure a free flow of innate intelligence through the body. The guidelines were skewed in favour of the agenda of the adulterated practice of medicalised chiropractors – the 'mixers' – who have divorced the epistemological foundations from the mechanistic practice of manipulation. This research demonstrates how scientifically constructed 'evidence' for an alternative therapy only works when the therapy has mutated into a medicalized version and divested itself of its alternative philosophy.

Rhetorics of evidence in biomedicine

I do not wish to discredit the notion of the RCT. In its purest ideological form, the concept of offering patients only therapeutic interventions that have been proven to work is unquestionably sensible and morally correct. Where the problems arise is the imperfection of the RCT tool as an arbiter of what works, because it measures the wrong things or the wrong populations. The real-world clinical context is different to the trial laboratory. The RCT can sometimes become a victim of hubris. Just being the 'gold standard' is not enough – it is still an imperfect tool. Even the most elegantly designed trial with statistically beneficial sample sizes and clever protocols for blinding usually measures only a subset of symptoms and therapeutic effects (those that are short term and easiest to measure). The production of scientific evidence is a social as well as a scientific process. There is no such thing as The Evidence, just competing bodies of evidence.

As part of a broader cultural movement towards the audit culture (Maguire *et al.*, 2001), 'evidence' has become an increasingly strong rhetoric in biomedicine. This is not without criticism from both within and without. There are, for example, ongoing extensive debates about EBM among biomedical practitioners. One explanation for its rise is that the NHS is becoming an increasingly managerial system. Greenhalgh (1999) argues that EBM is driven by those with managerial rather than clinical backgrounds. Overt rationing of health care services through the use of committees such as NHS trusts and the National Institute for Clinical Excellence (NICE) requires decisions about resource allocation to be based on evidence of efficacy and cost-effectiveness of treatments. The optimum evidence for this task is the 'gold standard' of the RCT, or preferably the Systematic Review of a number of RCTs, which has come to be positioned at the top of the evidence hierarchy (Lohr *et al.*, 1998).

Wolpe (2002) raises the paradox that many of the most powerful phenomena in orthodox medicine – the placebo effect, psychosomatic illness and spontaneous remission, which can account for large percentages of healing rates – get very little research attention. Mythological, ritualized and culturally embedded aspects of all healing systems, biomedicine included, can in themselves possess great healing potential. Orthodox medicine can be blind to such aspects of its own praxis in its claim to scientific legitimacy, and these elements are not studied in the RCT. Yet it is often these very aspects that attract patients to CAM. The rhetoric of evidence as encapsulated in the RCT represents only one, albeit powerful, formulation of evidence in biomedicine. What effect has this powerful evidence-based rhetoric had in the world of alternative medicine?

Evidence and alternative medicine

Alternative medicine in the past has shown little interest in producing RCT evidence. Its proponents are less embedded within a science-based epistemology, there is no money available, and there has been an awareness of the limitations of such methodology for studying complex individualized treatments (Long *et al.*, 2000). However, increasing integration requires alternative therapists to start to play the 'evidence' game. Alternative practitioners who take up research projects often want to use research for political ends, to validate therapies and to improve access by getting alternatives accepted in NHS settings. Most administrative units that hold budgets and allocate resources in primary care will not provide alternative medicine services to their constituency unless the proposer supports their request with RCT evidence.

Some biomedical researchers involved in the production of trials wish to quash the rise of alternative medicine, and RCT evidence can be used as a tool to discredit it and bar it from the NHS. RCT data are being used to limit the activities of non-medical complementary therapists.

In alternative models of healing, effectiveness is often constructed very differently. In homeopathy, short-term cures are only seen as appropriate to acute and minor illnesses. Homeopathy views treatment for chronic and serious illnesses extending over long timescales. The very publication of trials can act as a reformulation of the very nature of a therapy, generally in the direction of medicalization. Where homeopathy has been tested on a biomedically diagnosed disorder – rhinitis, for example (Schapowal, 2002) – it suggests to the readers that homeopathy can be used in a biomedicalized way, for medical conditions across a population of sufferers, ignoring the mental, spiritual and relational picture in favour of physical symptoms.

In a lay homeopathy clinic, I observed patients with rhinitis symptoms being prescribed very different remedies. One patient's nasal drip was accompanied by feelings of fear and distress about a recent mugging, unresolved grief from her parents' death and a metallic taste. Another patient with nasal drip reported menstrual problems, relationship issues and feelings of unexpressed anger. In the Schapowal (2002) trial, both would have been given the same remedy, Butterbur, yet neither was prescribed this remedy.

In homeopathy training, students are told that if a remedy does not match the total symptom picture, it is an inert substance. For a remedy to be active, the 'similimum', it has to have the most similar symptom picture to that of the patient. Under this logic, many of the prescriptions of Butterbur in the trial would have been inert and useless, in spite of the shared biomedical diagnosis of rhinitis.

After conducting an RCT, Elaine Weatherly Jones, a non-medical homeopath, reported a 'change of heart' on the usefulness of this method for researching such an individualized form of therapy (Weatherly Jones, 2004). Unusually, she interviewed the trial practitioners, who reported that the blinding procedure interfered with their normal practice routines, to produce a radically different version of their normal therapeutic practice.

The nature of evidence in anthropology

Although any one system of medicine covers a broad and varied range of practices and philosophies, contextualized accounts of practices and processes in specific circumstances are notably lacking in most forms of research. RCT research and survey research, for example, do not tend to investigate the detailed context in which health care was provided.

Just as the scientific laboratory method and the nature of population statistics have shaped the nature of RCT evidence, so too does anthropological method influence what constitutes evidence. Ethnographic research is conducted in everyday real-life settings and so can pay attention to the all-important contextual features of interaction.

Reality is seen as ever changing through a series of processes, formed by interactions and relationships between people, and always affected by the context in which social actions take place. The method utilizes an observer situated in the context, not researching from afar. The focus of research is neither wholly predetermined nor tightly structured. This allows for research to uncover issues of importance to participants that may have been ignored in the literature. Shifting the focus to the perspective of the actors involved, and seeking the native point of view, not mirroring the prior concerns of the academic community, can produce powerful new interpretations (O'Connor, 2002).

Ethnographic research recognizes that it is the interaction between a specific patient and their specific health care practitioner that needs to be looked at, as a system, and so would look at what happens in the actual interactions between them. Embodied and inter-subjective data are acceptable evidence in anthropology. Ethnographers pay attention to how people feel in their bodies and how they relate to each other. Action is analysed over long timescales; fieldwork extends for months, sometimes years. The anthropologist's main tool is her/himself. Thus the collection of evidence is not through randomization and standardization, but via personal, individual ways of knowing. This incorporates the utilization of the anthropologist's emotions, intuitions, relations with others and their own bodily responses (Turner, 2000). It also requires the anthropologist to account for their presence in the research through reflexivity, paying attention to the impact they have on the production and interpretation of data (Davies, 1999; Barry 2002a, b).

What works from homeopathy users' perspectives?

In an ethnography of homeopathy in South London I researched inside clinics (a homeopathic general practice, and a lay homeopath's low-cost clinic) and settings in the community: women's homes, educational classes and a support group (Barry, 2003). I observed the same people over two years and gained a processual view of engagement with homeopathy. I also incorporated my embodied experiences by attending homeopathic clinics as a patient and homeopathy classes as a student.

My research showed that a therapy's effectiveness, from the perspective of therapists and patients, was embedded in the development, over time, of a whole new set of beliefs about health, illness and the body, and about the nature of the healing process. For committed users, health is an ongoing inter-dependency with the social, physical and spiritual, and illness is an active and positive part of health. The healing process starts with health not sickness, and the body does the healing naturally. Ultimately, homeopathy helps, pharma-ceuticals hinder, and the user has primary responsibility for health care. The development of this new belief system about health was seen in itself as evidence of the power of homeopathy for many users (Barry, 2003).

Committed users and lay homeopaths shared notions of efficacy that involved evaluating (over much longer timescales) their health as embedded within and inseparable from a network of emotions and connectivity with others. The therapy was judged to be successful in many cases through perceived changes in family relations. One user judged the fact that her husband sought counselling for his depression as evidence for the effectiveness of her own homeopathic treatment. Homeopathy helped her come to terms with difficulties in adjusting to her second pregnancy and this, in turn, had linked effects of changing the communication between her and her partner, leading to a whole sequence of behavioural changes in the family. She explained this as working through quite physical responses (such as nausea) to remedies. She did not separate out physical and emotional effects. Her home-opath accepted this, unquestioningly, as matter-of-fact evidence of homeo-pathic therapeutic effect.

Gaining spiritual meaning through resonance with the homeopathic philos-ophy of treating mind, body and spirit was of particular importance to people who were struggling with transitions in their lives: divorce, bereavement or first experience of parenthood. Many of the women in the study who had had difficult experiences with orthodox medicine, often during pregnancy and childbirth, saw one aspect of the effectiveness of homeopathy as a way of being more in control of their own health care.

In evaluating the evidence for the success of these therapies, committed users stressed the importance of the individual relationship between their specific homeopath and themselves. They also drew on observations of their children's speedy and sometimes miraculous symptom response to remedies, or their own longer-term changes, as evidence that the homeopathy was work-ing. Evidence for them was the evidence of their own eyes and embodied experiences. Not that they ever used words such as 'evidence' or 'efficacy'. Users of homeopathy did not see a need for scientific testing and were happy with their own judgement of whether the treatment was working for them. Any existence of RCT proof that the remedy was efficacious was never sought. The science of biomedicine was perceived as old-fashioned and rejected in favour of the quantum and chaos theories of modern physics. Several referred to Capra's (1976) book on parallels between eastern mysticism and quantum physics as a rationale for favouring a more modern notion of scientific enquiry about healing.

Those who felt that homeopathy did not work for them tended to be those who remained tightly allied to biomedical notions of health and illness and did not change their views of the body. As a result of this view, they often were not compliant with homeopathic remedies. Interestingly, these were the only people who referred to scientific RCT evidence during the whole study, with a tendency to idolize science-based medicine. Laura, for example, declaimed: 'I believe that medicine is the most wonderful thing really. I think it is a God-given thing.' In spite of six months of homeopathy at a victim support clinic after she was mugged, she never came to believe in homeopathy and justified her continued attendance only because she felt it was like counselling.

Each of these pieces of ethnographic research contributes to a different notion of evidence in alternative medicine. Each produces a different answer to the question: 'Does it work?' The work of anthropologists has come much closer to investigating the power of alternative medicine as it is viewed by those who use it. What 'works' for alternative medicine users and their thera-pists does not just include relief from physical symptoms. It also includes changes in beliefs about health, healing and disease; the gaining of meaning for the illness experience in the context of the life story; bodily experiences and changed view of body-self; transcendent, transformational and spiritual heal-ing experiences; changed identity; and a powerful dialectical relationship with the therapist. None of these aspects of therapeutic effectiveness is measured within existing clinical trial research. While there are calls to include quality-of-life measures in RCT research more generally, such measures still do not incorporate any of the above.

Conclusion

Non-biomedically trained alternative practitioners have a knowledge system that is closer to that of anthropology than to science-based medicine; it is more grounded in the phenomenal world of everyday lived and embodied experience. In their view, the evidence needed is that which investigates not whether a therapy is working according to biomedical and scientific criteria, but whether it is making a difference to the bodies, beliefs, social and cultural experiences of its clients and whether patients keep coming back.

These two perspectives on evidence, the biomedical focus and the anthro-pological focus, are to some extent worlds apart. The goal of this chapter has been to attempt to raise questions about the suitability of the EBM approach, in spite of the power it holds in medical discourse. Social scientists can contribute to raising consciousness of this issue and offer alternative models of evidence such as the anthropological research presented here.

As the research community in alternative medicine has developed in recent years, it is beginning to ask questions of this nature, and qualitative and ethnographic research provides a powerful tool in this enterprise. Ethnographic research in alternative medicine is coming to be used politically as a challenge to the hegemony of a scientific biomedical construction of evidence. The introduction of ethnographic forms of evidence that represent the grounded experience of users and therapists of alternative medicine communities act as a critique of biomedical notions of evidence. Thus anthropological evidence can be used to open a debate about what one should be measuring as evidence of alternative medicine efficacy, and whether one should be measuring it at all.

Further reading

Dew, K. (2012) Evidence-based health care and complementary and alternative medicine. In A. Broom and J. Adams (eds) *Evidence-Based Health Care in Context: Critical Social Science Perspectives*. London: Ashgate.

Hansen, K. and Kappel, K. (2010) The proper role of evidence in complementary/ alternative medicine. *Journal of Philosophy and Medicine* 35(1): 7–18.

Keshet, Y. (2009) The untenable boundaries of biomedical knowledge: Epistemologies and rhetoric strategies in the debate over evaluating complementary and alternative medicine. *Health: The Interdisciplinary Journal for the Social Study of Health, Illness and Medicine* 13(2): 131–55.

References

Barry, C.A. (2002a) Multiple realities in a study of medical consultations. *Qualitative Health Research* 12(8): 1052–70.

Barry, C.A. (2002b) Identity and fieldwork: Studying homeopathy and Tai Chi 'at home' in South London. *Anthropology Matters* May (available at http://www.anthropologymatters.com/journal/2002/barry2002_identity.htm, accessed 17 January 2012).

Barry, C. (2003) The body, health, and healing in alternative and integrated medicine: An ethnography of homeopathy in South London. Unpublished PhD thesis, Brunel University.

Capra, F. (1976) *The Tao of Physics*. London: Fontana.

Davies, C.A. (1999) *Reflexive Ethnography: A Guide to Researching Selves and Others*. London: Routledge.

Greenhalgh, T. (1999) Narrative based medicine in an evidence based world. *British Medical Journal* 318: 323–25.

Lohr, K., Eleazer, K. and Mauskopf, J. (1998) Health policy issues and applications for evidence-based medicine and clinical practice guidelines. *Health Policy* 46: 1–19.

Long, A.F., Mercer, G. and Hughes, K. (2000) Developing a tool to measure holistic practice: A missing dimension in outcome measurement within complementary therapies. *Complementary Therapies in Medicine* 8: 26–31.

Maguire, M., Shore, C. and Wright, S. (2001) Comment: Audit culture and anthropology. *Journal of the Royal Anthropological Institute* 7(4): 759–63.

O'Connor, B. (2002) Personal experience, popular epistemology, and complementary and alternative medicine research. In D. Callahan (ed.) *The Role of Complementary and Alternative Medicine: Accommodating Pluralism.* Washington DC: Georgetown University Press, pp. 54–73.

Schapowal, A. (2002) Randomised controlled trial of butterbur and cetirizine for treating seasonal allergic rhinitis. *British Medical Journal* 324(7330): 144–8.

Turner, A. (2000) Embodied ethnography: Doing culture. *Social Anthropology* 8(1): 51–60.

Villanueva-Russell, Y. (2004) Evidence-based medicine and its implications for the profession of chiropractic. *Social Science and Medicine* 60(3): 545–61.

Weatherly Jones, E. (2004) Challenging the placebo controlled, double-blind trial. A change of heart after running trials of individualised homeopathy. Poster presented at 1st ACHRN conference: Diversity & Debate in Alternative and Complementary Medicine, Nottingham, July.

Wolpe, P.R. (2002) Medical culture and CAM culture: Science and ritual in the academic medical centre. In D. Callahan (ed.) *The Role of Complementary and Alternative Medicine: Accommodating Pluralism.* Washington DC: Georgetown University Press, pp. 163–71.

CHAPTER 22

Researching complementary and alternative treatments: The gatekeepers are not at home

VINJAR FØNNEBØ, SAMELINE GRIMSGAARD, HARALD WALACH, CHERYL RITENBAUGH, ARNE NORHEIM, HUGH MACPHERSON, GEORGE LEWITH, LAILA LAUNSØ, MARY KOITHAN, TORKEL FALKENBERG, HEATHER BOON AND MIKEL AICKIN

Introduction

Many physicians do not understand why large segments of their patients use CAM when research generally has failed to provide decisive evidence of efficacy. Patients seem to make these treatment choices based on the qualities of the provider, desire for 'individualized' treatments, and their perception of overall effectiveness rather than efficacy (Wilkinson *et al.*, 2002; Boon *et al.*, 2003; Schonekaes *et al.*, 2003).

There is apparently a 'gap' between the results of randomized controlled trials (RCT) showing little or no effect and the widespread use and reports of beneficial outcomes of CAM treatment (Launsø and Gannik, 2000; Fønnebø and Launsø, 2005). If we were to assume that patients are not completely misguided, then we would need to look closely at the research strategies utilized in the CAM field and try to understand the reasons for the gap.

The purpose of this chapter is therefore to explore the strengths and weaknesses of conventional biomedical research strategies and methods as applied

Source: Fonnebo, V., Grimsgaard, S., Walach, H. *et al.* (2007) Researching complementary and alternative treatments – the gatekeepers are not at home. *BMC Medical Research Methodology* 7: 7; S. Abridged version reprinted with permission of BioMed Central Ltd.

to CAM, and suggest a new research framework for assessing these treatment modalities.

Discussion

Gatekeeping and regulating CAM intervention use

A majority of CAM research to date has used the research strategy employed and developed by clinical pharmacologists to document, in a prescribed sequential pattern, the quality, dose, safety, efficacy and eventual effectiveness of a drug prior to its general release. In this model, governmental regulatory offices act as gatekeepers. Health insurers only reimburse for drugs meeting the appropriate criteria. An important principle in this model is that research determines which drugs are approved for generalized clinical use and are paid for by health insurers.

Previously, CAM researchers have largely assumed that these same pharmacological research methods and regulatory-reimbursement models can be followed in the evaluation of CAM. Much to the frustration of many clinical researchers, the availability of CAM treatments that are affordable with little or no reimbursement, however, does not seem to be amenable to the same rules as those we seek to apply to conventional medicine. Even if studies show that a CAM treatment has no effect, it does not necessarily disappear from the marketplace. We suggest that this is because the CAM market has had no statutory body (gatekeeper) that ensured the quality, safety, efficacy and effectiveness of CAM treatments before they appear on the 'market'. Furthermore, since few health insurers reimburse for CAM treatments, there are few financial gatekeepers. Millions of patients in developed countries have experienced the effect of CAM treatments provided in contrast to, or more likely in addition to, the care they have received in conventional medicine (Norheim and Fonnebo, 2000; Guthlin *et al.*, 2004; Hamre *et al.*, 2004; Steinsbekk and Ludtke, 2005; Witt *et al.*, 2005). The situation is therefore characterized by widespread patient experience of treatment outcomes combined with little research and no regulatory or financial gatekeeping activity.

Why is a different research strategy needed?

Research in conventional medicine therefore focuses on choosing the best tools for health professionals to use. These tools include drugs, diagnostic methods and surgical procedures, and employ a methodology often resulting in a one-size-fits-all therapeutic prescription. Conventional research may, however, have overlooked that the clinical effect of most therapies is overestimated when studied under optimal circumstances on susceptible, cooperative patients. Despite this, the randomized controlled trial is an important method when making decisions about tools to include in the toolbox of conventional medicine.

Because 'conventional' researchers have done most of the CAM research, it is not surprising that CAM research has travelled down the same path as conventional medicine. It has tested the specific efficacy of what conventional researchers believe to be the active components of a therapy, often discounting synergistic effects. In addition to providing a predominantly individualistic treatment approach, many CAM therapists hold that CAM treatments cannot be split up into parts that can be investigated separately. They argue that the total effect adds up to more than the sum of the parts.

If CAM is to be evaluated comprehensively, one needs to extend the research focus to all aspects of the treatment approach (Ritenbaugh *et al.*, 2003). To study only the specific effect of needling in acupuncture isolated from other interventions initiated by the acupuncturist, or the effect of a single, isolated homeopathic remedy separated from other aspects of homeopathic practice, is to neglect other potentially important components of these interventions (Lewith *et al.*, 2002; Wittman and Walach, 2002; Jonas, 2005; Paterson and Dieppe, 2005). Furthermore, clinical research teams should only venture into this area with a thorough contextual and philosophical understanding of the CAM treatment paradigm and its clinical use. Plunging into studies of efficacy that involve isolated detailed components of a treatment approach without thoroughly understanding its context is destined to failure and irrelevance, no matter what the results show. These issues point to the need for a different, and more complex, research strategy for the CAM field.

A suggested research strategy

The most important unique characteristics of CAM are the absence of gatekeepers and the complexity of individually tailored treatments. Our proposed strategy does not contain new methodological elements, but organizes existing elements in a way that is tailored to pragmatic clinical practice (see Figure 22.1 for more details). The strategy is not meant as a strictly chronological sequence defining when specific research phases should occur, but as a framework to guide CAM research, illustrating the necessary building blocks for a rigorous evidence base.

Phase 1: Context, paradigms, philosophical understanding and utilization (What is going on?)
The cornerstone of the suggested research strategy is to understand the process and assumptions within a particular therapy, often using an inductive research approach (Launso, 1999, 2000; Thomas *et al.*, 2001; Hanssen *et al.*, 2005; Launso and Rieper, 2005). Researchers need to understand what the treatment procedure is, how many variations there are, what philosophical foundations underlie it, its ideas about health and disease, its contextual

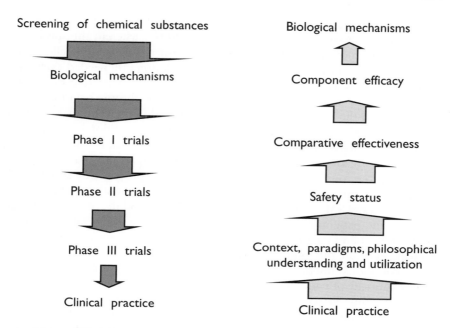

Screening of chemical substances

Biological mechanisms

Phase I trials

Phase II trials

Phase III trials

Clinical practice

Biological mechanisms

Component efficacy

Comparative effectiveness

Safety status

Context, paradigms, philosophical understanding and utilization

Clinical practice

Figure 22.1 Research strategies in drug trials and CAM (proposed). Phases that contrast the proposed phased research strategy in CAM (dark arrows) with that conventionally used in drug trials (light arrows).

framework and key treatment components. They also need to know how many and what segments of the patient population use it, and for what conditions.

Phase 2: Safety status (Is it safe?)

Safety issues are important in the treatment of any illness, but in the area of CAM they cannot be emphasized strongly enough. The inherent risks of the diseases or illnesses for which patients seek CAM are generally low. The treatments given should therefore carry a low risk of adverse effects. CAM treatments have often been claimed to be without risk, but adverse effects in CAM are more than occasional case reports (Norheim and Fonnebo, 1995). The methods of choice to study safety would be similar to the detection of adverse events associated with pharmaceutical treatments. The field of acupuncture has provided a thorough and rigorous risk assessment (Norheim and Fonnebo, 1995; Norheim, 1996; MacPherson *et al.*, 2001, 2004) based on these principles and the other fields within CAM need to follow suit (Thompson *et al.*, 2004; Endrizzi *et al.*, 2005; MacPherson and Liu, 2005).

Phase 3: Comparative effectiveness (What is the system effectiveness?)

Patients are seeking CAM as a treatment system. Research needs to examine the outcomes of these treatments both in combination with, and as alternative to, conventional care. Thus randomized, controlled pragmatic trials are needed (Hammerschlag, 1998; MacPherson, 2004), wherein the specifics of the system are not disassembled, but the system under study is allowed to function as it is clinically practised, including the urgently needed evaluation of cost-effectiveness (Thomas *et al.*, 2005). The pragmatic trial design has been used in the study of acupuncture treatment of chronic pain (Vickers *et al.*, 2004) and the methodology is also widely used in conventional medicine (Beresford *et al.*, 2006). In these trials, patients are randomly assigned to treatment alternatives, which may include alternative viable whole systems, conventional treatment or no treatment. The trials may also evaluate whole-system interventions that are implemented under protocols that specify individualized treatments based on specific patient characteristics, following the patterns of care found in the community. While blinding of the treatment providers and patients/subjects with regard to treatment allocation is usually not feasible, blinding of the outcomes evaluators can ensure an unbiased comparison of the outcome assessment.

It is considered unethical to include non-efficacious treatments in the real-world treatment of patients. Patients are, however, already using CAM treatments, and thus effectiveness studies can be employed to guide decisions about the necessity of studying the efficacy of specific components.

Included in this phase, and bordering on the next phase, would be studies to evaluate how limited a whole package of care can be while retaining its overall effectiveness. There are many components within a CAM treatment approach, but are there any that we can eliminate and at the same time retain or improve overall treatment effectiveness?

Phase 4: Component efficacy (What is the efficacy of a specific component of the therapy?)
This is the area that has received most attention and research money to date and, while it is important, it is not the starting point in our model. The methods of choice are often double-blind randomized controlled trials. It is, however, important to recognize that results from such research cannot be used to document or disprove the effectiveness of a 'whole-system' treatment.

Phase 5: Biological mechanisms (How can treatment outcomes be explained biologically?)
We want, and need, to understand the pathways and mechanisms through which treatments exercise their influence (Lewith *et al.*, 2005). We must, however, realize that treatment outcomes, both at the system and component level, can be documented before the biological mechanisms are understood. The most prominent example from conventional medicine is probably aspirin. The anti-inflammatory and pain-killing properties of aspirin were discovered long before it became known that aspirin influences prostaglandin synthesis.

Conclusion

CAM is not simply a new array of therapeutic tools that need to be evaluated; it presents other ways to think about disease and therapeutics, and consequently new ideas about how research should be strategically developed. Here we have suggested two ways of taking this forward. First, the absence of statutory and financial gatekeepers for CAM presents several issues that need to be considered closely. Secondly, the structure of CAM research should be different, in subtle but important ways. We have provided some suggestions for how this alternative research strategy could be structured, keeping in mind that the ultimate goal for all approaches to treatment is to provide effective medical interventions at reasonable cost and without harm.

Further reading

Jonas, W. (2005) Building an evidence house: Challenges and solutions to research in complementary and alternative medicine. *Research in Complementary Medicine* 12(3): 159–67.

Koithan, M., Verhoef, M., Bell, I., White, M., Mulkins, A. and Ritenbaugh, C. (2007) The process of whole person healing: 'Unstuckness' and beyond. *Journal of Alternative and Complementary Medicine* 13(6): 659–68.

Paterson, C., Baarts, C., Launso, L. and Verhoef, M. (2009) Evaluating complex health interventions: A critical analysis of the 'outcomes' concept'. *BMC Complementary and Alternative Medicine* 9: 18.

References

Beresford, S.A., Johnson, K.C., Ritenbaugh, C. *et al.* (2006) Low-fat dietary pattern and risk of colorectal cancer: The Women's Health Initiative Randomized Controlled Dietary Modification Trial. *Journal of the American Medical Association* 295: 643–54.

Boon, H., Brown, J.B., Gavin, A. and Westlake, K. (2003) Men with prostate cancer: Making decisions about complementary/alternative medicine. *Medical Decision Making* 23: 471–9.

Endrizzi, C., Rossi, E., Crudeli, L. and Garibaldi, D. (2005) Harm in homeopathy: Aggravations, adverse drug events or medication errors? *Homeopathy* 94: 233–40.

Fønnebø, V. and Launsø, L. (2005) Looking for new knowledge in the field of curing and healing. *Focus on Alternative and Complementary Therapies* 10: 13–14.

Guthlin, C., Lange, O. and Walach, H. (2004) Measuring the effects of acupuncture and homoeopathy in general practice: An uncontrolled prospective documentation approach. *BMC Public Health* 4: 6.

Hammerschlag, R. (1998) Methodological and ethical issues in clinical trials of acupuncture. *Journal of Alternative and Complementary Medicine* 4: 159–71.

Hamre, H.J., Becker-Witt, C., Glockmann, A., Ziegler, R., Willich, S.N. and Kiene, H. (2004) Anthroposophic therapies in chronic disease: The Anthroposophic Medicine Outcomes Study (AMOS). *European Journal of Medical Research* 9: 351–60.

Hanssen, B., Grimsgaard, S., Launso, L., Fonnebo, V., Falkenberg, T. and Rasmussen, N.K. (2005) Use of complementary and alternative medicine in the Scandinavian countries. *Scandinavian Journal of Primary Health Care* 23: 57–62.

Jonas, W.B. (2005) Building an evidence house: Challenges and solutions to research in complementary and alternative medicine. *Forsch Komplementarmed Klass Naturheilkd* 12: 159–67.

Launso, L. (2000) Use of alternative treatments in Denmark: Patterns of use and patients' experience with treatment effects. *Alternative Therapies in Health and Medicine* 6: 102–07.

Launso, L., Brendstrup, E. and Arnberg, S. (1999) An exploratory study of reflexological treatment for headache. *Alternative Therapies in Health and Medicine* 5: 57–65.

Launsø, L. and Gannik, D.E. (2000) The need for revision of medical research designs. In D.E. Gannik and L. Launsø (eds) *Disease, Knowledge and Society.* Copenhagen: Forlaget Samfundslitteratur.

Launso, L. and Rieper, J. (2005) General practitioners and classical homeopaths treatment models for asthma and allergy. *Homeopathy* 94: 17–25.

Lewith, G., Walach, H. and Jonas, W.B. (2002) Balanced research strategies for complementary and alternative medicine. In G. Lewith, W.B. Jonas and H. Walach (eds) *Clinical Research in Complementary Therapies: Principles, Problems, and Solutions.* London: Churchill Livingston, pp. 3–27.

Lewith, G.T., White, P.J. and Pariente, J. (2005) Investigating acupuncture using brain imaging techniques: The current state of play. *Evidence Based Complementary Medicine* 2: 315–19.

MacPherson, H. (2004) Pragmatic clinical trials. *Complementary Therapies in Medicine* 12: 136–40.

MacPherson, H. and Liu, B. (2005) The safety of Chinese herbal medicine: A pilot study for a national survey. *Journal of Alternative and Complementary Medicine* 11: 617–26.

MacPherson, H., Scullion, A., Thomas, K.J. and Walters, S. (2004) Patient reports of adverse events associated with acupuncture treatment: A prospective national survey. *Quality and Safety in Health Care* 13: 349–55.

MacPherson, H., Thomas, K., Walters, S. and Fitter, M. (2001) The York acupuncture safety study: Prospective survey of 34 000 treatments by traditional acupuncturists. *British Medical Journal* 323: 486–7.

Norheim, A.J. (1996) Adverse effects of acupuncture: A study of the literature for the years 1981–1994. *Journal of Alternative and Complementary Medicine* 2: 291–7.

Norheim, A.J. and Fonnebo, V. (1995) Adverse effects of acupuncture. *Lancet* 345: 1576.

Norheim, A.J. and Fonnebo, V. (2000) A survey of acupuncture patients: Results from a questionnaire among a random sample in the general population in Norway. *Complementary Therapies in Medicine* 8: 187–92.

Paterson, C. and Dieppe, P. (2005) Characteristic and incidental (placebo) effects in complex interventions such as acupuncture. *British Medical Journal* 330: 1202–05.

Ritenbaugh, C., Verhoef, M., Fleishman, S., Boon, H. and Leis, A. (2003) Whole systems research: A discipline for studying complementary and alternative medicine. *Alternative Therapies in Health and Medicine* 9: 32–6.

Schonekaes, K., Micke, O., Mucke, R. *et al.* (2003) Use of complementary/alternative therapy methods by patients with breast cancer. *Forsch Komplementarmed Klass Naturheilkd* 10: 304–08.

Steinsbekk, A. and Ludtke, R. (2005) Patients' assessments of the effectiveness of homeopathic care in Norway: A prospective observational multicentre outcome study. *Homeopathy* 94: 10–16.

Thomas, K.J., MacPherson, H., Ratcliffe, J. *et al.* (2005) Longer term clinical and economic benefits of offering acupuncture care to patients with chronic low back pain. *Health Technology Assessment* 9: iii–x.

Thomas, K.J., Nicholl, J.P. and Coleman, P. (2001) Use and expenditure on complementary medicine in England: A population based survey. *Complementary Therapies in Medicine* 9: 2–11.

Thompson, E., Barron, S. and Spence, D. (2004) A preliminary audit investigating remedy reactions including adverse events in routine homeopathic practice. *Homeopathy* 93: 203–09.

Vickers, A.J., Rees, R.W., Zollman, C.E. *et al.* (2004) Acupuncture for chronic headache in primary care: Large, pragmatic, randomised trial. *British Medical Journal* 328: 744.

Wilkinson, S., Gomella, L.G., Smith, J.A. *et al.* (2002) Attitudes and use of complementary medicine in men with prostate cancer. *Journal of Urology* 168: 2505–09.

Witt, C.M., Ludtke, R., Baur, R. and Willich, S.N. (2005) Homeopathic medical practice: Long-term results of a cohort study with 3981 patients. *BMC Public Health* 5: 115.

Wittman, W.W. and Walach, H. (2002) Evaluating complementary medicine: Lessons to be learned from evaluation research. In G. Lewith, W.B. Jonas and H. Walach (eds) *Clinical Research in Complementary Therapies: Principles, Problems, and Solutions*. London: Churchill Livingstone, pp. 93–108.

CHAPTER 23

Evidence-based complementary and alternative medicine: Promises and problems

IAN COULTER

Introduction

While there have been previous attempts by sociologists to discuss complementary and alternative medicine (CAM) and evidence-based medicine (EBM) (Willis and White, 2003), none has been from the insider's perspective of doing research in evidence-based complementary and alternative medicine, EBCAM. This chapter will focus on the process of establishing a US centre for EBM, reflecting some of the methodological challenges involved in such a project.

Setting up an EBM centre of CAM

In 2001, the National Center for Complementary and Alternative Medicine (NCCAM) released a request for proposals to establish an evidence-based practice centre (EPC) for complementary and alternative medicine (CAM). One successful centre proposal, the Southern California Evidence-Based Practice Center (SCEPC), was located at RAND, a major not-for-profit centre for health policy/health services research located in Santa Monica, California. This chapter is based on the experience gained from this work.

What is evidence-based practice?

In most discussions, EBP is viewed as defined within biomedical circles as 'the conscientious, explicit and judicious use of the current best evidence in

Source: Coulter, I. (2007) Evidence based complementary and alternative medicine: Promises and problems. *Forschende Komplementarmedizin* 14: 102–08. Abridged version reprinted with kind permission of Karger AG, Basel.

making decisions about the care of individual patients' (Coulter, 2001). In practice, 'evidence-based medicine constitutes the integration of individual clinical expertise with the best available external clinical evidence from systematic research' (Sackett, 1998). This is contrasted with tradition-based care (Niedrman and Badovinac, 1999), which is characterized as 'practical, prudent, and personal'. In traditional care, emphasis is placed on the accumulated knowledge and experience, adherence to accepted standards and opinion of experts and peers. EBP, in contrast, places a premium on using current evidence to solve clinical questions (Richards and Lawrence, 1998). At the very minimum, it involves reading current literature, being able to appraise the literature critically (Greenhalgh, 1997), being able to synthesize the literature or appraise syntheses, drawing conclusions that are relevant to clinical practice and applying the results of these processes to individual patients (Joskstad, 1998). Despite the great expectations held by some groups for EBP, there is little evidence to suggest that it results in better outcomes for patients or that those who are educated in EBP, in fact, practise better medicine (Morrison *et al.*, 1999; Dobbie *et al.*, 2000).

There is considerable debate about how much of clinical practice is actually evidence based. Initial estimates by the Office of Technology Assessment in 1979 and 1983 held that only about 10–20 per cent of medicine could claim to be evidence based. In 2001, an editorial in the *British Medical Journal* quoted a figure of 15 per cent for solid scientific interventions in medical interventions (Smith, 1991). The problem of establishing this figure is the need to define what will constitute 'evidence'. How this is done has a significant impact on the result (for a wider discussion of different perspectives of 'evidence', see Chapter 21 in this collection).

Towards evidence-based CAM

Because of the ideological nature over much of the debate about the evidence basis of CAM, it is necessary and prudent to acknowledge this context. Although the increasing popularity of CAM in western societies has been well documented, it should be noted that there have also been negative reactions among certain groups. This has led to the creation of one journal, the *Scientific Review of Alternative Medicine*, whose purpose is to examine the claims of CAM (Sampson, 1997). On the other hand, there is a suspicion among alternative health care providers that only those studies with negative results about CAM will be published in mainstream journals (Eskinazi and Muehsam, 1999), in stark contrast to traditional medicine, where there is a suspected bias against publishing negative results (Easterbrook *et al.*, 1991).

Many commentators have argued that CAM should be subjected to the same rules of evidence that are assumed to be held for medicine (Vickers *et al.*, 1997) and to the same methods of evaluation, such as assessment of clinical skills and safety evaluations (Lewith and Davies, 1996).

The position that EBP is the basis for integrating CAM and conventional medicine is fraught with difficulties and assumes that modern medicine is itself evidence based. Allopathic medicine could not meet such a strict criterion (Dalen, 1998). However, for some writers CAM is portrayed as having a 'free ride' by not having been subjected to the demands of science in the way medicine is (Angell and Kassirer, 1998). One has to wonder in what sense CAM has been given a free ride. For the most part, science has ignored the investigation of CAM. If it is meant as a criticism of the CAM community, then again one might question the fairness of the comment. The great research endeavours that are presumed to make biomedicine scientific have not been paid for by the medical profession, nor, in large part, conducted by the medical profession.

Furthermore, the experience at RAND has been, and the increasing publications about the efficacy of CAM would suggest, that the CAM community is only too willing to cooperate with researchers whose agenda is research and not political.

Practical work of the SCEPC

The SCEPC conducted a systematic literature review for CAM therapies. We completed nine systematic reviews of CAM. Prior to the SCEPC, RAND had completed two systematic reviews in chiropractic manipulation. The completed topics include manipulation for low-back pain, cervical manipulation, mind–body therapy for gastro-intestinal (GI) problems; Ayurvedic medicine for diabetes; S-Adenosyl-L-Methionine (SAMe) for depression, osteoarthritis and chronic liver problems; Coenzyme Q10, vitamin E and vitamin C for treating or preventing cardiovascular disease; and Coenzyme Q10, vitamin E and vitamin C for treating or preventing cancer.

Systematic reviews of CAM: What do the results show about the method?

While the results are too extensive to be reported fully here, the following brief discussion indicates the amount of literature that can be accessed even within CAM and the potential for producing systematic data on the effectiveness of particular CAM. The focus here is on the methods and the issues associated with this type of research. The publications of the evidence reports discussed here are available from AHRQ (http://www.ahrq.gov/clinic/evrptpdfs.htm).

Manipulation for low-back pain

We identified 1600 articles that focused on manipulation for low-back pain (Shekelle *et al.*, 1992, 1995; Coulter, 1996; Coulter *et al.*, 1996). Of these, we were able to conduct a meta-analysis on 29 RCTs and 9 trials with other therapy (Shekelle *et al.*, 1992, 1998; Coulter, 1998; Coulter *et al.*, 1995). For cervical manipulation, we identified 1100 articles and conducted a systematic review on 67 articles on efficacy and 14 RCTs. No meta-analysis was possible because of the heterogeneity in the studies (Coulter, 1996; Coulter *et al.*, 1996; Shekelle and Coulter, 1997).

Mind–body therapy for GI problems

We identified 4397 titles from which 1362 articles were selected for further review. There were 52 studies where there was a control or comparison group: biofeedback, hypnosis, relaxation, behavioural therapy, multimodal therapy, cognitive therapy, imagery and placebo. Because of the clinical heterogeneity it was not possible to conduct a meta-analysis. Most of the studies in the field of mind–body therapy have substantial methodological problems (Coulter *et al.*, 2002).

Ayurvedic medicine for diabetes

A total of 1311 potentially relevant titles were identified from all sources. Of these, 54 articles reported on the results of 62 studies in diabetes; 35 studies came from the western literature and 27 from the Indian literature. The designs of the 62 studies were varied. There were 7 RCTs and 10 controlled clinical trials (CCTs). There were 38 case series and 7 cohort studies. The report demonstrates the existence of a body of evidence evaluating Ayurvedic herbal interventions for diabetes. Furthermore, significant amounts of English-language literature relevant to this topic were available in India. Overall, the literature consisted of a few RCTs and CCTs with relatively low-quality scores as well as a larger number of case series (Hardy *et al.*, 2001).

S-Adenosyl-L-Methionine (SAMe)

An initial broad search of the literature found 1553 titles, of which 258 were judged to be RCTs, CCTs or systematic reviews (including meta-analyses); 89 articles met the criteria for inclusion. Of these, 38 focused on depression, 38 on liver disease and 13 on osteoarthritis. Interventions using SAMe were heterogeneous both for route of administration and dosage and the study populations also displayed considerable variability. The majority of the studies enrolled small numbers of patients and the quality of the studies varied widely. However, a sufficient range of studies with sufficiently homogeneous outcomes and disease states existed to perform meta-analyses of data on depression, osteoarthritis and cholestasis of pregnancy (Hardy *et al.*, 2002).

Coenzyme Q10, vitamin E and vitamin C for treating or preventing cardiovascular disease

Our literature search process identified 8173 titles, from which we found 144 unique trials (that is, those reporting data not duplicated in another publication) for cardiovascular disease. Of the reports, one third were judged to be of high quality (Shekelle *et al.*, 2004). Studies reporting on the outcomes of death, myocardial infarction and/or blood lipid levels were selected for further analysis. For the interventions of vitamin E alone and in combination with other antioxidants, sufficient numbers of studies existed to perform pooled analyses. We identified one meta-analysis of the effect of coenzyme Q10 and four studies were identified that assessed the effect of vitamin C (mostly in combination with other antioxidants) on clinical outcomes in patients with or at high risk for cardiovascular disease.

Coenzyme Q10, vitamin E and vitamin C for treating or preventing cancer

From the 8173 titles, we identified 432 articles for screening, of which 35 articles met the criteria for inclusion in the analysis for cancer (Coulter *et al.*, 2003). The studies identified varied greatly in quality. Sufficient numbers of homogeneous studies did not exist to permit a meta-analysis of the efficacy of vitamins C or E or coenzyme Q10 for the outcomes of death or new tumours. A meta-analysis was possible for polyps as an outcome. Additional qualitative reviews were done for studies that could not be pooled and for studies with intermediate outcomes (Coulter *et al.*, 2003).

Discussion

We have been able to identify some common problems across the CAM studies reviewed by SCEPC: the small number of good RCTs; the large number of observational studies; heterogeneity in study designs; heterogeneity in the clinical intervention in the trials; few trials receiving good-quality scores (due to lack of randomization, small sample sizes, being underpowered and inappropriate statistical methods); the large number of studies in languages other than English; accessing studies in non-traditional databases and in countries lacking the library infrastructures of developed countries; lack of studies testing a system of care as opposed to individual therapies within that system; and the lack of studies of effectiveness.

It is the last two issues that pose challenges for the advancement of EBCAM, but they are methodological challenges and not insurmountable ones. Although beyond the focus of this paper, they are being addressed in studies looking at observation studies and reviews (Concato *et al.*, 2000; Radford and Foody, 2001), in whole-systems research (Elder *et al.*, 2006), in new forms of evidence (such as non-hierarchical evidence) and in studies looking at effectiveness as opposed to efficacy studies (Gartlehner *et al.*, 2006).

We are now entering an important period in EBP. On the one side are those who see it as a process of privileging certain types of evidence over other forms (Djulbegovic *et al.*, 2000) and who look for reconciliation. On the other hand, there are those critics who see in it a form of intellectual fascism (Holmes *et al.*, 2006) and who would reject it entirely. The challenge for CAM is to recognize the limitations of EBP but not to 'throw the baby out with the bathwater'. There is much in EBP that clearly should be emulated by the CAM community, but only where it is appropriate. The challenge will be to establish where the boundaries are to be drawn.

Conclusion

The centre's results indicate that a lot more 'evidence' exists for CAM than one might expect. In fact, in many cases, such as low-back pain and manipulation, the number of RCTs now exceeds that found for many medical interventions. Where that evidence does exist, a good case can be made that they should be subjected to systematic reviews in the same way as mainstream medicine. This is both politically smart for those involved in CAM, but also academically smart in that it assembles the best kind of evidence. As the searches demonstrated, there are quite large bodies of literature that can be accessed and that are available. This does require considerable effort and resources.

What role do systematic reviews of CAM play? This can be seen in the review of manipulation of low-back pain. Prior to the RAND study, the general stance among many medical commentators was that manipulation had no role, had no efficacy. After the study, the question became for what conditions, for what type of patients and in whose hands does it have the best outcomes? This does not mean that the debate about manipulation has been resolved, but it does mean that the debate has moved in its focus. In that sense, the reviews allow the debate and the research to move to a new level of questions and more clinically significant questions.

Further reading

Adams, J. (2000) General practitioners, complementary therapies and evidence-based medicine: The defence of clinical autonomy. *Complementary Therapies in Medicine* 8(4): 248–52.

References

Angell, M. and Kassirer, J.P. (1998) Alternative medicine – the risks of untested and unregulated remedies. *New England Journal of Medicine* 339(12): 839–41.

Concato, J., Shah, N. and Horwitz, R.I. (2000) Randomized, controlled trials, observational studies, and the hierarchy of research designs. *New England Journal of Medicine* 342(25): 1887–92.

Coulter, I.D. (1996) Manipulation and mobilization of the cervical spine: The results of a literature survey and consensus panel. *Journal of Musculoskeletal Medicine* 4(4): 113–23.

Coulter, I.D. (1998) Efficacy and risks of chiropractic manipulation: What does the evidence suggest? *Integrative Medicine* 1(1): 61–6.

Coulter, I.D. (2001) Evidence-based dentistry and health services research: Is one possible without the other? *Journal of Dental Education* 65(8): 714–24.

Coulter, I.D., Favreau, J.T., Hardy, M.L., Morton, S.C., Roth, E.A. and Shekelle, P.G. (2002) Biofeedback interventions for gastrointestinal conditions: A systematic review. *Alternative Therapies in Health and Medicine* 8(3): 76–83.

Coulter, I.D., Hardy, M., Morton, S.C. *et al.* (2003) *Effect of the Supplemental use of Antioxidants Vitamin C, Vitamin E, and Coenzyme Q10 for the Prevention and Treatment of Cancer.* Evidence Report/Technology Assessment 75. AHRQ Publ No 03-E047.

Coulter, I.D., Hurwitz, E.L., Adams, A.H. *et al.* (1996) *The Appropriateness of Manipulation and Mobilization of the Cervical Spine.* Santa Monica, RAND, MR-781-CCR.

Coulter, I.D., Shekelle, P., Mootz, R. and Hansen, D. (1995) The use of expert panel results: The RAND panel for appropriateness of manipulation and mobilization of the cervical spine. *Journal of Topics in Clinical Chiropractic* 2(3): 54–62 [reprinted with permission RAND/RP-592].

Dalen, J.E. (1998) 'Conventional' and 'unconventional' medicine. Can they be integrated? *Archives in Internal Medicine* 158: 2179–81.

Djulbegovic, B., Morris, L. and Lyman, G.H. (2000) Evidentiary challenges to evidence-based medicine. *Journal of Evaluation in Clinical Practice* 6: 99–109.

Dobbie, A.E., Schneider, F.D., Anderson, A.D. *et al.* (2000) What evidence supports teaching evidence-based medicine? *Academic Medicine* 75(12): 1184–5.

Elder, C., Aickin, M., Bell, I.R. *et al.* (2006) Methodological challenges in whole systems research. *Journal of Alternative and Complement Medicine* 9: 843–50.

Eskinazi, D. and Muehsam, D. (1999) Is the scientific publishing of complementary and alternative medicine objective? *Journal of Alternative and Complementary Medicine* (6): 587–94.

Easterbrook, P.J., Berlin, J.A., Gopalan, R. *et al.* (1991) Publication bias in clinical research. *Lancet* 337: 867–72.

Gartlehner, G., Hansen, R.A., Nissman, D., Lohr, K.N. and Carey, T.S. (2006) A simple and valid tool distinguished efficacy from effectiveness studies. *Journal of Clinical Epidemiology* 59(10): 1040–48.

Greenhalgh, T. (1997) Assessing the methodological quality of published papers. *British Medical Journal* 315: 305–08.

Hardym M.L., Coulter, I.D., Morton, S.C. *et al.* (2002) *S-adenosyl-L-methionine (SAMe) for Treatment of Depression, Osteoarthritis and Liver Disease.* Evidence Report/Technology Assessment 64. AHRQ Publ No 02- E034.

Hardy, M., Coulter, I., Venuturupalli, S. *et al.* (2001) *Southern California Evidence-Based Practice Centre/RAND. Ayurvedic Interventions for Diabetes Mellitus: A*

Systematic Review. Evidence Report/Technology Assessment 41. Rockville MD: USDHHS Agency for Healthcare Research and Quality. AHRQ Publ No 01-E040.

Holmes, D., Murray, S.T., Perron, A. and Rail, G. (2006) Deconstructing the evidence for evidence-based discourse in health sciences: Truth, power and fascism. *International Journal of Evidence-Based Healthcare* 4: 180–86.

Joskstad, A. (1998) Evidence-based healthcare: Avoiding ivory tower research? *Evidence-Based Dentistry* 1(1): 5–6.

Lewith, G. and Davies, P. (1996) Complementary medicine: The need for audit. *Complementary Therapies in Medicine* 4: 233–6.

Morrison, J.M., Sullivan, F., Murray, E. and Jolly, B. (1999) Evidence-based education: Development of an instrument to critically appraise reports of educational interventions. *Medical Education* 33: 890–93.

Niedrman, R. and Badovinac, R. (1999) Tradition-based dental care and evidence-based dental care. *Journal of Dental Research* 78(7): 1288–91.

Radford, M.J. and Foody, J.M. (2001) How do observational studies expand the evidence base for therapy? *Journal of the American Medical Association* 286(10): 1228–30.

Richards, D. and Lawrence, A. (1998) Evidence based dentistry. *Evidence-Based Dentistry* 1(1): 7–10.

Sackett, D.L. (1998) Evidence-based medicine. *Spine* 23(10): 1085–6.

Sampson, W. (1997) Why a new alternative medicine journal? *Scientific Review of Alternative Medicine* 1: 4–6.

Shekelle, P., Adams, A.H., Chassin, M.R., Hurwitz, E.L., Phillips, R.B. and Brook, R.H. (1992) *The Appropriateness of Spinal Manipulation of Low-Back Pain: Indications and Ratings by an all Chiropractic Expert Panel*. Santa Monica, RAND, R-4025/3-CCR/FCER.

Shekelle, P. and Coulter, I.D. (1997) Cervical spine manipulation: Summary report of a systematic review of the literature and a multidisciplinary expert panel. *Journal of Spinal Disorders and Techniques* 10(3): 223–8.

Shekelle, P., Coulter, I.D., Hurwitz, E.L. and Genovese, B. (1995) *The Appropriateness of Spinal Manipulation for Low-Back Pain: Data Collection Instruments and a Manual for Their Use*. Santa Monica, RAND, R-402515-CCR/FCER.

Shekelle, P., Coulter, I.D., Hurwitz, E.L. *et al.* (1998) Congruence doctrine decisions to initiate chiropractic spinal manipulation for low back pain and appropriateness criteria in North America. *Annals of Internal Medicine* 124: 9–17.

Shekelle, P.G., Morton, S.C., Jungvig, L.K. *et al.* (2004) Effect of supplemental Vitamin E for the prevention and treatment of cardiovascular disease. *Journal of General Internal Medicine* 14: 380–89.

Smith, R. (1991) Where is the Wisdom …? *British Medical Journal* 303: 798–99.

Vickers, A., Cassileth, B., Ernst, E. *et al.* (1997) How should we research unconventional therapies? *International Journal of Technology Assessment in Health Care* 13: 111–21.

Willis, E. and White, K. (2003) Evidence-based medicine and CAM. In P. Tovey, G. Easthope and J. Adams (eds) *The Mainstreaming of Complementary and Alternative Medicine: Studies in Social Context*. London: Routledge, pp. 49–63.

CHAPTER 24

Indirect risks of complementary and alternative medicine

JON WARDLE AND JON ADAMS

Introduction

A discussion of issues of safety and risk around complementary and alternative medicine (CAM) has primarily revolved around issues of direct risk, including adverse events (such as the potential hepatotoxicity of CAM products or potential CAM–drug interactions) and the monitoring of these events (pharmacovigilance). Yet the development of a broader public health agenda for CAM (Adams, 2008) provides an opportunity for a new focus on the inherent indirect health risks associated with these medicines – representing a novel, innovative approach to the consideration of risk and safety in CAM.

Indirect risks associated with product variability

The generic interchangeability that exists in pharmaceutical medicines does not apply to CAM. There may be significant safety and efficacy profiles between different manufacturers' nominally 'identical' CAM and even between different batches of the same CAM product (Basch *et al.*, 2005). Moreover, while regulatory mechanisms usually focus on simple principles such as good manufacturing processes, they rarely extend to other issues affecting CAM product quality, such as growing and manufacturing methods relating to raw materials.

Such risks are compounded by the fact that both the public and health practitioners are generally unaware of the unregulated nature of the CAM industry (Ashar *et al.*, 2008). Additionally, many poorer-quality CAM products are substantiated via claims to evidence pertaining to higher-quality formulations.

The opportunity costs associated with this variability are clear. A poor-quality preparation of a CAM product can expose the consumer to economic risk (incurring financial losses with no therapeutic benefit) and also present opportunity costs if the patient is using the poor-quality substitute of an otherwise effective CAM, or even instead of a high-quality CAM.

This variability also makes it difficult to develop comprehensive or accurate post-market surveillance, or to develop effective regulatory and legislative solutions to the direct risk of CAM products (Basch *et al.*, 2005). As most of these solutions are often based on frameworks designed for pharmaceutical medicines, they inherently make an assumption of comparing different products as 'like for like', a situation that is not applicable to CAM.

Practitioner variability

False consultations

The confusing situation that often surrounds practitioner training and accreditation can give rise to the phenomenon of 'false consultations'. Consumers may erroneously believe that they are getting advice from a trained professional when they purchase CAM from pharmacies or health food stores (HFS). HFS are rarely obliged to employ qualified staff, although some do, and most pharmacies defer CAM questions to relatively untrained 'vitamin consultants' or similar positions (Mills *et al.*, 2003b; Lin *et al.*, 2005). Although issues surrounding CAM training are important at all levels, they are magnified in the retail HFS and pharmacy environments by virtue of their accessibility to the public.

Consumers may also be unduly put at risk due to statements made by an unqualified person, who may appear qualified by virtue of their position. For example, a Canadian study of health advice from HFS for HIV patients found that even though two-thirds of employees had no health training, over 75 per cent made product suggestions, only 25 per cent asked whether the patient was taking medication and only 19 per cent recommended visiting a physician (Mills *et al.*, 2003a).

Pharmacies are often seen as superior to HFS as sources of objective information, as they are required to have trained pharmacists on hand (where patients may seek further CAM information) and are bound by more professional guidelines than HFS. However, regulations governing conventional therapeutic goods sales rarely apply to CAM, even in a pharmacy setting. Additionally, few pharmacists exhibit confidence in their CAM knowledge or feel prepared to make clinical judgements on CAM (Kwan *et al.*, 2006) and over 90 per cent of pharmacists have no formal training in CAM (Semple *et al.*, 2006), with manufacturer training being the primary source of training for over a quarter of pharmacists (Semple *et al.*, 2006). Over a quarter of pharmacies sell CAM without any access to CAM information whatsoever. Pharmacies have also been demonstrated to be just as guilty as HFS of promoting false claims relating to CAM (Harvey *et al.*, 2008).

Poor CAM knowledge among conventional providers

False consultations are not limited to retail settings, and may also include consultations with conventional practitioners, who, although qualified in their own discipline, may have little knowledge of CAM. The unregulated nature of much of the CAM practitioner education and practice sector, poor levels of CAM training among conventional practitioners, the propensity towards self-prescription and the lack of easy access to sources of reputable CAM information may also pose further economic risk through inappropriate or injudicious use of otherwise effective remedies.

More worrying still, despite often feeling ill prepared or unable to make clinical judgements in relation to CAM, few health professionals believe that further specific training is warranted or required to practise CAM (Brown *et al.*, 2008). Such attitudes may increase both direct and indirect risks to the patient, if clinicians feel automatically 'qualified' to practise CAM by virtue of their conventional health training.

Conventional practitioners' poor knowledge of CAM may also become a greater issue as CAM-specific policy increases. For example, the introduction of health warning labels on CAM in Canada is expected to generate more CAM questions from patients for conventional providers (Boon and Kachan, 2007).

Variability in CAM practitioner training

The extraordinary variability of CAM practitioner training is also an area of great public health consequence. Variability in training may mean that CAM practitioners may not appropriately identify clinical situations requiring referral, and may not know the limitations of their therapies or appropriately assess the risk of their treatments. When combined with the generally unregulated nature of CAM, this proffers many risks to the patient (Lin *et al.*, 2005). CAM practitioners may not even be aware of the risks of their therapies. While professional resources and reporting regimes mean that neurologists are made aware of one out of every two vertebral artery dissections associated with spinal manipulation, chiropractors are made aware of only one in forty-eight through mechanisms available to them (Haldeman *et al.*, 2002). This may lower the perceived risk of their therapies and be reflected in their communication of risks to patients. Risks are magnified by the fact that a large proportion of the population now rely on a CAM practitioner as their primary provider (Grace *et al.*, 2006). CAM practitioners may also offer advice on conventional medicines, even though they may not necessarily have the competence to do so (MacPherson *et al.*, 2004).

Risk of financial exploitation (economic risk)

Conflict of interest in product sales

Some commentators have highlighted a potential conflict of interest due to the lack of separation between the prescription and sale of CAM by practitioners in the clinical encounter (Parker *et al.*, 2010). In Australia, 98 per cent of naturopaths have a dispensary in their clinic, and 78 per cent sell pre-packaged (rather than extemporaneous) products directly to their patients (Smith *et al.*, 2005). This is not limited to CAM practitioners: conventional medical practitioners often view the integration of CAM as a business opportunity, rather than solely its health benefits (Slomski, 1999; Smith, 2006). This potential conflict of interest may encourage some practitioners to prescribe products or deliver services primarily for financial gain and clearly offers incentive for practitioners to over-service patients.

While the obvious solution would be to transfer dispensing of prescribed CAM to third parties such as pharmacies, as often occurs in conventional medicine, this may not reduce exposure to this risk. Many pharmacies also view CAM as a business opportunity, to the point where some now rely on CAM for nearly two-thirds of their revenue (Offord, 2006). Clinic sales aren't always nefarious: many practitioners hold on to their sales function to ensure that their patients are given high-quality products, and that there is no risk of brand substitution by pharmacists or HFS employees when filling prescriptions. Until adequate infrastructure, policies and procedures are developed so that patients can easily access good-quality CAM, and procedures developed so that CAM practitioners can be assured that patients filling prescriptions externally will be likely to receive the specific recommended formulations without interference from third parties, it is likely that any move to dissuade CAM practitioners from selling products will fail.

Over-utilization and over-servicing of diagnostic tools

Economic risk through over-servicing during the clinical encounter may occur due to a lack of training. This may lead to the over-utilization of diagnostic tests such as 'functional pathology' or chiropractic X-rays by CAM practitioners (Grace *et al.*, 2006). This use, when combined with the variability in CAM practitioner training, may also result in opportunity costs borne through misdiagnosis (Seely and Mills, 2006). The issue of over-servicing is not isolated to CAM and may not always be nefarious in nature. For example, it may also be representative of the lack of training or specific guidelines on the appropriate use and prioritization of CAM services.

The commercialization of CAM

Such financial risks may go unnoticed, as there seems to be little public perception of CAM services as commercial transactions; rather, they are seen as altruistic exchanges, with CAM practitioners viewed as offering a more ethical and caring approach to patients (Siahpush, 1998). In combination with the fact that CAM products are often perceived as the safer, 'natural' alternatives to synthetic or high-technology products, this may obscure some of the less palatable commercial and corporate realities of much of the CAM sector (Collyer, 2004). The commercial focus of CAM may be entrenched even at a government level, as CAM may be seen more as a growth industry with potential broader national benefits (job creation, new industry development and) than as an issue that has a direct impact on public health.

Lack of reporting mechanisms

Non-disclosure of CAM use is reported as widespread (see Chapter 15 for details). However, when patients do choose to report harm there may be few avenues to do so, resulting in many valid complaints going unreported. One of the arguments for regulating CAM practitioners in Ontario was the diffi-culty often observed in seeking recourse for poor treatment from CAM prac-titioners, as any harm was often seen as 'poor judgment on [their] part, not poor practice on the part of the practitioner, unless they physically harm you' (Vogel, 2010).

Additionally, the proliferation of self-regulatory bodies – who may not be obliged or able to take further action – can also make it difficult for patients to identify avenues for directing complaints against practitioners. This results in many instances of practitioner-induced harm going unreported. This can be reversed with the implementation of a clear complaints mechanism. For example, the registration of Chinese medicine practitioners in Australia resulted in a fivefold increase in complaints against practitioners once a single accountable complaints authority had been established (Lin *et al.*, 2005).

Confusing or non-existent reporting regimes also limit the availability of adverse events data in relation to CAM products and result in significant under-reporting of CAM adverse events (Myers and Cheras, 2004). CAM practitioners have also consistently reported that they are often unaware of the proper channels for reporting adverse events (Lin *et al.*, 2005). Patients may not only be unaware of channels for reporting adverse events, but also be reluctant to do so (Barnes *et al.*, 1998).

Even once safety issues are uncovered, the lack of communication infra-structure may mean that distributors of these products are unaware of the potential risks. HFS in Canada were unaware of new laws banning kava and were selling it two months after official notification (Mills *et al.*, 2003b).

And even two years after the US Food and Drug Administration had issued warnings and import alerts for products containing aristolochic acid, these were still widely available for purchase on US websites (Gold and Slone, 2003).

In addition to posing barriers to appropriate safety measures, lack of such infrastructure compounds risks. It makes the investigation of CAM more difficult. For example, the lack of gatekeeper and regulatory bodies may mean that treatments are widespread before they even become known to researchers (see Chapter 25 for details). Some commentators have suggested that the reluctance to develop appropriate or regulatory or legislative arrangements to incorporate appropriate CAM may in fact be creating legal barriers to patients receiving the best treatment for their condition (Ruggio and DeSantis-Then, 2009).

Conclusion

Although there are clear indirect (and direct) risks associated with CAM use, with over 500 systematic reviews demonstrating CAM therapies that do more good than harm (Ernst *et al.*, 2006), there is also clear potential for positive incorporation. Although not appreciating the risks of CAM can pose a safety issue for CAM users, there is also an inherent danger that these risks can be over-hyped, potentially denying patients valid treatment options (Moyad, 2010). The solutions are not difficult, and simply require policy and research attention in the area that is commensurate with the contemporary use of CAM (for example in developing minimum standards of training, appropriate levels of regulation and clear infrastructure for communication).

Looking at the indirect risks of CAM is a novel, fruitful approach that suggests a variety of areas that require attention. Nevertheless, developing solutions to the problems of indirect risk require a new paradigm – one that appreciates a more complex and multifactorial picture of CAM and the safety and risk issues surrounding it and that requires a multidisciplinary approach able to meet the challenges associated with CAM use.

Further reading

Jacobsson, I., Jonsson, A., Gerden, B. and Hagg, S. (2009) Spontaneously reported adverse reactions in association with complementary and alternative medicine substances in Sweden. *Pharmacoepidemiology and Drug Safety* 18(11): 1039–47.

References

Adams, J. (2008) Utilising and promoting public health and health services research in complementary and alternative medicine: The founding of NORPHCAM. *Complementary Therapies in Medicine* 16: 245–6.

Ashar, B., Miller, R., Pichard, C. *et al.* (2008) Patients' understanding of the regulation of dietary supplements. *Journal of Community Health* 32: 22–30.

Barnes, J., Mills, S., Abbot, N., Willoughby, M. and Ernst, E. (1998) Different standards for reporting ADRs to herbal remedies and conventional OTC medicines: Face-to-face interviews with 515 users of herbal remedies. *British Journal of Clinical Pharmacology* 45(5): 496–500.

Basch, E., Servoss, J. and Tedrow, U. (2005) Safety assurances for dietary supplements: Policy issues and new research paradigms. *Journal of Herbal Pharmacotherapy* 1: 3–15.

Boon, H. and Kachan, N. (2007) Natural health product labels: Is more information always better? *Patient Education and Counseling* 68(2): 193–9.

Brown, J., Morgan, T., Adams, J. *et al.* (2008) *Complementary Medicines Information Use and Needs of Health Professionals: General Practitioners and Pharmacists.* Sydney: National Prescribing Service.

Collyer, F. (2004) Corporatisation and commercialisation of CAM. In P. Tovey, G. Easthope and J. Adams (eds) *The Mainstreaming of Complementary and Alternative Medicine: Studies in a Social Context.* London: Routledge.

Ernst, E., Pittler, M. and Boddy, K. (2006) *The Desktop Guide to Complementary and Alternative Medicine.* Edinburgh: Elsevier Mosby.

Gold, L. and Slone, T. (2003) Aristolochic acid, an herbal carcinogen, sold on the Web after FDA alert. *New England Journal of Medicine* 349: 1576–7.

Grace, S., Vemulpad, S. and Beirman, R. (2006) Training in and use of diagnostic techniques among CAM practitioners: An Australian study. *Journal of Alternative and Complementary Medicine* 12(7): 695–700.

Haldeman, S., Carey, P., Townsend, M. and Papadopoulos, C. (2002) Clinical perceptions of the risk of vertebral artery dissection after cervical manipulation: The effect of referral bias. *The Spine Journal* 2(5): 334–42.

Harvey, K., Korczak, V., Marron, L. and Newgreen, D. (2008) Commercialism, choice and consumer protection: Regulation of complementary medicines in Australia. *Medical Journal of Australia* 188(1): 21–5.

Kwan, D., Hirschkorn, K. and Boon, H. (2006) U.S. and Canadian pharmacists' attitudes, knowledge, and professional practice behaviors toward dietary supplements: A systematic review. *BMC Complementary and Alternative Medicine* 6: 31.

Lin, V., Bensoussan, A., Myers, S. *et al.* (2005) *The Practice and Regulatory Requirements of Naturopathy and Western Herbal Medicine.* Melbourne: Department of Human Services.

MacPherson, H., Scullion, A., Thomas, K. and Walters, S. (2004) Patient reports of adverse events associated with acupuncture treatment: A prospective national survey. *Quality and Safety in Health Care* 13: 348–55.

Mills, E., Singh, R., Kawasaki, M. *et al.* (2003a) Emerging issues associated with HIV patients seeking advice from health food stores. *Canadian Journal of Public Health* 94(5): 363–6.

Mills, E., Singh, R., Ross, C., Ernst, E. and Ray, J. (2003b) Sale of kava extract in some health food stores. *Canadian Medical Association Journal* 169: 1158–9.

Moyad, M. (2010) Under-hyped and over-hyped drug–dietary supplement interactions and issues. *Urologic Nursing* 30(1): 85–7.

Myers, S. and Cheras, P. (2004) The other side of the coin: Safety of complementary and alternative medicine. *Medical Journal of Australia* 181(4): 222–5.

Offord, L. (2006) Grab a slice of the wellness pie. *Australian Journal of Pharmacy* 87(1040): 48–9.

Parker, M., Wardle, J., Weir, M. and Stewart, C. (2010) Medical merchants: Conflict of interest, office product sales and notifiable conduct. *Medical Journal of Australia* 194(1): 34–7.

Ruggio, M. and DeSantis-Then, L. (2009) Complementary and alternative medicine: Longstanding legal obstacles to cutting edge treatment. *Journal of Health & Life Sciences Law* 2(4): 137: 139–70.

Seely, D. and Mills, E. (2006) Diagnostic accuracy among the allied health professions: Commentary on Grace et al.', *Journal of Alternative & Complementary Medicine* 12(7): 701–02.

Semple, S., Hotham, E., Rao, D., Martin, K., Smith, C. and Bloustien, G. (2006) Community pharmacists in Australia: Barriers to information provision on complementary and alternative medicines. *Pharmacy World Science* 28: 366–73.

Siahpush, M. (1998) Postmodern values, dissatisfaction with conventional medicine and popularity of alternative therapies. *Journal of Sociology* 34: 58–70.

Slomski, A. (1999) Doctors are selling the fountain of youth. *Medical Economics* 76(15): 94.

Smith, C., Martin, K., Hotham, E., Semple, S., Bloustien, G. and Rao, D. (2005) Naturopaths practice behaviour: Provision and access to information on complementary and alternative medicines. *BMC Complementary and Alternative Medicine* 5(15).

Smith, P. (2006) Investigation launched into drug kickbacks. *Australian Doctor* September 28.

Vogel, L. (2010) 'Hodge-podge' regulation of alternative medicine in Canada. *Canadian Medical Association Journal* 182(12): E569–E570.

CHAPTER 25

The liberalization of regulatory structure of complementary and alternative medicine: Implications for consumers and professions

MICHAEL WEIR

Introduction

Over the past 30 years there has been a rapid development in the regulatory structure for complementary and alternative medicine (CAM) in many western countries. Focusing primarily on Australia (with reference and in comparison to Canada and the United States), this chapter argues that the reform of the regulatory structure since the 1970s, a development driven by economic imperatives among a number of complex factors (for discussion of wider societal changes linked to CAM, see Chapters 1 and 2), has resulted in CAM no longer being subject to overly restrictive legislative restrictions. The implications of this liberalization of regulatory structure for consumers, CAM therapists, orthodox medicine and patients are also considered.

Over the past 40 years in most jurisdictions there has been a dramatic liberalization in the regulatory structure for CAM and an acknowledgement of the role of CAM in health care. This has occurred at a time when the popularity of CAM has burgeoned, caused partly by dissatisfaction with aspects of orthodox medicine, but also based on the values expressed in CAM. The emphasis of CAM on the whole person and not just disease and a stress on a partnership model of health care involving active participation by the client have provided a contrast in therapeutic approach to orthodox medicine (Crellin and Ania, 2002). CAM has a focus on the treatment of chronic disease for which orthodox medicine does not always provide effective treatment (Crellin and Ania, 2002). In a postmodern world where there is ready access to medical and health information, the position of the expert medical doctor has been eroded. This has meant that orthodox medicine does not enjoy the same ascendancy that it enjoyed in previous generations and CAM has become an attractive option for many health care consumers (Weir, 2005: 47).

The practice of medicine provision in Australia

Legislation in some states in Australia until recent years contained provisions that penalized 'the practice of medicine' or 'medical treatment' by persons who were not registered medical practitioners (Weir, 2005: 154). For non-registrants, the failure to define 'the practice of medicine' properly in this legislation meant that unregistered CAM practitioners risked prosecution for performing standard procedures if these activities were deemed to constitute medical practice. This had a chilling impact on CAM practice (Weir, 2005: 165). In addition, in some jurisdictions there were specific provisions that made it an offence to treat some health conditions such as cancer unless the person was a medical practitioner (for instance the Medical Practice Act 1992 (NSW) s108). These provisions have now been repealed, though they are now reflected in the New South Wales *Code of Conduct for Unregistered Health Practitioners* clause 5, which states that a health practitioner must not hold himself or herself out as qualified, able or willing to cure cancer and other terminal illnesses.

Registered health practitioner scope of practice provisions in Australia

The scope of practice provisions for registered CAM practitioners, chiropractors and osteopaths provided some difficult regulatory problems for unregistered CAM practitioners. Until recent years some state legislation limited 'the practice of chiropractic' to registered chiropractors, with exemptions for osteopaths, medical practitioners and physiotherapists. Some statutory definitions of 'the practice of chiropractic' were very broad and had the potential to proscribe many harmless therapies. The most problematic definition was in Queensland, which defined 'chiropractic' as 'the manipulation, mobilization and management of the neuromusculoskeletal system of the human body' (s 4 Chiropractors and Osteopaths Act 1979 (Qld)). This very broad and ill-defined description effectively encompassed procedures well beyond standard chiropractic practice and had the potential to proscribe standard practices by unregistered CAM practitioners. The Chiropractors Board of Queensland tended to enforce this provision only when unregistered practitioners were involved in spinal manipulation.

In Queensland and New South Wales, legislation relevant to physiotherapy included in the definition of 'physiotherapy' the provision of massage. Other than facial massage or massage provided as part of a training regime (which was exempt), this scope of practice definition meant that therapeutic massage as performed by unregistered practitioners was potentially illegal (Physiotherapists Act 1964 s 26 (2) (Qld); Physiotherapists Registration Act 1945(NSW) s 26(2)(e)). These provisions were repealed in Queensland in 2001 and in New South Wales in 2002 (Physiotherapists Registration Act 2001(Qld) s 216). Accordingly, until early in the twenty-first century, unregistered CAM practitioners in Australia were required to tread a wary path between regulatory restrictions in relation to the practice of medicine, chiropractic and physiotherapy, with the restrictions varying substantially between states.

A process of liberalization: 1990s

The Australian regulatory regime began to liberalize in the 1990s as part of the Competition Review that arose out of the Hilmer Report (The Report of the Independent Committee of Inquiry into National Competition Policy (1993)). The Hilmer Report recommended a review of state legislation to avoid anti-competitive provisions.

This process included a review of professional legislation with the potential to limit competition. The review required that any anti-competitive provision needed to be justified on the basis of the public interest (protection from injury). The use of broad scope of practice provisions over 'the practice of chiropractic' was abandoned for the more limited control of high-velocity spinal manipulation, as this practice was considered to provide a risk of injury to patients. In Queensland in 2001 the broad chiropractic scope of practice provision was deleted and replaced with controls over high-velocity manipulation (Section 120A Chiropractors Registration Act 2001). New South Wales made a similar provision (Section 10AC Public Health Act 1991).

The statutory scope of practice for physiotherapy was either abolished or limited to controls in a handful of states over the use of certain equipment, such as electro-physical treatments in New South Wales and Western Australia (Section 10 AD Public Health Act 1991 and s 20 A Public Health (General) Regulation 2002 NSW; Physiotherapists Act 2005 (WA) s 83).

The National Law

The next stage of the liberalization of the regulatory structure had its origin in Australia after the signing of the Intergovernmental Agreement for a National Registration and Accreditation Scheme for the Health Professions on 26 March 2008. This agreement resulted in the enactment of almost identical health profession legislation in each state and territory and the establishment of a national registration and accreditation system ('the National Law'). This scheme commenced on 1 July 2010.

Significant in this new regulatory scheme is that there are now no 'scope of practice' provisions applying to health professionals in any Australian jurisdiction.

The National Law does create offences for unregistered persons undertaking particular activities and describes three restricted acts that must only be performed by medical practitioners or specified registered health professions. The restricted act relevant to CAM is 'performing manipulation of the cervical spine'. This restricted act is defined in section 123 of the National Law: 'manipulation of the cervical spine means moving the joints of the cervical spine beyond a person's usual physiological range of motion using a high velocity, low amplitude thrust'. This definition is significantly narrower than the definitions of spinal manipulation that are familiar from repealed legislation, as it is limited to the cervical spine, which is normally defined to include the neck region of the spine containing the first seven vertebrae (Drake *et al.*, 2010: 58).

Accordingly, in relation to CAM the limits on practice that resulted from statutory scope of practice provisions or limits on the use of certain types of equipment have now been removed. Significantly, the National Law from 1 July 2012 will regulate TCM and acupuncture nationally.

The United States: a strict regulatory structure

The US model of regulation for CAM and orthodox medicine exhibits many similarities to the position in Australia, although there are some important distinctions. Most state jurisdictions in the United States still define 'medical practice' very broadly in their medical practice statutes to encompass most matters related to healing, and limit those acts to registered medical doctors (Cohen *et al.*, 2007: 27). There is a practice of enforcing these provisions against CAM practitioners (Cohen *et al.*, 2007: 28).

In contrast to Australia, the US regulatory structure provides for the licensing or statutory acknowledgement of a wide variety of CAM practitioners in statutes that define and thereby protect their statutory scope of practice. In the United States there is statutory regulation in some states for acupuncture, chiropractic, osteopathy, massage therapy, naturopathy and homoeopathy (Weir, 2005: 210; Cohen *et al.*, 2007: 30).

The US regulatory structure favours registered CAM modalities, as they are provided with some certainty in relation to their practice and protection from scrutiny while being carried out within their scope of practice, which is normally closely defined (Cohen *et al.*, 2007: 30). The protection afforded by statutory regulation is subject to scrutiny in some cases where a trespass into the practice of medicine has occurred, as has arisen for chiropractors offering nutritional advice (Cohen *et al.*, 2007: 30). The practice of an unregistered professional who has not yet obtained the endorsement of statutory regulation may be restricted and subject to proactive legislative enforcement.

The harsh nature of medical licensing legislation has meant that some states provide statutory protection for certain health practices, with some limitations. For example, in Rhode Island unlicensed health care practices such as the Alexander technique, rolfing, homeopathy and naturopathy are permitted if notice is given to the patient that the state has not adopted any educational or training standards for unlicensed health practitioners (Cohen *et al.*, 2007: 29). Similar provision is made in California (2002 Cal. Stat.820).

Canada: A liberal regulatory structure

The position in Canada reflects a generally more liberal stance towards CAM and in some provinces, similar to in Australia, the regulatory structure became much more accommodating for CAM from the early 1990s. In Ontario the omnibus legislation, the Regulated Health Professions Act 1991 (O) (RHPA), regulates health professions including chiropractic and massage therapy. Naturopaths are not regulated by the RHPA but by the Drugless Practitioners Act 1990 (O), as natural healing methods made the articulation of common standards of practice difficult (Weir, 2005: 56).

The RHPA regulates both practitioners and professional practice (Bohnen, 1994: 1). Each regulated profession also has a separate statute that should be read with the RHPA, or in some cases a statute that includes other professions such as osteopaths and physicians under the Medicine Act (O) (Bohnen, 1994: 10).

These modality-specific statutes define a scope of practice and any authorized acts of that profession (Bohnen, 1994: 10). This scope of practice provides a frame of reference or context for the performance of their authorized 'controlled acts' (Bohnen, 1994: 10). The heart of the professional regulation model is found in section 27 of the RHPA, which specifically defines 13 'controlled acts'. It is an offence for a person to perform a controlled act in the course of providing health services to an individual unless that person is authorized to do so by a health profession act, or the performance of the controlled act has been delegated to the person by an authorized person (s27 RHPA).

The process of reform is ongoing. In 2007 Ontario passed the Homoeopathy Act to regulate the practice of homeopathy in the province. The statutory regulation of homeopaths is rare. To date this legislation has not been enacted, although there is in place a Transitional Council of the College of Homeopaths of Ontario that is currently undertaking the drafting of regulations that will apply to this profession when the legislation commences (refer to www.collegeofhomeopaths.on.ca, accessed 31 May 2011).

British Columbia

British Columbia regulates health professions through the Health Professions Act 1996 (RSBC) (HPA). Health professions regulated under the HPA include orthodox medicine, physiotherapy, chiropractic, podiatry, acupuncture, naturopathy and massage therapy. The practice of medicine or an offer to practise medicine is confined to registered medical doctors (Medical

Practitioners Act 1996 (BC) s 81). Naturopaths are designated health professionals in British Columbia under the Naturopathic Physicians Regulation of the HPA:

> Naturopathic medicine means the art of healing by natural methods or therapeutics, including the first aid treatment of minor cuts, abrasion and contusions, bandaging, taking of blood samples, and the prescribing or administering or authorized preparations and medicines. (Naturopathic Physicians Regulation regulation 1)

Massage therapists are permitted to practise under the Massage Therapists Regulation of the HPA. The definition of massage therapy is broad, but does not include any form of medical electricity. This regulation preserves for massage therapists titles such as 'massage therapist' and 'registered massage practitioner' (Massage Therapists Regulation, regulation 3). Only massage therapists can practise massage therapy unless they are authorized by another statute or regulation (Massage Therapists Regulation, regulation 3).

Acupuncturists are permitted to practise under the Traditional Chinese Medicine Practitioners and Acupuncturists Regulation. Acupuncture is defined as:

> an act of stimulation, by means of needles, of specific sites on the skin, mucous membranes or subcutaneous tissues of the human body to improve health or alleviate pain, laser acupuncture, magnetic therapy or acupressure and moxibustion (JIU) and suction cup (Ba Guan). (Chinese Medicine Practitioners and Acupuncturists Regulation, regulation 1)

> Only an acupuncturist or TCM practitioner can insert acupuncture needles under the skin for the purpose of practising acupuncture unless that practitioner is permitted by some other statute or regulation (Traditional Chinese Medicine Practitioners and Acupuncturists Regulation (BC) r1, Regulation 4).

The significance of the British Columbia Regulation on TCM and acupuncture is that it provides both protection of title and scope of practice provisions for acupuncture and TCM. It acknowledges TCM by providing that (subject to the entitlements of other registered practitioners) only a TCM practitioner, acupuncturist or herbalist can make a traditional Chinese medicine diagnosis, and only a TCM practitioner or acupuncturist may insert acupuncture needles under the skin.

Implications of the liberalization of the regulatory structure

The liberalization of the regulatory structure evidenced particularly in Canada and Australia and to some extent in the United States provides some opportunities and challenges. The liberalization in Australia was born out of a movement to increase competition in the economy and in other jurisdictions to deal with the burgeoning demand for CAM from consumers. This process will allow the establishment and development of new modalities, for example different forms of massage, manipulation and ingestive modalities, that previously ran the real risk of falling foul of the broad and somewhat vague and broad scope of practice legislation. The narrower and better-focused legislation now applying in many jurisdictions will no longer have such a chilling effect on innovation and expansion of the frontiers of CAM. This may in turn lead to a greater acceptance of CAM, as it cannot be said that these practices are limited to a small number of registered health practitioners or medical doctors. A less restrictive legislative regime is likely to lead to greater variety in the potential therapies available to the consumer.

The process of liberalization has increased the number of registered CAM practitioners beyond the long-established chiropractors and osteopaths. Across a number of jurisdictions TCM practitioners, massage therapists and naturopaths have or will shortly be granted registered status. The advantage of registration for the consumer is the reliance on the fact that the practitioner has been assessed as having the required level of training and education. A consumer will be able to expect that generally a registered health practitioner will be subject to a statutory obligation to complete continuing professional education and to statutory disciplinary procedures. In this sense, the level of uncertainty in assessing the quality of CAM health practices is reduced by the statutory registration process (Weir, 2005: 309). The process of registration will also increase the prestige of the profession, although at the price of becoming subject to statutory ethical and practice parameters, continuing professional education and higher costs for registration (Weir, 2005: 302). The process of registration of CAM will also allow greater freedom for registered professionals, including medical doctors, to refer to CAM practitioners, as it is likely to be less problematic from the medical profession's perspective to refer to a registered health professional as against an unregistered health professional. This process may also accelerate the process of colonization of CAM modalities by orthodox medicine, which has already occurred in regard to acupuncture (Weir, 2005: 58).

The liberalization of the regulatory structure will also potentially expose consumers to unregistered and poorly trained practitioners providing therapies that were previously controlled; that is, non-cervical spinal manipulation, and in some jurisdictions use of heat, cold or other physiotherapy electrical equipment. To the extent to which the previous legislation protected against injury from the use of those modalities, the consumer may now be exposed to practitioners who have limited training and generally unenforceable ethical obligations. This issue is of particular importance in regard to CAM and health care generally, where there is always a degree of uncertainty from the consumer's perspective as to what is or is not valid and competent health practice (Weir, 2005: 305–06).

Further reading

Cohen, M.H., Ruggie, M. and Micozzi, M. (2007) *The Practice of Integrative Medicine: A Legal and Operational Guide.* New York: Springer.

Dimond, B. (1998) *The Legal Aspects of Complementary Therapy Practice: A Guide for Health Care Professionals.* Edinburgh: Churchill Livingstone.

Kelner, M., Wellman, B., Welsh, S. and Boon, H. (2006) How far can complementary and alternative medicine go? The case for chiropractic and homeopathy. *Social Science and Medicine* 63: 2617–27.

Timmermans, K. (2003) Intellectual property rights and traditional medicine: Policy dilemmas at the interface. *Social Science and Medicine* 57: 745–56.

Weir, M. (2011) *Complementary Medicine: Ethics and Law,* Sydney: Allen and Unwin.

References

Bohnen, L.S. (1994) *Regulated Health Professions Act: A practical Guide.* Ontario: Canada Law Book Inc.

Cohen, M.H., Ruggie, M. and Micozzi, M. (2007) *The Practice of Integrative Medicine: A Legal and Operational Guide.* New York: Springer.

Crellin, J. and Ania, F. (2002) *Professionalism and Ethics in Complementary and Alternative Medicine.* New York: Haworth Press.

Drake, R.L., Vogl, A.W. and Mitchell, M. (2010) *Gray's Anatomy for Students.* Edinburgh: Churchill Livingstone.

Weir, M. (2005) *Alternative Medicine: A New Regulatory Model.* Melbourne: Australian Scholarly Publishing.

Traditional, complementary and integrative medicine in perspective

Introduction

As discussed elsewhere in this collection (see Introduction for details), TCIM has attracted the attention of a growing number of scholars across a wide range of disciplines and fields. As a consequence, TCIM has not only been increasingly subject to analysis via rigorous methodology and through the lens of a range of 'critical' perspectives (undoubtedly a positive development), but it has in turn begun to offer new insights and directions for broader disciplines looking to refine, revise and refresh their curricula and gaze. In this section we focus on three such disciplinary perspectives, all relatively newly emerging, in the shape of health geography, public health and health economics.

In Chapter 26 Andrews and colleagues overview the historical engagement of geography with first traditional medicine and then more recently complementary and alternative medicine, both providing a review of geographical issues relating to CAM and also proposing a number of areas for future enquiry within health and medical geography.

Moving attention to traditional medicine in low-income countries, Hollenberg and colleagues consider the potential for traditional medicine to play a more central role in global health research and practice/provision. As the authors note, traditional medicine is often the first type of care sought by millions of people worldwide, yet its potential contribution to the well-being of patients and communities remains under-appreciated. In response, Hollenberg and colleagues argue that the inclusion of traditional medicine as a core focus within global health and within overall health care provision is crucial for the sake of the vast number of people and communities impoverished around the world, many of whom are not able to access professional biomedical services.

If TCIM is to be more systemically supported and integrated within health care systems (via any of the many models of integration outlined in the Introduction to Section 6 and in Chapter 18), one crucial line of argument will need to address the potential costs and benefits of incorporation and integration with reference to a solid evidence base. Disappointingly, this is an area of study that has not attracted significant attention within the agenda of the wider CAM research community; until relatively recently, that is. With the advance of collaborative approaches to research and also the widening of the CAM research gaze to include public health and health services research perspectives and methodologies, a growing number of studies have begun to emerge subjecting a range of CAM to economic methodological analysis. However, as Doran and colleagues explain in Chapter 28, the future growth in this area is dependent on establishing the clinical effectiveness of CAM – a line of research that has been advancing of late, but for which much more research effort is also required. Furthermore, as Section 7 illustrates, notions of evidence and efficacy are themselves far from straightforward with regard to TCIM and have been and remain topics of contestation and debate within the wider health research community.

CHAPTER 26

The geography of complementary and alternative medicine

GAVIN J. ANDREWS, JEREMY SEGROTT, CHI WAI LUI AND
JON ADAMS

Introduction

Prior to the emergence of complementary and alternative medicine (CAM) in many advanced industrial societies during the 1980s, geographers focused their research efforts on its 'predecessor', 'traditional medicine'. However, the need for geographers to research CAM, rather than traditional medicine, was first highlighted by Anyinam (1990), and the emergence of the 'geography of health' as a distinct area of investigation (Kearns, 1993) has involved a far more comprehensive engagement with CAM by contemporary geographers.

Geographical issues and literature

Place and healing

Some geographers have sought to investigate the construction and meaning of the spaces and places in which CAM therapies are performed. A key focus of this work is to think through how the characteristics of places such as the therapist's clinic might have therapeutic qualities, promote the healing process and help constitute the performance of CAM therapies. Williams (1998) and Andrews (2003), for instance, have applied Gesler's concept of the therapeutic

Source: Andrews, G., Adams, J. and Segrott, J. (2009) Complementary and alternative medicine (CAM): Production, consumption, research. In T. Brown, S. McLafferty and G. Moon (eds) *A Companion to Health and Medical Geography*. Oxford. Abridged version reprinted with kind permission of John Wiley & Sons Ltd (Wiley-Blackwell).

landscape to CAM to explore how the places where CAM is practised may produce feelings of health and well-being or promote healing. Williams suggests that practitioners create therapeutic landscapes, both because of the physical attributes of the spaces in which they deliver care and due to the strong inter-personal relationships that are built within them. In this sense, through the work they do, CAM practitioners can create 'authentic' or 'caring' environments that promote the healing process and CAM clients may come to attach particular meanings to the clinics where they receive treatment, and a sense of place can develop (Gesler, 1992; Williams, 1998; Andrews, 2003).

Imagination and visualization

Some work has taken the concept of therapeutic landscapes in new directions by considering how such landscapes might not only comprise physical settings, but also include places and spaces in the imagination (Andrews, 2004; Williams, 1998). These authors explore the ways in which many CAM therapists purposefully use imagination and visualization in their work, asking clients to visualize their own bodies as well as to imagine distant spaces as part of the healing process.

Alongside work on the role of place and its links with the construction of meaning and subjective experience in the practice of CAM, geographical studies have also examined the spaces in which CAM is performed, and how such spaces are produced, arranged and contested. One key focus of such work is the space of the clinic, in which encounters between practitioners and clients take place. Doel and Segrott (2004: 728), for example, explore the materialization of CAM and the importance of materials within therapeutic practice. Using a poststructuralist approach, they view CAM less in terms of unified therapies and more in terms of unique events in which practice depends on the articulation of bodies and materials: 'What takes place is always unexpected. It is always an event: a singular articulation of heterogeneous materials and practices with a unique consistency that is specific to each encounter.'

The authors describe three kinds of materials within the practice of CAM: 'signature materials' that 'exemplify the specificity of each therapy', such as aromatherapy's essential oils; 'supplementary materials' that enable practice to 'take place' and include the spatial setting itself and equipment such as the treatment couch and the 'marginalia' of waiting room furnishing, patient records and name plates. Each enactment of CAM requires a unique articulation of such materials, particularly given the ways in which the selection of aromatherapy oils (for instance) will be tailored to the individual client. Doel and Segrott also highlight a tension between the ongoing professionalization and regulation of CAM modalities that seeks to achieve greater standardization and accountability among practitioners, and the will of many CAM practitioners to retain their clinical autonomy and the individualized nature of their practice.

Drawing on the work of Fournier (1999), they suggest that the clinical autonomy of CAM is being governed 'at a distance' through the creation of generalizable 'work identities' and ways of being professional. This generaliz-able professionalism focuses on the margins of practice, such as the importance of note taking, the ethics and aesthetics of advertising, and the creation of a professional image. Such an image is to be achieved in large part through attending to space – to the ambience of the clinic (clean towels, good-quality couches) and the furnishing of the waiting room (comfortable seating and the presentation of a diverse set of objects, from framed qualification certificates to potted plants). As Doel and Segrott suggest, therefore, professionalization takes place through the regulation of micro-geographies and the ways in which previ-ously functional and neglected marginal materials are arranged in such spaces.

At another level, Andrews (2004) focuses on design features to explore the ways in which therapists seek to create a particular 'ambience' or 'feel' in their clinics. Andrews describes how clinics were designed and decorated to exert a subtle calming effect. The use of plush furniture, pastel colours, natural light, indoor foliage, water fountains, scents and 'new age' posters gave them a distinct 'spiritual' feel. However, in their study of the collaboration between CAM practitioners and biomedical professionals in a hospital setting, Mizrachi and colleagues (2004) suggest that spatial arrangements of this kind can reflect broader structures and inter-professional relationships: 'alternative practitioners copy the structure and symbols of the dominant [biomedical] professional group in the hospital' as a way of gaining legitimacy and recognition. They argue that such isomorphism is not only 'present in the dress code of alternative practitioners, which resemble that of physicians or nurses' and the 'furnishings and decor of their clinical settings, which are generally similar to those of their biomedical colleagues', but also in the professional conduct of some CAM prac-titioners, who even refer to their clients as 'cases' (Mizrachi *et al.*, 2004: 37).

The spatial diffusion of places

While the delivery of therapies by professional practitioners in private clinics remains important and commonplace, recent years have seen the diffusion of CAM into a range of new spaces, particularly through the increased consump-tion of self-treatment remedies and materials. Homeopathic preparations, aromatherapy oils, acupuncture pens, crystals and a bewildering array of manuals, self-help books, CDs and other sources of information are all now freely available (though only to those with the financial means). Wiles and Rosenberg (2001: 221) suggest that the growth in the use of CAM is linked to the growing importance of health and the body in western society and to the 'constant (re)formulation and negotiation of situated identities'. They suggest that CAM consumption takes place within a range of everyday geog-raphies and that the study of CAM should be situated within the 'geographies of consumption'. The newly dispersed geography of CAM therefore takes place in domestic space, workspace, retail space and the mass media (including magazines and the internet) alongside the therapist's clinic.

Exploring one such space, Doel and Segrott (2003) explore the mass mediation of CAM by health and lifestyle magazines and its displacement into consumer culture. As they note, 'the media … situate and enact CAM in terms of particular performances in specific settings, often in relation to everyday spaces such as the home and the workplace rather than medicalized spaces such as hospitals and clinics' (Doel and Segrott, 2003: 742). CAM is frequently presented as a 'de-differentiated' form of consumption, which extends beyond the treatment of discrete illness. The mass mediation of CAM presents it variously as a means of dealing with the diffuse disease of everyday life or as a pleasurable and sensuous form of consumption in which experiencing CAM may be an end in itself. In this sense, CAM comprises a diverse collection of materials and practices that readers can utilize to deal with almost every aspect of daily life (energy imbalances, stress, pollution in the environment and so on). Furthermore, Doel and Segrott argue that 'what CAM demonstrates above all else is not only the drawing of such things as experience, place and health into the orbit of the medical, but the dispersal of the medical itself' (2003: 744). Geographically, what this means is that CAM potentially enters every kind of conceivable space.

Future enquiry

Although geographers have now started to take an interest in CAM, there remains much more to be discovered. As we have indicated above, CAM is not only about health and health care: it is a much wider social and cultural phenomenon and has a central place in many people's everyday lives. With regard to social issues, there is a need for geographical research to examine the consumption of CAM in different social groups, their circumstances, experiences and outcomes. These groups could be demographically defined and involve age, income or ethnicity, for example. Otherwise they could relate to lifestyle or social situation and include sexuality or disability. In terms of production, there is also a need to consider the social character of providers, businesses and sectors.

With regard to cultural issues, research needs to examine the many identities associated with CAM production and consumption. These include spiritual and 'alternative' lifestyle cultures and consumer cultures, ranging from individuals and groups desperately seeking solutions to pressing health problems to those for which CAM is a status leisure activity. Future research also needs to locate CAM in local and regional cultures and specific versions of contemporary urbanism and rurality (Andrews *et al.*, 2004). Similarly, a historical perspective is required to investigate how CAM might contribute to the gradual 'becoming' and 'making' of places and exist as a source of historical contestation and struggle. Here, one potentially important area for research is the transportation of traditional medicine to places in the developed world. Postcolonial theory, with its sensitivity to diversity and critical understanding of the power relations and processes involved in the creation and oppression of the 'other', needs to be used in understanding how traditional medicines might be morphed into CAM in western cultural contexts.

Many political, policy and economic considerations also arise with CAM that have spatial dimensions. With regard to policy, still to be explored geographically are the regulation and training of CAM providers in places, the legal status of various modalities in places, the extent to which care is publicly provided or market driven, and a range of geographically defined policies with respect to CAM. With regard to economic issues, a number of fields of research can be identified. Traditional spatial analysis might map the flows of private and public finance associated with CAM and the factors that affect these flows. A closely aligned strand of research would model and map the macro-scale distributive features of labour markets from the international to the local level. Meanwhile, a more critical line of research, again focused on work, could investigate workplaces and their performative labour relations (Andrews and Evans, 2008). Indeed, therapists' workplaces may be complex constructions involving spatial routines, practices and power relationships. With regard to consumption, research questions might focus, for example, on the consumption experience of the 'clinic' and the situated experiences and negotiation of care. More generally, there is a need to acknowledge that CAM is female dominated in its production (Andrews and Hammond, 2004) and in some forms of consumption (Andrews, 2002). Hence, future research needs also to account for the ways in which gender interacts with specific places of CAM.

Finally, researching CAM in the above ways might contribute towards the development of health geography. At one level it has the potential to further expand the subdiscipline's growing understanding of health, especially with regard to notions of wellness, well-being and happiness. At another level, understanding geographies in the production of CAM might help the subdiscipline to engage far more deeply and critically with health care, including the nature of health work, workplaces, work practices and concepts in care (Andrews and Evans, 2008).

Further reading

Adams, J., Sibbritt, D. and Lui, C. (2011) The urban–rural divide in complementary and alternative medicine use: A longitudinal study of 10,638 women. *BMC Complementary and Alternative Medicine* 11: 2.

Robinson, A. and Chesters, J. (2008) Rural diversity in CAM usage: The relationship between rural diversity and the use of complementary and alternative medicine modalities. *Rural Society* 18(1): 64–75.

Wardle, J., Adams, J. and Lui, C. (2010) A qualitative study of naturopathy in rural practice: A focus upon naturopaths' experiences and perceptions of rural patients and demands for their services. *BMC Health Services Research* 10: 185.

Wardle, J., Adams, J., Magalhaes, R. and Sibbritt, D. (2011) The distribution of complementary and alternative medicine (CAM) providers in rural New South Wales, Australia: A step towards explaining high CAM use in rural health?' *Australian Journal of Rural Health* 19(4): 197–204.

Wardle, J., Lui, C. and Adams, J. (2011) Complementary and alternative medicine in rural communities: Current research and future directions. *Journal of Rural Health* doi.1111/j.1748-0361.2010.003848.x.

References

Andrews, G.J. (2002) Private complementary medicine and older people: Service use and user empowerment. *Ageing and Society* 22: 343–68.

Andrews, G.J. (2003) Placing the consumption of private complementary medicine: Everyday geographies of older peoples' use. *Health and Place* 9: 337–49.

Andrews, G.J. (2004) (Re)thinking the dynamics between healthcare and place: Therapeutic geographies in treatment and care practices. *Area* 36: 307–18.

Andrews, G.J. and Evans, J. (2008) Understanding the reproduction of health care: Towards geographies in health care work. *Progress in Human Geography* 32(6): 759–80.

Andrews, G.J. and Hammond, R. (2004) Small business private complementary medicine: Therapists' employment profiles and their pathways to practice. *Primary Health Care Research and Development* 5: 40–51.

Andrews, G.J., Wiles, J. and Miller, K.L. (2004) The geographical study of complementary medicine: Perspectives and prospects. *Complementary Therapies in Nursing and Midwifery* 10: 175–85.

Anyinam, C. (1990) Alternative medicine in western industrial countries: An agenda for medical geography. *Canadian Geographer* 34: 69–76.

Doel, M.A. and Segrott, J. (2003) Beyond belief? Consumer culture, complementary medicine, and the disease of everyday life. *Environment and Planning D: Society and Space* 21: 739–59.

Doel, M.A. and Segrott, J. (2004) Materializing complementary and alternative medicine: Aromatherapy, chiropractic, and Chinese herbal medicine in the UK. *Geoforum* 35: 727–38.

Fournier, V. (1999) The appeal to 'professionalism' as a disciplinary mechanism. *The Sociological Review* 47: 280–307.

Gesler, W. (1992) Therapeutic landscapes: Medical issues in the light of the new cultural geography. *Social Science and Medicine* 34: 735–46.

Kearns, R. (1993) Place and health: Towards a reformed medical geography. *The Professional Geographer* 45: 139–47.

Mizrachi, N., Shuval, J.T. and Gross, S. (2004) Boundary at work: Alternative medicine in biomedical settings. *Sociology of Health and Illness* 27: 20–43.

Wiles, J. and Rosenberg, M. (2001) 'Gentle caring experience.' Seeking alternative health care in Canada. *Health and Place* 7(3): 209–24.

Williams, A. (1998) Therapeutic landscapes in holistic medicine. *Social Science & Medicine* 46(9): 1193–203.

CHAPTER 27

Repositioning the role of traditional medicine as essential health knowledge in global health: Do they still have a role to play?

Daniel Hollenberg, David Zakus, Tim Cook and Xu Wei Xu

Introduction

One of the most widespread observations by critically informed scholars today is that the majority of evidence models for traditional medicine (TM) have consistently relied on laboratory and outcome studies of mechanisms of action and strictly controlled design models that are considered as at the top of the evidence-based medicine pyramid. Of particular consequence is that within this pyramid, internally consistent TM paradigms and explanatory models, on the whole, do not fit and are discounted as legitimate knowledge (Hollenberg and Muzzin, 2008). The hegemony of biomedical knowledge is also felt, for example, in the Cochrane Review online database of TM research, where meta-analyses of TM studies conclude that nearly all TM modalities reviewed are clinically ineffective or 'require more research'. It is not surprising, then, that the dominance of biomedical modes of enquiry into TM has left important pockets of TM completely unexplored, marginalized or poorly researched. One of these pockets is the role of TM in global health. Global health is understood to refer to health care important to populations around the world, especially for

Source: Hollenberg, D., Zakus, D., Cook, T. and Wei Xu, X. (2008) Re-positioning the role of traditional, complementary and alternative medicine as essetnail health knowledge in global health: Do they still have a role to play? *World Health and Population* 10(4): 62–74. Abridged version reprinted with kind permission of Wiley-Blackwell; Longwoods Publishing.

those most vulnerable and marginalized from the formal health system, with relevance to diverse aspects of health, illness, disease and wellness.

Despite having entered the limelight once again in the international health arena, TM remains stigmatized in a way that is not an accurate or fair representation of its full potential for the health of world populations. We are proposing that a shift is required to view TM more legitimately as an essential health resource for both local communities and wider populations alike. In focusing on the potential and future roles of TM, we represent a group of like-minded scholars and health care practitioners who recognize the importance of TM in international and global health.

TM is neither a pure and untapped resource that will become the 'new' primary health care technique to rid the world of disease, nor merely a vehicle to be appropriated by biomedical knowledge, with TM having no richly detailed and clinically effective health knowledge of its own. It is clear that TM does have merit, both in the context of primary health care and as clinically effective traditional health knowledge. In certain contexts TM clearly has the ability to affect physical disease categories in ways that closely resemble a biomedical 'cure', and that could be recognized by both biomedical doctors and traditional healers alike. Yet biomedically recognized forms of TM represent only a part of what TM would consider 'effective'. For TM, the amelioration of suffering is at times a complex interplay between the relief of physical symptoms and health on multiple other levels that include changes to psycho–emotional–spiritual states and reintegration with one's family or community. Perhaps baffling to biomedicine, TM often recognizes that there could exist 'healing without cure' and that healing can comprise multiple and intricate processes (Waldram, 2000).

The purpose of this chapter is thus (a) to re-examine the role of TM in the context of global health by highlighting specific areas where it can be viewed as important; (b) to draw on these examples to reposition TM critically as legitimate and essential knowledge for global health initiatives today; and (c) to discuss, by drawing on a more critical theoretical perspective, the inherent challenges to TM that are restricting it from being viewed as an essential part of international health projects. The majority of the discussion that follows will largely focus on TM in non-western health care settings, as it is TM in particular that has been most overlooked in global health.

Since 1978, a major part of TM has been recognized by the World Health Organization (WHO) as important for advances in global health. Recent TM policy documents have been generated (for example WHO, 2002, 2008) emphasizing the role of TM in health care systems. At the same time, the main prevention approach for major global diseases such as HIV/AIDS enacted by development leaders, including UNAIDS, the WHO and most aid organizations, is increased access to biomedical forms of drug-based treatment, such as antiretroviral (ARV) drugs, not TM. Critically informed anthropologists question why the 'evidence' and/or science of TM is not included in international development policy and projects.

As Kaboru *et al.* (2008) comment, what remains to be resolved is how this consistent biomedical orientation to large-scale international health projects will operate in various non-western targeted countries, where biomedical health care is out of reach financially to many, and staff are in short supply, overwhelmed or simply non-existent.

In certain areas of health care policy dealing with TM (see for example WHO, 1990; UNAIDS, 2000), TM is viewed as a targeted resource discussed as part of scaling-up efforts to control diseases such as HIV/AIDS and malaria. The main approach, continuing to reflect a biomedical bias towards TM, is to retrain traditional health practitioners (HPs) to deliver biomedical primary health care skills and services, such as public health education and counselling, and condom distribution in the case of HIV infections (see Peltzer *et al.*, 2006; UNAIDS, 2000). Although biomedical training for traditional HPs remains important, in the minority are new approaches that focus on biomedical HPs and traditional HPs learning together and from each other (see Kaboru *et al.*, 2006) and working together for the general good of their shared populations.

Even with focused efforts towards a more balanced approach to the professional interface between biomedical and traditional HPs, negative biomedical attitudes towards TM continue to surface among biomedical HPs, even in China, where TCM is protected by government policy and is a big part of shared tradition. An optimistic argument has been proposed by some commentators to suggest that the ongoing criticism by biomedical HPs working with traditional HPs reflects a critical awareness process full of conflict and tension, which it is hoped could adapt biomedical HPs so that they become reflective and capable of questioning their own assumptions, and also become more open to new perspectives (see Kaboru *et al.*, 2008: 121). In the professions literature, biomedical HPs are naively portrayed as simply reacting from their perspective of strong professional values that are resistant to new perspectives (Hall, 2005).

Repositioning the role of TM from marginalization to importance in global health

TM in particular has a long history in precolonial indigenous nations of treating a wide array of primary health care concerns, extending from first-aid-type treatment for broken bones and burns to treatment for acute physical symptoms associated with infectious diseases such as diarrhoea. Much TM knowledge was lost through the direct actions of colonial powers that banned use of TM in the nineteenth and twentieth centuries, when western medicine was professionalizing and expanding globally. However, numerous TM traditions and a great deal of health knowledge have re-established themselves and are now essential aspects of health care systems in their countries of origin. For example, in countries such as China, India, Vietnam, Japan, Korea, Nepal,

Thailand and various countries in Africa (such as Ghana), and in many other countries and regions, significant aspects of TM are directly integrated at national levels of health care systems (see WHO, 2002).

As will be discussed below using various examples, TM has provided and continues to provide direct forms of primary health care to global communities. By drawing on local resources, TM also provides important care to communities with low physician-to-population ratios and little access to western biomedicine.

Examples of TM and their potential use in global health

The efficacy of TM can be interpreted in a number of different ways, depending on one's theoretical orientation and what one counts as legitimate and illegitimate knowledge. The marginalization of TM also happens in a number of simultaneously occurring ways. TM is overlooked for its potential impact, recognized in only a limited fashion and ignored when biomedical results are produced. In the section that follows, we focus on the last category of biomedical forms of TM evidence that have been ignored and under-used in international health. Biomedical TM evidence represents only one type of 'evidence' that has been marginalized in international health projects, in addition to other evidence types that include different kinds of healing, from physical to spiritual levels. We have chosen the most biomedically amenable forms of TM evidence to highlight that even when TM is 'proven', it is largely ignored.

For the purposes of our discussion, then, the main strengths of TM that have been overlooked in the context of global health can be generally categorized into two main areas: (1) direct symptom management and reversal of acute diseases; and (2) health promotion, management and prevention related to illness and disease and maintaining well-being. These two related strengths of TM can be viewed as an integral part of primary health care in which TM is used to treat between 60 and 80 per cent of the global burden of disease (Kaboru *et al.*, 2006).

Discussion: Theorizing about challenges to TM in global health

Although WHO documents have possibly expanded the awareness of TM in the international health community, the response to TM that can be viewed in the international biomedical health literature continues to reflect a reductionist biomedical bias. Moreover, it is fair to say that the majority of policy issues involving TM as endorsed by the WHO have yet to be widely implemented by international health projects 'on the ground', also a likely symptom of the continued biomedical bias against TM. This lack of engagement can be repeatedly observed even with the renewed emphasis on TM by new leaders in the WHO. While stating that 'traditional medicine can also help prevent so-called modern lifestyle diseases such as diabetes, heart disease and mental disorders', WHO leaders insist that 'Many traditional medicines have an inadequate evidence base when measured by these [biomedical] standards' (Schearf, 2008). For example, health researchers around the world who are working directly with TM in HIV/AIDS patient populations are frustrated with this contradictory agenda (see Kaboru *et al.*, 2006).

From the pervasive conservative biomedical tradition that has 'invaded' international health policymaking, TM is viewed colonially as a resource only to be cautiously explored for its potential benefit to increase the effectiveness of biomedical primary health care techniques. From the biomedical perspective, the inherent challenge of TM is how to use a valuable resource while attempting to tame or restrict its 'wild', uncontrollable qualities (such as perceived side-effects and misguiding patients to ineffective treatments). Biomedical critics of TM are quick to ask that if TM can treat infectious diseases like malaria and HIV/AIDS, why has there not been an eradication of these diseases worldwide? The main response to this critique is that while TM is certainly not a 'cure-all' for infectious disease and drugs are certainly important, TM *can* have efficacy in locally embedded contexts. At the same time, however, the widespread therapeutic effect of local knowledge has been marginalized through colonization, with the overall consequence that TM is under-valued in today's biomedical and international health communities.

The inherent biomedical bias against TM has additional consequences that directly affect relationships between patients and traditional and biomedical HPs. Just as with CAM in more industrialized nations, patients using TM are hesitant to disclose their use of TM when consulting a biomedical HP, such as in a more formal primary health care clinic. Relations between biomedical and traditional HPs have historically been strained, with little communication and cross-referral, similar to tensions between biomedical HPs and CAM providers.

Establishing policy solutions for TM in global health?

Although there are many challenges ahead to repositioning TM as an essential resource in international health, it is useful to consider a different approach that might be taken in the future. We propose that at the outset, TM must be considered on its own as a legitimate and coherent system of locally embedded healing knowledge with relevance to the local communities in which it is used. Although this stance does not preclude its wider application to global populations (such as the use of the TCM herb *Artemisia* for malaria), TM can be most effectively used at the community level in which it originated and is practised. While TM is certainly not a panacea, substantial areas of health and wellness can be maintained with its use. TM also has the inherent strength of being able to work with or alongside other health measures and does not need to be altered by a biomedical agenda. For example, modified and culturally sensitive public health measures such as clean water, effective housing and shelter and access to viable food sources form an ecological system that promotes the efficacy of TM and the health of communities in which it is practised. Evidence already exists demonstrating that when TM is altered and/or synthesized for its component parts, not only does it become less effective, it also contradicts the bio-ethical tenet of non-maleficence by causing increased harm in patient populations (that is, increased side-effects and/or pathogen resistance, such as *artemisinin* for malaria).

Viewing TM as both legitimate and clinically effective health knowledge repositions TM in ways in which it has not previously been widely viewed. For example, this perspective moves past a purely ethnographic viewpoint that classifies TM as only a cultural practice without clinical benefit. It also reconceptualizes TM as having a healing benefit, not only as a vehicle for biomedical retraining. Some scholars are combining TM, activism and 'ecological' perspectives in the development community. For example, Trickett (2002) proposes movement away from macro-level international health campaigns towards ecological community-level interventions that directly address community issues by engaging the community context and create interventions by enhancing local resources; but without changing or appropriating them, as Pigg (1995) has cautioned.

Thus, the best way forward could be to forge partnerships between traditional HPs who practise TM and biomedical HPs associated with international primary health care projects. Policy makers have already imagined how partnerships could operate (Kaboru *et al.*, 2006), despite these professional patterns of interaction having yet to be implemented in many areas of the world.

Modified degrees of international policy intervention could also be implemented to recognize when an operational TM system requires little or no assistance from biomedical primary health care and, also, when biomedical HPs could be useful, based on community input. Many of these challenges and scenarios mirror developments in integrative medicine where biomedical and CAM practitioners are working together in the same clinic (see Hollenberg, 2006, 2007). Although far from resolving the above challenges, IM in more industrialized health care settings and countries has identified ideals that while perhaps utopian, include such concepts as 'trust', 'respect' and establishing a 'seamless continuum of care'.

It should also be re-emphasized that a handful of countries, as pointed out by the WHO, have established systems of TM and biomedicine that already work alongside each other and are at times approaching patterns of integration. For example, China has fully functional TCM–western IM hospitals. Although there are advances here, even China has not escaped the effect of the biomedical marginalization of TCM (see Scheid, 2002), pointing to the need to reposition TM as essential knowledge.

Conclusion

TM is often the first type of care sought by millions of people worldwide, although its place in the national and government-funded health systems of most countries is marginal, and its potential contribution to the well-being of patients and communities is under-appreciated and hardly recognized. For the sake of the vast number of people and communities impoverished around the world and their severe lack of professional biomedical services, it is important to reconsider the place of TM in overall health care and to begin to recognize its value for people worldwide.

Further reading

Adams, J. (2008) Utilising and promoting public health and health services research in complementary and alternative medicine: The founding of NORPHCAM. *Complementary Therapies in Medicine*, 16: 245–6.

Bodeker, G. and Burford, G. (eds) (2007) *Traditional, Complementary and Alternative Medicine: Policy and Public Health Perspectives*. London: Imperial College Press.

Wardle, J. and Oberg, E. (2011) The intersecting paradigms of naturopathic medicine and public health: Opportunities for naturopathic medicine. *Journal of Alternative and Complementary Medicine* (in press).

References

Hall, P. (2005) Interprofessional teamwork: Professional cultures as barriers. *Journal of Interprofessional Care* 19(1): 188–96.

Hollenberg, D. (2006) Uncharted ground: Patterns of professional interaction among complementary/alternative and biomedical practitioners in integrative health care settings. *Social Science and Medicine* 62: 731–44.

Hollenberg, D. (2007) How do private CAM therapies affect integrative health care settings in a publicly funded health care system? *Journal of Complementary and Integrative Medicine* 4(1). Available at http://www.bepress.com/jcim/vol4/iss1/5 (accessed 9 October 2008).

Hollenberg, D. and Muzzin, L. (2008) Epistemological challenges to integrative medicine. Unpublished manuscript.

Kaboru, B.B., Falkenberg, T., Ndubani, P. *et al.* (2006) Can biomedical and traditional health care providers work together? Zambian practitioners' experiences and attitudes towards collaboration in relation to STIs and HIV/AIDS care: A cross-sectional study. *Human Resources for Health* 4(16): 1–8.

Kaboru, B.B., Ndubani, P., Falkenberg, T. *et al.* (2008) A dialogue-building pilot intervention involving traditional and biomedical health providers focusing on STIs and HIV/AIDS care in Zambia. *Complementary Health Practice Review* 13(2): 110–26.

Peltzer, K., Mngqundaniso, N. and Petros, G. (2006) A controlled study of a HIV/AIDS/STI/TB intervention with traditional healers in KwaZulu-Natal, South Africa. *AIDS Behaviour* 10: 683–90.

Pigg, S.L. (1995) Acronyms and effacement: Traditional medical practitioners (TMP) in international health development. *Social Science and Medicine* 41(1): 47–68.

Schearf, D. (2008) WHO promotes Chinese model for integrated traditional medicine. *WHO Chinese Medicine Report.* Available at http://www.voanews.com/english/2008-11-17-voa26.cfm (accessed 18 November 2008).

Scheid, V. (2002) *Chinese Medicine in Contemporary China: Plurality and Synthesis.* Durham, NC: Duke University Press.

Trickett, E.J. (2002) Context, culture, and collaboration in AIDS interventions: Ecological ideas for enhancing community impact. *Journal of Primary Prevention* 23(2): 157–74.

UNAIDS (2000) Collaboration with traditional healers in HIV/AIDS prevention and care in Sub-Saharan Africa: A literature review. In *UNAIDS Best Practice Collection Geneva. Joint United Nations Programme on AIDS.* Geneva: UNAIDS.

Waldram, J.B. (2000) The efficacy of traditional medicine: Current theoretical and methodological issues. *Medical Anthropology Quarterly* 14(4): 609–25.

World Health Organization (1990) *Global Programme on AIDS and Traditional Medicine. Report of a WHO Consultation on Traditional Medicine and AIDS: Clinical Evaluation of Traditional Medicines and Natural Products.* Geneva, Switzerland: WHO.

World Health Organization (2002) *Traditional Medicine Strategy 2002–2005.* Geneva: WHO.

World Health Organization (2008) *Beijing Declaration, Adopted by the WHO Congress on Traditional Medicine, Beijing, China, 8 November 2008.* Geneva: WHO. Available at http://www.who.int/medicines/areas/traditional/TRM_BeijingDeclarationEN.pdf (accessed 10 November 2008).

CHAPTER 28

Review of economic methods used in complementary and alternative medicine

CHRISTOPHER DORAN, DENNIS CHANG, HOSEN KIAT AND
ALAN BENSOUSSAN

Introduction

In spite of the growing body of evidence on the quality and effectiveness of CM (Ernst, 2000; Cherkin *et al.*, 2003; Herman *et al.*, 2005; Debas *et al.*, 2006; White and Ernst, 2000), there is a dearth of evidence examining the economics of CM and, in particular, evidence relating to economic evaluation. There are two types of economic evaluation: partial and full (Drummond *et al.*, 2005). Partial evaluations are limited in scope because they focus on either costs or consequences but not both. Full economic evaluations compare both the costs and the consequences (or outcomes) of competing health care interventions, demonstrate whether the new intervention represents value for money, and present results as an incremental cost-effectiveness ratio that provides policymakers with the information required to justify expenditure decisions.

There are three types of full economic evaluation: cost-effectiveness analysis (CEA), cost–utility analysis (CUA) and cost–benefit analysis (CBA) (Drummond *et al.*, 2005). All types of analysis use a similar method for measuring and valuing the resources used in an intervention. The social perspective considers resource use from all potential stakeholders such as the government, health care providers and patients themselves. A third payer perspective is narrower and considers resources used specifically from the viewpoint of the health care insurer. The distinguishing feature between

Source: Doran, C., Chang, D., Kiat, H. and Bensoussan, A. (2010) Review of economic methods used in complementary medicine. *Journal of Alternative and Complementary Medicine* 16(5): 591–5. Abridged version reprinted with kind permission of Mary Ann Liebert, Inc.

245

analyses is how consequences are measured (and valued). In CEA, the consequence is measured in a unit natural to the intervention (for example, number of urinary tract infections prevented or life years saved). In CUA, the consequence is expressed as a more final outcome measure that considers changes to both quality and quantity of life as a result of the intervention. Common utility measures include the quality-adjusted-life-year (QALY) and the disability-adjusted-life-year. In a CBA, the consequences are measured, and then valued, in monetary terms, with results expressed as a ratio of costs to benefits. Drummond *et al.* (2005) provide a good overview of each technique.

Methods

A literature review of peer-reviewed publications identified 14 economic evaluations of CM (Herman *et al.*, 2005). The authors noted several possible explanations for the paucity of such evidence. First, consumers already spend considerable amounts of money on CM despite the limited scientific evidence of its efficacy. Secondly, economic evaluations have typically been required for the incorporation of new procedures and therapies under traditional financing mechanisms. Given that CM has traditionally fallen outside public funding, there has, perhaps, been little need to justify value for money (Herman *et al.*, 2005). In addition, some commentators have further suggested that the current application of economic evaluation techniques may be limited in CM given the inability of these techniques to capture accurately both the absolute magnitude of process-related benefits from CM and their magnitude relative to conventional treatment (Meenan 2001, 2005).

While CBA is considered to be the 'gold standard' in economic evaluation (Drummond *et al.*, 2005), the application of this technique in evaluating health care interventions is somewhat limited. This is due to the ethical issues surrounding the valuation of health improvement and ultimately human life (Ryan *et al.*, 2003; Meenan, 2005). However, a recent advance in the economics literature is the development of tools to translate underlying preferences and outcomes (both process and final) into monetary terms. The most common measure of benefit in monetary terms is willingness to pay (WTP) (Donaldson and Shackley, 2003) and there are two commonly accepted techniques to estimate WTP: contingent valuation methods (CV) and discrete choice experiments (DCE).

CV is a decision-based approach in which individuals are presented with a choice between not having a good or service and having the good or service but forgoing a certain amount of money. The WTP is equivalent to the money that they are willing to forgo to have the good or service (Donaldson and Shackley, 2003). It is important to note that WTP measures have also been criticized, as they are strongly influenced by an individual's ability to pay. DCE, on the other hand, is an attribute-based measure of benefit based on the assumption that any good or service can be described by its characteristics (or attributes), and the extent to which an individual values a good or service depends on the levels of these characteristics (Ryan and Gerard, 2003). The technique is also decision based and involves presenting choices to individuals that vary with respect to the level of attribute. The key feature of WTP assessments derived using DCE is the fact that process attributes can be factored into the decision-making process. WTP implicitly allows consumers to trade all relevant utility components with each other and with health. Another feature of DCE is that results can be used to produce utility estimates for alternatives with different attribute levels. These utilities can then be used in a CUA as the common outcome measure to compare two interventions (Ryan and Gerard, 2003; Ryan *et al.*, 2003).

Given that there is a range of economic methods available, the purpose of this research is to review the economic methods that have been used in CM. It is envisaged that such a review may shed light on the current state of play that economics can, and may, play in advancing the scientific rigour of CM.

Results

A total of 148 articles were located (later reduced to 43 articles after closer examination of each abstract to ensure that studies adopted some type of economic method). After closer inspection of these 43 studies, all related to traditional economic evaluations, with no studies identified exploring alternative economic methods. The economic evaluation studies were further scrutinized to remove partial economic evaluations. This left 15 full economic evaluations, which were then grouped into CM domains as defined by the US National Institutes of Health: biologically based practices; manipulative and body-based approaches; mind–body medicine; alternative medical systems; and energy medicine (NCCAM, 2007).

A summary of the key features of the 15 economic evaluations are provided in Table 28.1. Three articles related to the manipulative and body-based practices domain, five to the whole medical systems domain and seven to the biologically based practices domain. No full economic evaluations were identified for the domains of mind–body medicine, alternative medical systems or energy medicine.

In the manipulative and body-based practices domain, three studies conducted CUA: Korthals-deBos *et al.* (2004) compared physiotherapy, manual therapy and general practitioner (GP) care for patients with neck pain; Williams *et al.* (2004) compared osteopathy and GP care for patients with spinal pain; and van Tubergen *et al.* (2002) compared combined spa therapy, exercise therapy and usual care in patients with ankylosing spondylitis. All three evaluations were conducted alongside randomized controlled trials (RCT). Costs were collected prospectively using cost diaries completed by the

Table 28.1 Findings from literature review of economic methods used in complementary medicine

Country	Complementary medicine treatments against comparator of usual care (patient group)	Economic approach, study design (N)	Perspective, year	Economic outcome	Key finding	Ref.
Manipulative and body-based practices						
Netherlands	Physiotherapy versus manual therapy (patients with neck pain)	CUA, RCT (183)	Social, 1997–98	QALY	Manual therapy is the dominant treatment	15
Wales	Primary care osteopathy (patients with spinal pain)	CUA, RCT (187)	NHS, 1999–00	QALY	Primary care osteopathy may be a cost-effective addition to usual GP care	16
Netherlands	Combined spa therapy and exercise therapy (patients with ankylosing spondylitis)	CUA, RCT (120)	Social, 1999	QALY	Combined therapy is cost-effective	17
Whole medical systems						
Germany	Acupuncture (patients with chronic low-back pain, headache, pain of the knee, hip or neck)	CUA, RCT (8496)	Social, 2000–05	QALY	Acupuncture is cost-effective	18
USA	Hyperbaric oxygen (patients with severe foot ulcers from diabetes)	CUA, modelling (1000)	Social, 2001	QALY	Hyperbaric oxygen is cost-effective	19
UK	Acupuncture (patients with chronic low-back pain)	CUA, RCT (239)	NHS, 2001–02	QALY	Acupuncture is cost-effective	20
Germany	Acupuncture (patients with chronic neck pain)	CUA, RCT (201)	NHS, 2002–03	QALY	Acupuncture is cost-effective	21
UK	Acupuncture (patients with chronic headache)	CUA, RCT (401)	NHS, 2002–03	QALY	Acupuncture is cost-effective	22

Biologically based practices

Country	Intervention	Method	Perspective, year	Outcome	Conclusion	Ref
USA	Vitamin supplementation (folic acid and cyanocobalamin) (patients between 35 and 84 years)	CUA, population modelling	Health care, 1997	QALY	Vitamin supplementation may be cost-effective among many population subgroups and could have major epidemiological benefit from primary and secondary prevention of CHD	23
Italy	n-3 3 polyunsaturated fatty acids (PUFA) (patients with recent myocardial infarction (MI))	CEA, follow-up study (5664)	Third-party payer, 1999	Life years gained	n-3 PUFA is cost-effective compared with other drugs used in the routine care of secondary prevention after MI	24
Sweden	Calcium and vitamin D3 (women aged 50 years and over)	CUA, population modelling	Health care and social, 2000	QALY	Calcium and vitamin D3 are cost-effective for the 50- and 60-year-old cohorts and women with identified osteoporosis or a maternal family history of hip fracture	25
Canada	Concentrated cranberry tablets versus cranberry juice (women aged between 21 and 72 years)	CEA, RCT (150)	Social, 2000	Urinary tract infection	Cranberry tablets are the most cost-effective option for prevention of urinary tract infection	26
Australia	High-dose zinc and antioxidants (patients aged 55 years and over)	CUA, population modelling	Third-party payer, 2001	QALY	High-dose zinc and antioxidants should be further assessed for possible implementation	27
Australia	Photodynamic therapy (PDT) (patients with reasonable and poor visual acuity)	CUA, population modelling	Health care, 2003	QALY	PDT is moderately cost-effective for those with reasonable visual acuity but less cost-effective for those with initial poor visual acuity	28
Scotland	Multivitamin and multimineral supplementation (patients aged 65 years and over)	CUA, RCT (910)	NHS, 2003	QALY	Multivitamin and multimineral supplementation was dominant	29

CUA, cost–utility analysis; CEA, cost-effectiveness analysis; RCT, randomized controlled trial; QALY, quality-adjusted-life-year; CHD, coronary heart disease; NHS, National Health Services, UK.

patient (Korthals-deBos *et al.*, 2004) or clinical records (Williams *et al.*, 2004; van Tubergen *et al.*, 2002). QALY was used as the primary outcome measure, and all studies reported that the intervention treatment was cost-effective compared to usual care. Korthals-deBos *et al.* (2004) found manual therapy to be a dominant treatment (that is, less costly and more effective than either physiotherapy or GP care).

As highlighted in Table 28.1, five full economic evaluations (that is, CUA) were identified in the domain of whole medical systems. The studies involving acupuncture incorporated prospective data collection alongside a RCT, while Guo *et al.* (2003) developed a decision tree model to follow a hypothetical cohort of 1000 patients with severe foot ulcers from diabetes. QALY was reported as the primary economic outcome and all of the studies reported that the intervention treatment was cost-effective compared to usual care. For acupuncture treatment, all of the authors concur that acupuncture should be considered an option in the medical care of patients with chronic pain. Thomas *et al.* (2005) further suggest that more research is required to look at other forms of care in comparison to acupuncture, such as massage, chiropractic or physiotherapy.

The majority of full economic evaluations identified were in the biologically based practices domain. The review identified seven articles that examined a range of treatment alternatives across several countries. Franzosi *et al.* (2001) compared n-3 polyunsaturated fatty acids to usual care in patients after myocardial infarction; Tice *et al.* (2001) compared vitamin supplementation (folic acid and cyanocobalamin) in women aged between 35 and 84 years; Willis (2002) compared calcium and vitamin D3 to usual care in women aged 50 years and over; Hopley *et al.* (2004b) compared high-dose zinc and antioxidants to no screening or treatment in women aged 55 years and over; Hopley *et al.* (2004a) compared photodynamic therapy to usual care for the general population; Stothers (2002) compared cranberry products as a prophylaxis against urinary tract infections in women aged between 21 and 72 years; and Kilonzo *et al.* (2007) compared multivitamin and multimineral supplementation to usual care for patients aged 65 years and over. Five of the studies conducted a CUA and used QALY as the primary economic outcome, with the exception of Franzosi *et al.* (2001) and Stothers (2002), which adopted a CEA and used life years gained and urinary tract infections prevented, respectively, as the primary economic outcome. Three of the studies collected cost data prospectively: Franzosi *et al.* (2001) alongside a follow-up study, and Stothers (2002) and Kilonzo *et al.* (2007) alongside a RCT. The remaining studies used modelling techniques and relied on secondary data. A consistent finding across all studies was that the intervention treatment was cost-effective compared to usual care. Only one study suggested otherwise, finding that the use of multivitamin and multimineral supplements is not cost-effective for use in older people (Kilonzo *et al.*, 2007).

Discussion

This research has reviewed the economic methods that have been used in CM. Using a comprehensive search strategy, the literature review identified a total of 15 full economic evaluations. No evidence was found of CM research that had used alternative economic methods such as contingent valuation or discrete choice experiments. From those 15 economic evaluations, despite variations in project design and underlying methodologies, the overall results suggest that the CM interventions, as evaluated in these studies, are cost-effective compared to their respective conventional care interventions.

As health care costs continue to rise, decision makers, both consumers and policymakers, must allocate increasingly scarce resources towards those treatments that offer the best value for money. With the advent of guidelines on conducting economic evaluations that facilitate methodological consistency and scientific rigour, involving prospective data collection alongside an RCT, the opportunity now exists to promote a wider uptake of economic evaluation techniques in CM. However, it is worth noting that while the evidence base of CM has increased over the past decade, the majority of these medicines and therapies have not been comprehensively evaluated clinically. Without proven clinical effectiveness, it is meaningless to conduct economic studies on these interventions. This explains, at least partially, why the number of existing economic studies of CM remains small.

Given the high level of CM use in the community, it is important that more attention be devoted to developing a better understanding of the economic rationale for certain consumers preferring CM over conventional medicine. The recent advances in the development of tools to translate underlying preferences and outcomes into monetary terms provide a further opportunity to advance the science behind CM.

The implementation of high-quality economic research on CM does require a strong commitment by researchers, practitioners and manufacturers, as well as sustained financial support. Nevertheless, this commitment is essential if the public and health care providers are to have sufficient information to realize the full social and economic benefits of CM.

Further reading

Ford, E., Solomon, D., Adams, J. and Graves, N. (2010) The use of economic evaluation in CAM: An introductory framework. *BMC Complementary and Alternative Medicine* 10: 66.

Solomon, D., Ford, E., Adams, J. and Graves, N. (2011) The potential of St. Johns Wort for the treatment of depression. The economic perspective. *Australian and New Zealand Journal of Psychiatry* 45(2): 123–30.

References

Cherkin, D., Eisenberg, D., Sherman, K.J. *et al.* (2003) A review of the evidence for the effectiveness, safety, and cost of acupuncture, massage therapy, and spinal manipulation for back pain. *Annals of Internal Medicine* 138: 898–906.

Debas, H.T., Laxminarayan, R. and Straus, S.E. (2006) Complementary and alternative medicine. In D. Jamison, W.H. Mosley, A.R. Measham and J.L. Bobadilla (eds) *Disease Control Priorities in Developing Countries.* New York: Oxford University Press.

Donaldson, C. and Shackley, P. (2003) Willingness to pay for healthcare. In A. Scott, A. Maynard and R. Elliott (eds) *Advances in Health Economics.* Chichester: John Wiley & Sons Ltd.

Drummond, M.F., Sculpher, M., Torrance, G.W., O'Brien, B.J. and Stoddart, G.L. (2005) *Methods for the Economic Evaluation of Health Care Programmes.* Oxford: Oxford University Press.

Ernst, E. (2000) Prevalence of use of complementary and alternative medicine: A systematic review. *Bulletin of the World Health Organization* 78: 252–7.

Franzosi, M.G., Brunetti, M., Marchioli, R. (2001) Cost-effectiveness analysis of n-3 poly-unsaturated fatty acids (PUFA) after myocardial infarction. *Pharmacoeconomics* 19: 411–20.

Guo, S., Counte, M.A., Gillespie, K.N. and Schmitz, H. (2003) Cost-effectiveness of adjunctive hyperbaric oxygen in the treatment of diabetic ulcers. *International Journal of Health Technology Assessment in Health Care* 19: 731–7.

Herman, P.M., Craig, B.M. and Caspi, O. (2005) Is complementary and alternative medicine (CAM) cost-effective? A systematic review. *BMC Complementary and Alternative Medicine* 5: 11.

Hopley, C., Salkeld, G. and Mitchell, P. (2004b) Cost utility of photodynamic therapy for predominantly classic neovascular age related macular degeneration. *British Journal of Ophthalmology* 88: 982–7.

Hopley, C., Salkeld, G., Wang, J.J. and Mitchell, P. (2004b) Cost utility of screening and treatment for early age related macular degeneration with zinc and antioxidants. *British Journal of Ophthalmology* 88: 450–54.

Kilonzo, M.M., Vale, L.D., Cook, J.A. *et al.* (2007) A cost–utility analysis of multivitamin and multimineral supplements in men and women aged 65 years and over. *Clinical Nutrition* 26: 364–70.

Korthals-de Bos, I., Hoving, J., van Tulder, M. *et al.* (2003) Cost effectiveness of physiotherapy, manual therapy, and general practitioner care for neck pain: Economic evaluation alongside a randomised controlled trial. *British Medical Journal* 326: 911.

Meenan, R. (2001) Developing appropriate measures of the benefits of complementary and alternative medicine. *Journal of Health Services Research and Policy* 6: 38–43.

Meenan, R. (2005) Applicability of discrete-choice methods to economic evaluations of complementary and alternative medicine. *Expert Review of Pharmacoeconomics and Outcomes Research* 5: 479–87.

National Center for Complementary and Alternative Medicine (2007) *What Is CAM?* Bethesda, MD: NIH.

Ryan, M. and Gerard, K. (2003) Using discrete choice experiments in health economics: Moving forward. In A. Scott, A. Maynard and R. Elliott (eds) *Advances in Health Economics.* Chichester: John Wiley and Sons Ltd.

Ryan, M., Watson, V. and Amaya-Amaya, M. (2003) Methodological issues in the monetary evaluation of benefits in healthcare. *Expert Review of Pharmacoeconomics and Outcomes Research* 3: 717–27.

Stothers, L. (2002) A randomized trial to evaluate effectiveness and cost effectiveness of naturopathic cranberry products as prophylaxis against urinary tract infection in women. *Canadian Journal of Urology* 9: 1558–62.

Thomas, K., MacPherson, H., Thorpe, L. *et al.* (2005) Longer term clinical and economic benefits of offering acupuncture care to patients with chronic low back pain. *International Journal of Health Technology Assessment in Health Care* 9: 1–109.

Tice, J.A., Ross, E., Coxson, P.G. *et al.* (2001) Cost-effectiveness of vitamin therapy to lower plasma homocysteine levels for the prevention of coronary heart disease: Effect of grain fortification and beyond. *Journal of the American Medical Association* 286: 936–43.

Van Tubergen, A., Boonen, A., Landewe, R. *et al.* (2002) Cost effectiveness of combined spa–exercise therapy in ankylosing spondylitis: A randomized controlled trial. *Arthritis and Rheumatism* 47: 459–67.

White, A. and Ernst, E. (2000) Economic analysis of complementary medicine: A systematic review. *Complementary Therapies in Medicine* 8: 111–18.

Williams, N.H., Wilkinson, C., Russell, I.T. *et al.* (2004) Cost–utility analysis of osteopathy in primary care: Results from a pragmatic randomized controlled trial. *Family Practice* 21: 643–50.

Willis, M.S. (2002) The health economics of calcium and vitamin D3 for the prevention of osteoporotic hip fractures in Sweden. *International Journal of Health Technology Assessment in Health Care* 18: 791–807.

Witt, C., Brinkhaus, B., Reinhold, T. and Willich, S. (2006) Efficacy, effectiveness, safety and costs of acupuncture for chronic pain: Results of a large research initiative. *Acupuncture in Medicine* 24(S1): 33–9.

Wonderling, D., Vickers, A.J., Grieve, R. and McCarney, R. (2004) Cost effectiveness analysis of a randomised trial of acupuncture for chronic headache in primary care. *British Medical Journal* 328: 747.

Future agendas: Key debates and themes

Introduction

In this final section of the reader, authors reflect on a selection of issues imperative to the future of TCIM in terms of practice and research developments and the relationship between these two spheres (specifically in relation to practitioners-as-researchers [Chapter 30] and the capacity-building needs of practitioners and academics in the CAM research community [Chapter 31]). As the collection here attests, there have been many advances in understanding and investigating TCIM over recent decades, with a plethora of increasingly good-quality research literature now available to scholars and practitioners on this area.

In Chapter 29, Coulter reflects on contemporary integrative medicine and offers a personal perspective on a way forward for the field. As Coulter identifies, the advancement of integrative medicine must face a number of challenges (also see Chapters 18 and 19 for detailed overviews of similar challenges facing attempts to integrate the different forms of health care), yet, he also argues, few movements within the context of CAM (at least within western societies) offer the excitement and opportunities of integrative medicine. Agreement or disagreement with this perspective will no doubt depend in part on the location and vantage point of the reader; as the work of Hsiao and colleagues (Chapter 18) and more forcefully that of Fan and Holliday (Chapter 19) illuminates, it is critical that we not overlook or underestimate the political and cultural mangle in which collaborative practice and integration must operate.

Rewinding to the work of Fonnebo and colleagues (Chapter 22), we are reminded of the importance of clinical effectiveness studies mirroring the pragmatic clinical realities of CAM. This is a theme that also runs through the arguments of Wardle and Seely (Chapter 30) with regard to the challenges and issues facing the TCIM practitioner base in a drive to engage with research and/or participate in the research process. Ultimately, as Adams also suggests (Chapter 31), TCIM practitioners represent one huge but in many cases untapped resource with which to advance the capacity of TCIM research and ensure that the findings of investigation into TCIM sufficiently reflect practice realities and effectively feed into health care practice and policy.

The prospect of producing a stronger, increasingly rigorous evidence base for TCIM across a broad spectrum of agendas and concerns (including but also widening well beyond clinical context to include public health, health services research and other major contributions) and building on the successes of the CAM research community to date should not be underestimated. However, as Adams (Chapters 31) and others in the field stress, such a prospect does not simply rely on critical, innovative thinking and sound, rigorous methodology, but also on an ability to continue to attract and retain good-calibre practitioners and academics as part of a growing and sustainable research community. The CAM research community (both as individuals and as a collective) will need to rise to these challenges if all populations in diverse parts of the globe are to benefit fully from the potential of TCIM in helping treat illness and maintain health, based on a broad and substantial evidence base gleaned from rigorous, scientific study.

CHAPTER 29

The future of integrative medicine: A commentary on complementary and alternative medicine and integrative medicine

IAN COULTER

Introduction

In the history of CAM in western societies, few movements offer the excitement and opportunities of integrative medicine (IM). To the extent that IM signals a new relationship between biomedicine and CAM, for the first time we are seeing CAM such as chiropractic, naturopathy, acupuncture and massage therapy being practised in settings from which they have been historically excluded (such as hospitals). In 2003 a national survey of 1007 hospitals in the United States documented that 16 per cent provided IM and over 27 per cent offered some form of CAM (Larson, 2005).

In the United States, chiropractors are now to be found throughout the Veterans Administration hospitals and clinics and military treatment facilities (Lisi *et al.*, 2009), and in general hospital where even 20 years ago they would never have been found. Indeed, CAM and IM have increasingly been seen as part of US health care and reimbursed by managed care entities, insurance carriers and hospital providers (Pelletier *et al.*, 1997).

Not all of this is due to IM. Chiropractors were finding their way into such settings independent of IM, although there is no doubt that under IM, more CAM groups are finding themselves in such places as medical schools and academic health centres (Bhattacharya, 1998). However, not all groups seem to welcome CAM equally into academic health centres. Such groups as acupuncture, traditional Chinese medicine and massage seem to be preferred to others such as chiropractic, naturopathy and homeopathy. A version of IM is also developing that is not dependent on the inclusion of CAM. In many settings it is politically and strategically advantageous to use the umbrella of IM to introduce CAM. This can be seen most clearly in centres treating cancer patients, where CAM is being used as an adjunctive therapy. In departments of paediatric oncology at prestigious universities such as UCLA, it is now possible to find acupuncture and massage therapy. This would have been almost inconceivable a decade ago.

Despite this achievement, there are some challenges facing CAM and its inclusion in IM. Bell *et al.* (2002) assert that care that simply combines biomedicine with CAM is not integrative, instead arguing that true IM 'represents a higher order system of care that emphasizes wellness and healing of the entire person (bio-psycho-socio-spiritual dimension) as primary goals, drawing on both conventional and CAM approaches in the context of a supportive and effective physician–patient relationship' (Bell *et al.*, 2002: 133).

It should be noted that while current IM in the US may be driven by many factors, integration of CAM and biomedicine is predominantly being driven by patients as they combine both approaches to treatment (Pelletier *et al.*, 1997; Ni *et al.*, 2002; Barnes *et al.*, 2004; Wolsko *et al.*, 2004). Larson (2005), in a national survey of 1007 hospitals in the United States, documented patient demand as the most significant factor (83 per cent) for incorporating IM/CAM. To the extent that this is being driven by patients, we can expect that the pressures to maintain such developments will continue. But is it necessarily all good news for CAM?

The definitional problem

In this commentary I define IM as a process in which integration or convergence between biomedicine and CAM occurs without necessarily implying the degree of integration, the nature of the integration or the process by which it is achieved. However, the definition of integrative health care can range from simply incorporating CAM into conventional medicine to the notion that integrative health care constitutes a new form of medical practice (Bell *et al.*, 2002; Maizes *et al.*, 2002; Boon *et al.*, 2004). It is not always clear that it necessarily includes CAM. A single definition, or set of definitions, for IM has been difficult to establish even for leading entities that shape health care policy and practice (Ullman, 2009).

Why is the definition important? If IM is defined as a new form of 'medicine' it might once again exclude CAM. Even the term integrative medicine as opposed to integrative health care is problematic. Some within the CAM field do not see themselves as practising *medicine* (for instance massage therapy) but health care. Politically it will be easier to develop IM within university settings if in fact it does not insist on CAM inclusion. There are few university-based programmes in chiropractic, naturopathy or homeopathy except where they are CAM universities (which many of the chiropractic colleges now term themselves).[1] One could predict that introducing a school or faculty of integrative medicine into a university academic health science centre might be an easier sell than introducing a school of CAM.

Types of integration

There are three possible approaches to the integration of CAM and biomedicine: incorporate those CAM therapies that have passed rigorous scrutiny (evidenced-based therapies) into biomedicine and biomedical practice; incorporate those CAM therapies that have passed the test of time into biomedicine and biomedical practice (for example acupuncture); incorporate selected CAM therapies that are licensed/CAM providers that are credentialled or licensed. CAM can be adopted (co-opted) into biomedicine itself as largely adjunctive therapy without its philosophical elements. It may be that the first option more accurately describes what is happening in university-based centres.

The question that must be asked here is whether this is a process of integration or co-optation. Unless there is genuine joint management of patients, can we really talk about integration? Khorsan *et al.* (2010), in a review of over 10 000 articles on IM, found that few studies focused on the incorporation of a collaborative and integral partnership of an integrated health care system. That is, the integration of conventional (allopathic) medicine and CAM – involving shared management of the patient, shared patient care, shared practice guidelines and shared common values and goals to treat the well-being of the whole person – is not found in the literature.

To call it *integrative* implies some process in which integration or convergence occurs that may or not be true. Even if true, this does not capture the nature of the integration or the process by which it has been achieved (Hyman, 2005).

Strategies for integration

Centres of IM differ in the type of staff who primarily deliver and manage the care (e.g. physicians, nurses, specially trained CAM providers); sources of revenues (e.g. fee for service, health insurance, philanthropy, research grants); type of delivery setting (e.g. teaching hospital, non-profit or for-profit hospital, community clinic); type of care they provide (e.g. primary care, adjunctive, maintenance care after conventional medical care is not effective); and in

---

[1] In Australia there are chiropractic programmes in universities and this is also true in Europe, but this is the exception not the rule. In the United States only one college is based in a traditional university.

strategic approaches to integrating CAM into biomedicine (e.g. incorporating only those CAM therapies and providers who are credentialled or licensed already). IM care can be delivered in vastly different ways and in vastly different settings and with vastly different therapies (Coulter and Khorsan, 2011). In the United States, integrative medicine is being developed in a highly individualistic manner.

Some of these settings have been traditionally off limits to CAM providers and raise serious questions about differences in licensing, registration, educational accreditation, malpractice insurance, primary contact status and ability to diagnose; the very things that highlight the extreme variation among the groups that have been collectively termed CAM. IM therefore has the potential to drive a serious wedge between those CAM groups that will make it in and those that will not.

Paradigms

As Coulter (2004) has noted, CAM and biomedicine are based on two distinct paradigms, and have distinct philosophical foundations, a priori assumptions and metaphysical beliefs that are considered by many to be incommensurable, incomparable and contradictory. The challenge is whether IM will acknowledge and respect the philosophical basis of CAM. Cassidy (1995) notes that the different paradigms reflect two different ways of constructing reality in our society: reductionism by biomedicine and holism by CAM. These paradigmatic differences are recognized by the public. And this is the challenge for CAM participating in IM. Will the groups have to 'sell their soul' to participate? Will such things as acupuncture be practised only as a therapy devoid of any of its philosophical basis in traditional Chinese medicine? Will yoga be separated from its basis in Ayurvedic medicine? Will chiropractic be practised without any reference to innate intelligence? For most groups this might mean abandoning the vitalism that the CAM groups all share in one form or another.

At the most fundamental level, an IM clinic brings together those who offer a service (biomedical providers) and those who offer what can be perceived as an adjunctive or competitive service (IM/CAM providers), those who regulate integration (administrators) and those who seek a service (IM/CAM patients). Each of these stakeholder groups has a distinct stake in integrative medicine and many of these may be in conflict. Moreover, integrating an IM clinic into a hospital setting requires a change not only in the attitudes of medical staff, but also in the relationship between CAM providers and the hospital. There must also be an acceptance by the patients with regard to the use of CAM. Thus, from a social and cultural perspective, for CAM to be fully integrated it must become a seamless part of a social nexus uniting these numerous stakeholders, not all of whom will be committed to it and many of whom have been strong opponents of CAM.

Integration of CAM and IM will continue to face challenges, including historical professional animosity; changes in work environment infrastructure; culture and relationships; economic competition; the lack of clearly agreed principles on which to base integration at organizational and health care system levels; and the variation in organizational models that exist. In some settings chiropractic will be part of the team; in others it will never be invited to participate. It may be excluded because of the animosity of the medical staff. It may be included because its practitioners are licensed, are covered by insurance, have malpractice insurance and represent the most frequently requested CAM by the public and consequently may generate the most income. A telling example is provided in California, where in two IM clinics that are about 20 miles apart, one includes chiropractic and one does not. When asked, the director of the latter said that she would not dare bring chiropractic into what is a very prestigious medical centre because of hostile medical opposition. In the former, a community-based clinic, the director said: 'This is a patient-centered care facility and chiropractic was the most requested by the patients and they also do the most billing for us.'

The EBP trap

One common strategy that is proposed for integrating CAM is to include those therapies for which there is an evidence base. IM represents a rather recent but emerging field (Coulter, 2007). For example, the report prepared for the IOM conference on IM notes that both clinical effectiveness and cost-effectiveness are required 'to formulate evidence-based policy' (Sox and Greenfield, 2009: 3). However, while there is an increasing body of literature on the clinical effectiveness of CAM and a much smaller literature on cost-effectiveness, there is a much smaller evidence base at the moment for IM. CAM research represented about 0.02 per cent[2] in 2009 of the NIH budget and its inclusion in NIH as a separate section dates only from 1992.

There are two problems with using evidence as the basis for inclusion. The first is that the standard being applied to CAM could not in fact be met by medicine, even currently when about 20 per cent of treatment is considered to be evidence base. Furthermore, no other professions had to meet this standard prior to being accepted into universities or hospital settings. The second problem is that for some groups there is a body of literature about efficacy and effectiveness, but for others there is no such body of evidence, simply because no one has yet bothered to create it. Again, this will create two classes of CAM providers: those thought to be evidence based and those who are not.

---

2   Personnel correspondence with staff of NCCAM 2010.

Financial sustainability

Of all the problems that confront IM in the United States, the most compelling is financial viability or sustainability. Although no data exist for this, it is likely that a great number of such programmes have ceased to exist because they failed to develop a sustainable financial model (Coulter *et al.*, 2008). Many of the existing institutional programmes have been funded through philanthropy and/or grants. Others have offered the CAM services as a way of attracting or retaining patients. This can be seen in some cancer treatment centres, where the CAM is adjunctive therapy. There are many financial barriers to a successful IM clinic, one of which is insurance. While an increasing number of insurance plans incorporate CAM, they tend to be selective in what they will cover. They also vary in the amount of payment they will make per visit and the number of visits they will reimburse. Since CAM treatments for the most part tend to be much longer than visits for biomedicine, this is seldom recognized in the insurance reimbursement.

Traditionally, CAM providers have operated with a fee-for-service model. However, this is not the model that exists within many of the institutions. So to introduce this model into such centres can set up a comparison that hurts the CAM. Coulter *et al.* (2007) found in their study of a hospital-based IM programme that patients resented paying for a CAM service when they could go to another service in the hospital, such as physical therapy, and have it covered by insurance.

To the extent that IM may involve a variety of services, it can be an expensive option. This constitutes another significant challenge, providing IM to the under-serviced population. Because of this numerous models have been developed. Dovey (2001) suggests that the medical institutional models of integration that have been implemented can be delineated into five types. The most prevalent type, the 'virtual' model, characterizes 75 per cent of hospital-based programmes. This model is also known as a 'clinic without walls', as CAM services are dispersed throughout a hospital or medical system; it requires little internal restructuring and reduces costs, as it typically draws on existing medical staff to add on complementary services (for instance, physical therapists provide therapeutic massage). In contrast, consultatory models, either focused on a particular medical specialis, or more generalized, rely on referrals from staff physicians to in-house CAM providers, with the referring physicians maintaining responsibility for these patients. Dovey (2001) suggests that the third model of primary care integrating CAM and biomedicine is the least common because it positions IM/CAM providers in direct competition with staff physicians. The fourth model, fitness or wellness centres, may provide a funnel system for CAM providers, as does the increasingly popular fifth model, the health spa, which, while more closely aligned to the hotel and service industries, caters to high-end clients willing to pay out of their own pocket for high-end CAM services in a retreat-like environment.

Vohra *et al.* (2005) used content analysis of their notes from site visits to nine successful IM programmes in North America. These programmes, few of which were financially profitable, institutionalized two or more 'pillars' of integration: clinical care, education or research. Twelve key themes related to successful integration were identified: a flexible, low-cost, small start-up; hiring top clinicians; containing costs by hiring within; keeping the clinical component broad but the research pillar focused; establishing and tracking evaluation benchmarks; documenting utilization; having the team in place before formally opening the clinical component; keeping administration lean; making use of electronic record keeping; investing in high-end scalable information technology; and giving priority to revenue-generating space.

The way forward

CAM is more than simply a set of therapeutic interventions. CAM is offered within a distinct health encounter, and within usually a distinct philosophy of health and health care, both of which may have a direct and indirect impact on the efficacy of such interventions. At the most fundamental level, an IM clinic brings together those who offer a service (biomedical providers) and those who offer what can be perceived as an adjunctive or competitive service (IM/CAM providers), those who regulate integration (administrators) and those who seek a service (IM/CAM patients). Each of these stakeholder groups has a distinct stake in integrative medicine and many of these may be in conflict. Moreover, integrating an IM clinic into a hospital setting requires a change not only in the attitudes of medical staff but also in the relationship between CAM providers and the hospital. There must furthermore be acceptance on the part of the patients with regard to the use of CAM. Thus, from a social and cultural perspective, for CAM to be fully integrated it must become a seamless part of a social nexus uniting these numerous stakeholders, not all of whom will be committed to it and many of whom will have been strong opponents of CAM.

Further reading

Fortney, L., Rakel, D., Rindfleisch, J. and Mallory, J. (2010) Introduction to integrative primary care: The health-orientated clinic. *Primary Care* 37(1): 1–12.

Maizes, V., Rakel, D. and Niemiec, C. (2009) Integrative medicine and patient-centered care. *Explore: The Journal of Science and Healing* 5(5): 277–89.

References

Barnes, P.M., Powell-Griner, E., McFann, K. and Nahin, R.L. (2004) Complementary and alternative medicine use among adults: United States. *Advance Data* 343: 1–19.

Bell, I.R., Caspi, O., Schwartz, G.E. *et al.* (2002) Integrative medicine and systemic outcomes research: Issues in the emergence of a new model for primary health care. *Archives of Internal Medicine* 162(2): 133–40.

Bhattacharya, B. (1998) Programs in the United States with complementary and alternative medicine education: An ongoing list. *Journal of Alternative and Complementary Medicine* 4(3): 325–35.

Boon, H., Verhoef, M., O'Hara, D., Findlay, B. and Majid, N. (2004) Integrative healthcare: Arriving at a working definition. *Alternative Therapies in Health and Medicine* 10(5): 48–56.

Cassidy, C.M. (1995) Social science theory and methods in the study of alternative and complementary medicine. *Journal of Alternative and Complementary Medicine* 1(1): 19–40.

Coulter, I.D. (2004) Integration and paradigm clash. In P. Tovey, G. Easthope and J. Adams (eds) *The Mainstreaming of Complementary and Alternative Medicine: Studies in Social Context.* London: Routledge, pp. 103–22.

Coulter, I.D. (2007) Evidence based complementary and alternative medicine: Promises and problems. *Forsch Komplementarmed* 14(2): 102–08.

Coulter, I.D., Ellison, M.A., Hilton, L., Rhodes, H. and Ryan, G. (2007) *Hospital-Based Integrative Medicine: A Case Study of the Barriers and Factors Facilitating the Creation of a Center,* RAND MG-591-NCCAM.

Coulter, I., Hilton, L., Ryan, G., Ellison, M. and Rhodes, H. (2008) Trials and tribulations on the road to implementing integrative medicine in a hospital setting. *Health Sociology Review* 17(4): 368–85.

Coulter, I.D. and Khorsan, R. (2011) Complementary alternative and integrative medicine: Current challenges for outcomes measurement. In J. Magnabosco and R. Manderscheid (eds) *Outcomes Measurement in the Human Services: Cross-Cutting Issues and Methods.* Washington, DC: National Association of Social Workers Press.

Dovey, D. (2001) *Basic Principles of Complementary/Alternative Medicine: Clinicians' Complete Guide to Complementary/Alternative Medicine.* St Louis, MI: Moseby, pp. 5–7.

Hyman, M.A. (2005) Finding the right medicine: Skillful means. *Alternative Therapies in Health and Medicine* 11(2): 10–12.

Khorsan, R., Coulter, I.D., Crawford, C. and Hsiao, A. (2010) Systematic review of integrative health care research: Randomized control trials, clinical controlled trials, and meta-analysis. *Evidence-Based Complementary and Alternative Medicine* 2011: 1–10.

Larson, L. (2005) Integrating integrative medicine – a how-to guide. *Trustee* 58(10): 14–16, 21–22.

Lisi, A.J., Goertz, C., Lawrence, D.J. *et al.* (2009) Characteristics of Veterans Health Administration chiropractors and chiropractic clinics. *Journal of Rehabilitation Research and Development* 46(8): 997–1002.

Maizes, V., Schneider, C., Bell, I. and Weil, A. (2002) Integrative medical education: Development and implementation of a comprehensive curriculum at the University of Arizona. *Academic Medicine* 77(9): 851–60.

Ni, H., Simile, C. and Hardy, A.M. (2002) Utilization of complementary and alternative medicine by United States adults: Results from the 1999 national health interview survey. *Medical Care* 40(4): 353–8.

Pelletier, K.R., Marie, A., Krasner, M. and Haskell, W.E. (1997) Current trends in the integration and reimbursement of complementary and alternative medicine by managed care, insurance carriers, and hospital providers. *American Journal of Health Promotion* 12(2): 112–23.

Sox, H.C. and Greenfield, S. (2009) Comparative effectiveness research: A report from the Institute of Medicine. *Annals of Internal Medicine* 151(3): 203–05.

Ullman, D. (2009) A review of a historical summit on integrative medicine. *Evidence Based Complementary and Alternative Medicine* 7(4): 511–14.

Vohra, S., Feldman, K., Johnston, B., Waters, K. and Boon, H. (2005) Integrating complementary and alternative medicine into academic medical centers: Experience and perceptions of nine leading centers in North America. *BMC Health Services Research* 5: 78.

Wolsko, P.M., Eisenberg, D.M., Davis, R.B. and Phillips, R.S. (2004) Use of mind–body medical therapies. *Journal of General Internal Medicine* 19(1): 43–50.

CHAPTER 30

The challenges of traditional, complementary and integrative medicine research: A practitioner perspective

JON WARDLE AND DUGALD SEELY

Introduction

As in any health practice, traditional complementary and integrative medicine (TCIM) practitioners will see clinical results that provide insights and clues to guide optimal patient care. However, good care also requires exploring external sources of information beyond clinical practice, and applying this knowledge in a way that enhances patient care. Such external information sources may include traditional knowledge, anecdotes from other practitioners and informal inter-professional networks. However, as the broader health care world moves into a more 'evidence-based' paradigm, scientific research and knowledge transfer will need to play an ever larger role in TCIM practice.

Issues with TCIM research

The TCIM community has argued that typical research evaluation techniques do not often accurately represent clinical TCIM practice (Mason *et al.*, 2002). The scientific community, however, has argued that TCIMs need to be evaluated like any other therapies. Both arguments are valid. What is required is research that accurately reflects and evaluates TCIM as it is practised in real-world settings. A key consideration of clinical research that accurately evaluates the practice in question is model validity. Model validity implies that the application of research does indeed reflect the care provided in real-life settings and the philosophical basis of the system explored (Lewith *et al.*, 2002).

A major issue with TCIM research is that much of the research performed by those with intimate knowledge of the therapies – such as TCIM practitioners – often lacks scientific rigour due to insufficient methodological or research training. Likewise, much of the research performed by experienced researchers may not have adequate model validity and accurately evaluate TCIM treatments due to lack of knowledge or experience of the therapies themselves. For example, while acupuncture texts document that auricular acupuncture can treat tachycardia, but generally has little effect on normal heart rates, a randomized controlled trial (RCT) that failed to lower heart rates in healthy volunteers has been used to dismiss claims that auricular acupuncture could be effective in lowering heart rate (White and Ernst, 1999). Just as medical interventions are only effective when used appropriately, evaluation of TCIM requires collaboration with someone with intimate knowledge of TCIM to ensure model validity.

Some TCIM practitioners may also be motivated to enter research to 'prove' that their particular therapies work. This approach can lead to intentional or unintentional bias and methodological flaws that reduce scientific rigour and objectivity. Ample preparation and collaboration with methodological experts can help reduce the potential for these problems to arise. Additionally, TCIM practitioners may not fully appreciate the methods and types of data to be collected in clinical practice that contribute to sound and unbiased results. For example, TCIM practitioners may not understand the importance of using validated outcome measures in clinical research, or, even if they do, may not have the research experience to identify the most appropriate validated tool (a database of outcome measures can be found at www.outcomesdatabase.org).

Incorporating evidence-based principles into practice

TCIM practitioners also require skills that allow them to engage with and critically appraise research findings – and to translate these into improved clinical outcomes for their patients – if TCIM is to be incorporated more broadly into the evidence-based world.

David Sackett, the 'grandfather' of the evidence-based medicine movement, suggested that '(g)ood doctors use both individual clinical expertise and the best available external evidence, and neither alone is enough' (Sackett, 1996). Without incorporating the clinical expertise of the practitioner, practice risks becoming tyrannized by evidence. Even excellent external evidence may be inapplicable to, or inappropriate for, an individual patient, failing to recognize the contribution of the individual and the confounding role of multiple factors.

However, without current best evidence, practice risks becoming rapidly out of date, to the detriment of good patient care. The development of new information can assist practitioners in prioritizing choice of therapeutic options based on risk–benefit ratios. New information may also help make practitioners aware of novel therapies or procedures that fit within the scope of TCIM. Moreover, evidence can also make practitioners aware of harms that have previously not been considered.

The nature of evidence in TCIM practice

Most research to date has focused on narrowly applied clinical and experimental trials that have explored safety, efficacy and mechanism of action. However, studies are required that also examine the effectiveness of TCIM therapies. Whereas efficacy refers to whether interventions work under ideal conditions – that is, '*Can* this work?' – effectiveness refers to whether the intervention works under 'real-life' conditions as would be experienced in clinical practice – that is, '*Does* this work?' While efficacy remains important, these areas of research form only part of the TCIM research equation. The World Health Organization Traditional Medicine Strategy, for example, outlines a broad research agenda that looks beyond issues of clinical efficacy (World Health Organization, 2002).

As implied above, a focus on classic research designs such as RCTs may not always be methodologically appropriate for the evaluation of TCIM (Mason *et al.*, 2002). Modern interpretation and utilization of evidence-based RCTs often fail to recognize the complexities of real-world clinical settings, for example by the wholesale exclusion of 'real-world' variables such as patients with co-morbid conditions (Fortin *et al.*, 2007). Although the pressure to rely only on 'gold-standard' RCTs is often overwhelming, evidence-based practice relies on 'best available evidence', which may include all levels of evidence (Mills *et al.*, 2002).

Additionally, RCTs are not a homogenous entity in and of themselves and can be split between 'explanatory' and 'pragmatic' RCTs (Thorpe *et al.*, 2009). Explanatory RCTs are the 'classic' RCT favoured for reductionist evaluation in the biomedical model, which tests for efficacy under highly controlled settings within a highly selected population. Pragmatic trials, on the other hand, test for effectiveness in 'real-world' clinical settings in comparatively flexible conditions and participants. These may form the basis of 'whole practice' investigations. Examples of this type of whole-practice trial include a series of RCTs conducted by one of the authors that incorporated semi-individualized naturopathic treatments to treat the conditions of low-back pain (Szczurko *et al.*, 2007), rotator-cuff tendonitis (Szczurko *et al.*, 2009) and anxiety (Cooley *et al.*, 2009).

Non-clinical research may also be valuable for TCIM. Public health and health services research may critically examine the professional status and role of TCIM practitioners in the broader health setting, which may help to highlight the potential of and opportunities for incorporating TCIM therapies and practitioners into the broader health system (Wardle and Oberg, 2011).

However, broader research questions relevant to the development of TCIM as a field also need to be complemented by research that is directly relevant to TCIM practice 'at the coalface'.

Benefits of TCIM practitioner research involvement

There are numerous benefits for TCIM practitioners in engaging with research. Benefits to practitioners themselves include the assumption of valuable new clinical skills and knowledge with which to treat patients, as well as developing skills to enable them individually and critically to assess new developments in their fields. This may build their development and understanding of their discipline – or of medicine/TCIM more broadly. Exposure to new ideas may also renew enthusiasm in TCIM for those clinicians who feel as though their practice has become 'stale'. For those who do choose to move into research or academia more tangible benefits may exist, for example providing alternative sources of income to clinical practice.

Building research capacity among TCIM practitioners also has broader benefits for TCIM. TCIM practitioner clinical expertise is invaluable to good TCIM study design – who better to help design research studies in TCIM practice than those who actually practise TCIM? Beyond this, building research capacity among TCIM practitioners expands TCIM research, as many researchers without such a background may simply be uninterested in evaluating TCIM.

Practitioners of any persuasion have obligations to ensure that patients receive the best available treatment. Involvement in research can be an excellent complement to practice, providing a reflexivity that is beneficial to patient care (Zick and Benn, 2004; Steinsbekk, 2007). Some commentators have even suggested that practitioners may be ethically obliged to participate in research in order to comply fully with their duty of care to patients and ensure that they are able to have access to the best available treatment (Ives *et al.*, 2009).

Benefits to TCIM of increased practitioner involvement

The evolution and growth of a profession require the development of an evidence base. This requires not only clinical evidence, but broader public health and health services research to identify the role that TCIM can play in health care delivery. The legitimacy of any profession arguably depends on its ability to take a critically self-reflexive approach. In a health care world where evidence-based practice is becoming more important, building the evidence base of TCIM therapies is imperative to ensuring their ready inclusion in contemporary health care.

Research has a role in bridging the gap between conventional health care and TCIM. It offers a common language and approach for rigorous comparison of

TCIM and conventional treatment options (Fonnebo *et al.*, 2007) and provides data for the development of clinical guidelines (Shekelle *et al.*, 1999). However, it is also a major factor in conventional provider or health service manager decisions to refer to TCIM or to integrate TCIM practitioners into treatment plans or services (Maha and Shaw, 2007).

Broader research engagement may also be an indicator of a profession's maturity. Higher research involvement generally increases involvement in academic settings, which may have positive policy and integration implications. Additionally, the development of networks beyond the internal TCIM group – for example fostering collaborations – may facilitate positive change in both internal (TCIM) and external (non-TCIM) culture in relation to TCIM integration.

Challenges

Despite the obvious benefits of collaboration, there remain significant barriers. Most practitioners have a focus on clinical outcomes. This is understandable, given that the primary goal of most TCIM practitioners is to facilitate improved health in their patients, not to facilitate research. Combined with the traditionally marginalized nature of TCIM, this can make engaging practitioners difficult. Some TCIM practitioners may also be distrustful of research, particularly those without scientific worldviews (Boon, 1998). As in any multidisciplinary environment, inter-personal tensions may exist that affect research projects when collaborative arrangements between researchers and TCIM practitioners are formed.

Difficulties exist in engaging TCIM practitioners in research even when they are supportive. For example, a survey of US naturopaths found that although 40.7 per cent would recommend that their patients participate in a research project, only 25.5 per cent would support recruiting from their own clinics (Weber and McCarty, 2007).

This may be due in part to TCIM practitioners seeing research as relevant to how the public and the broader health system view TCIM, but not necessarily relevant to clinical practice. Moreover, although incoming students of some TCIM disciplines have a strong interest in research, some studies suggest that interest in research may diminish as students mature into clinicians (Wayne *et al.*, 2010).

Research literacy among TCIM practitioners is also often limited (Leung *et al.*, 2005). Busy TCIM practitioners may also prioritize clinical encounters over keeping up with fast-paced changes in the literature, or even if they do exhibit interest, may find it difficult to keep up while maintaining a busy patient load. Further methodological and research design training may not be possible without severe disruption to their clinical practice (Verhoef *et al.*, 2010).

How can practitioners become involved?

TCIM practitioners do not need personally to design and conduct studies to become more involved in the research process. TCIM practitioners may choose to develop collaborative arrangements with researchers, for example through networks such as the Network of Researchers in the Public Health of CAM (www.norphcam.org).

Another way in which TCIM practitioners may become more actively involved in the research process is through 'lower-hierarchy' research activities such as writing up case reports or case series. Although these provide informal observations that are uncontrolled, are not subject to scientific method, cannot be independently confirmed and are considered anecdotal, they are often regarded as an invitation to more rigorous scientific research (Vandenbroucke, 2001). However, many TCIM therapies lack even these lower hierarchies of evidence. A set of guidelines developed and published for naturopathic doctors is readily applicable for TCIM practitioners in general (Leung and Seely, 2009).

Encouraging organized data collection in practice can also engage practitioners in the research process. Development of a systematic approach to practice is essential, as is effectively documenting information when developing an evidence base for a profession. Documenting aspects of clinical practice through practitioner-based research development is also important for identifying an appropriate role for TCIM in broader health care settings (Steinsbekk, 2007). Practitioners may formalize this relationship via involvement in a practice-based research network (PBRN), which involves researchers and clinicians in a collaborative research community that focuses on clinical problems. Ongoing PBRN data collection itself may be analysed to offer valuable clinical or professional insights, or the collaboration may be used to facilitate clinical trials that actively involve TCIM practitioners in clinical practice. The Naturopathic Practitioners Research Institute is an example of a mature TCIM PBRN, and information on current studies can be found on its website (www.nprinstitute.org).

Importance of collaboration

Rigorous TCIM research requires the active collaboration of experienced TCIM practitioners (Pearson and Chesney, 2007; Adams and Wardle, 2009). Involving TCIM practitioners in collaborative research work is a win–win scenario. Skills acquired in clinical practice may not always translate effectively to the research field, and working closely with established researchers can provide methodological expertise and rigour. Meanwhile, experienced researchers may be divorced from clinical applications or distanced from practice issues and working with an experienced practitioner can help to ground and contextualize studies with grass-roots realities.

Through developing collaborative arrangements with researchers, practitioners can become involved in research while still committing primarily to practice. Moreover, aligning with methodological experts may allow TCIM practitioners to demonstrate objectivity in research studies with which they are involved as a counterweight to possible criticism – even if such criticism is unfounded.

Conclusion

Research is an essential component of modern medicine. Not only does the involvement of practitioners in research enrich research itself, it also proffers tangible benefits to the patient, TCIM practitioner and TCIM professions. As the health care world moves towards an integrated model of evidence-based health care, it is essential that TCIM practitioners take a more proactive attitude to research and the application of methods that accurately reflect and test their therapies. This contribution to rigorous evaluation can come either through analysis and implementation in practice, or through more active participation in developing a strong evidence base for TCIM.

Further reading

Leung, B. and Seely, D. (2009) Guidelines to case report writing for naturopathic doctors. *International Journal of Naturopathic Medicine* 4(1): 50–54.

Steinsbekk, A. (2007) The practitioner as researcher: Research capacity building within the ranks of CAM. In J. Adams (ed.) *Researching Complementary and Alternative Medicine*. London: Routledge.

Verhoef, M.J., Mulkins, A., Kania, A., Findlay-Reece, B. and Mior, S. (2010) Identifying the barriers to conducting outcomes research in integrative health care clinic settings – a qualitative study. *BMC Health Services Research* 10: 14.

References

Adams, J. and Wardle, J. (2009) Engaging practitioners in research. *Journal of Complementary Medicine* 8: 5.

Boon, H. (1998) Canadian naturopathic practitioners: Holistic and scientific world views. *Social Science and Medicine* 46: 1213–25.

Cooley, K., Szczurko, O., Perri, D. *et al.* (2009) Naturopathic care for anxiety: A randomized controlled trial. *PLoS ONE* 4: e6628.

Fonnebo, V., Grimsgaard, S., Walach, H. *et al.* (2007) Researching complementary and alternative treatments: The gatekeepers are not at home. *BMC Medical Research Methodology* 7: 7.

Fortin, M., Soubhi, H., Hudson, C., Bayliss, E. and van Den Akker, M. (2007) Multi-morbidity's many challenges. *British Medical Journal* 334: 1016–17.

Ives, J., Draper, H., Damery, S. and Wilson, S. (2009) Do family doctors have an obligation to facilitate research? *Family Practice* 26: 543–8.

Leung, B. and Seely, D. (2009) Guidelines to case report writing for naturopathic doctors. *International Journal of Naturopathic Medicine* 4: 50–54.

Leung, B., Verhoef, M. and Dryden, T. (2005) Mentorship programs within a network to build research literacy and capacity in complementary and alternative medicine (CAM) Practitioners. *Journal of Complementary and Integrative Medicine* 2: 9.

Lewith, G., Walach, H. and Jonas, W. (2002) Balanced research strategies for complementary and alternative medicine. In G. Lewith, H. Walach and W. Jonas (eds) *Clinical Research in Complementary Therapies: Principles, Problems and Solutions.* Edinburgh: Churchill Livingstone.

Maha, N. and Shaw, A. (2007) Academic doctors' views of complementary and alternative medicine (CAM) and its role within the NHS: An exploratory qualitative study. *BMC Complementary and Alternative Medicine* 7: 17.

Mason, E., Tovey, P. and Long, A. (2002) Evaluating complementary medicine: Methodological challenges of randomised controlled trials. *British Medical Journal* 325: 832–4.

Mills, E., Hollyer, T., Guyatt, G., Ross, C., Saranchuk, R., Wilson, K. for the Evidence-Based Complementary and Alternative Medicine Working Group (2002) Teaching evidence-based complementary and alternative medicine: 1. A learning structure to clinical decision changes. *Journal of Alternative and Complementary Medicine* 8: 207–14.

Pearson, N. and Chesney, M. (2007) The CAM education program of the National Centre for Complementary and Alternative Medicine: An overview. *Academic Medicine* 82: 921–6.

Sackett, D. (1996) Evidence based medicine: What it is and what it isn't. *British Medical Journal* 312: 71–2.

Shekelle, P., Woolf, S., Eccles, M. and Grimshaw, J. (1999) Clinical guidelines: Developing guidelines. *British Medical Journal* 318: 593–6.

Steinsbekk, A. (2007) The practitioner as researcher: Research capacity building within the ranks of CAM. In J. Adams (ed.) *Researching Complementary and Alternative Medicine.* London: Routledge.

Szczurko, O., Cooley, K., Busse, J. *et al.* (2007) Naturopathic care for chronic low back pain: A randomized trial. *PLoS ONE* 2: e919.

Szczurko, O., Cooley, P., Mills, E., Zhou, Q., Perri, P. and Seely, D. (2009) Naturopathic treatment of rotator cuff tendonitis amongst Canada Post workers: A randomized controlled trial. *Arthritis Rheum* 61: 1037–45.

Thorpe, K., Zwarenstein, M., Oxman, A. and Al, E. (2009) A pragmatic-explanatory continuum indicator summary (PRECIS): A tool to help trial designers. *Canadian Medical Association Journal* 180: E47–57.

Vandenbroucke, J. (2001) In defense of case reports and case series. *Annals of Internal Medicine* 134: 330–34.

Verhoef, M., Mulkins, A., Kania, A., Findlay-Reece, B. and Mior, S. (2010) Identifying the barriers to conducting outcomes research in integrative health care clinic settings – a qualitative study. *BMC Health Services Research* 10: 14.

Wardle, J. and Oberg, E. (2011) The intersecting paradigms of naturopathic medicine and public health: Opportunities for naturopathic medicine. *Journal of Alternative and Complementary Medicine* in press.

Wayne, P., Hammerschlag, R., Savetsky-German, J. and Chapman, T. (2010) Attitudes and interests toward research among students at two colleges of acupuncture and alternative medicine. *Explore* 6: 22–28.

Weber, W. and McCarty, R. (2007) Interest of naturopathic physicians in pediatric research. *Journal of Alternative and Complementary Medicine* 14: 445–6.

White, A. and Ernst, E. (1999) The effect of auricular acupuncture on the pulse rate: An exploratory randomised controlled trial. *Acupuncture in Medicine* 17: 86–88.

World Health Organization (2002) *WHO Strategy for Traditional Medicine 2002–2005.* Geneva: World Health Organization.

Zick, M. and Benn, R. (2004) Bridging CAM practice and research: Teaching CAM practitioners about research methodology. *Alternative Therapies in Health and Medicine* 10: 50–56.

CHAPTER 31

Research capacity building in traditional, complementary and integrative medicine: Grass-roots action towards a broader vision

JON ADAMS, DAVID SIBBRITT, ALEX BROOM, JON WARDLE, AMIE STEEL, VIJAY MURTHY AND JANE DALEY

Introduction

Developing capacity to undertake health research effectively is an integral component of national and global health research systems (Lansang and Dennis, 2004) and is essential to producing a sound evidence base for decision making in policy and practice (Cooke, 2005). Moreover, research capacity building (RCB) – nurturing and producing sustainable increased capacity for future research endeavours – is important for all health research fields and TCIM is no exception (Andrews, 2006; Adams, 2007). There is currently a great opportunity to embrace RCB in relation to TCIM in order to help develop an evidence base and a stronger and more robust research culture among scholars and practitioners alike.

This chapter explores the needs and opportunities surrounding RCB in TCIM with reference to an ongoing programme developed over recent years by the Network of Researchers in the Public Health of Complementary and Alternative Medicine (NORPHCAM). While this programme is focused on public health and health services research, the approach and strategy of the NORPHCAM capacity-building programme provide insights relevant to the wider international TCIM research community.

The NORPHCAM experience: Context and aims

The NORPHCAM network was founded in 2008 with two overarching aims: to promote and conduct rigorous public health and health services research on traditional medicine, complementary and alternative medicine and integrative health care and to facilitate and directly promote RCB in the TCIM field. Recent years have seen growth in the volume and quality of TCIM scholarship (particularly around CAM) and a number of initiatives in the United Kingdom, United States and Canada have begun to address the issue of capacity building in this field (Lewith *et al.*, 2006). Yet, as the National Center for Complementary and Alternative Medicine (NCCAM) programme in the United States has identified, there is much work to be undertaken around capacity building for the TCIM field (NCCAM, 2011). The NORPHCAM Executive has also identified such a gap and NORPHCAM was partly established as a capacity-building venture to address these RCB needs directly with reference to TCIM public health/health services research and beyond. The NORPHCAM RCB programme has been devised and refined with the input and aid of many professional organizations working in partnership with practitioner-based representatives to maintain practice and practitioner relevance.

Challenges facing RCB in TCIM

One major difficulty facing attempts to foster research capacity in TCIM has been related to the somewhat fragmented resources and disparate researchers in the field. A number of TCIM-specific university schools and departments, research centres and other institutions have evolved across a number of countries. Nevertheless, it remains that a substantial and significant proportion of researchers conducting empirical study into TCIM are located in organizational units whose research is broadly disciplinary (that is, units and centres of public health, pharmacy, health services research, health economics and so on) and in which TCIM is but one of a spectrum of research interests competing for attention and resources. This does pose challenges for those seeking to identify and motivate the full capacity of expertise available to the TCIM field and has to date partly led to a fragmented RCB approach for TCIM.

Meanwhile, such circumstances have also helped (and will continue to help) support an influx of researchers to the TCIM field who can be primarily identified as methodologists: heavily grounded in disciplinary perspective(s) and equipped with rigorous methodological and research design training (Andrews, 2006). Such recruits have the potential to transform TCIM scholarship into a truly robust, rigorous field that will attract the attention (and funding) of national and international grant agencies. A number of crucial RCB challenges relate specifically to this issue: a need to attract and retain more methodologists to the TCIM field; and, of equal importance, a need for such methodologists to work in close collaboration with colleagues who possess TCIM-specific expertise (for example practitioners) to ensure that enquiry is appropriate to TCIM practice realities and needs and can feed into policy and practice development (see Chapter 30 for more details relating to the research needs of practitioners).

Maximizing the potential of TCIM practice and research for the benefit of patients, providers and policymakers requires a concerted effort on behalf of a number of interested stakeholders. However, as the next section of this chapter will outline, there are very real practical steps that the 'grass roots' of the TCIM research community can undertake to achieve short-term advances towards developing human resource development in the context of a systems and long-term perspective (Lansang and Dennis, 2004).

What do we need to do?

RCB endeavours involve developing enabling environments with particular reference to leadership, career structure, critical mass, infrastructure, information access and interfaces between research producers and users (Lansang and Dennis, 2004). Ultimately, many aspects of RCB in TCIM demand a national or international coordinated effort (including government involvement) in order to establish infrastructure and ongoing funding. However, we should not restrict ourselves to relying on others beyond the TCIM field and there is much that can be achieved at the grass-roots level (Andrews, 2006). The NORPHCAM RCB programme has begun to make inroads around a number of activities that help highlight the practical steps towards developing capacity at the local, grass-roots level of the TCIM research community.

The NORPHCAM RCB programme

One large untapped research resource is obviously the extensive practitioner networks representing the wide array of modalities and therapies included in TCIM. Many TCIM practitioners lack research evaluation skills (Wye and Digby, 2008) – this is not too surprising given their focus on practice and extensive workload, nor unusual; the same could certainly be said of many general practitioners and other conventional primary health care providers (Farmer and Weston, 2002). However, as acknowledged in other health care fields, one crucial pathway to gaining professional legitimacy and elevated status is to build a research evidence base for practice (Adams and Smith, 2003) and robust TCIM studies are more likely if research teams include *both* therapists and academics (House of Lords, 2000).

To clarify, this does not necessarily refer exclusively to studies of efficacy, but can and should also include gathering empirical evidence and understanding about related issues (for example examining practitioner decision making, the patient–provider interface and communication and the drivers and motivations for consumption and provision).

NORPHCAM has followed the lead of Farmer and Weston (2002) in terms of developing a 'whole-system approach' to capacity building for both practitioners and academics. A whole-system approach 'allows [participants] at any stage to enter the system at an appropriate level and then progress to a higher level of research capacity' (Farmer and Weston, 2002: 1141). In line with this approach, NORPHCAM has initiated a number of distinct but inter-related RCB activities that enable practitioners and academics interested in TCIM (whether conventional or complementary in training and affiliation) to enter the capacity-building programme at different levels and to progress 'up' levels and activities as and when appropriate.

Promoting research literacy
The initial level RCB activities (primarily aimed at practitioners) include 'introductory' workshops on a range of topics directly tailored to practitioner needs. For example, NORPHCAM currently offers a suite of workshops/short courses built around initial research skills and literacy (for example workshops on 'How to search research literature via databases' and 'How to read and appraise research reports'). These early-stage training sessions are aimed at not only identifying and encouraging practitioners who wish to actively develop a research side to their career, but also help meet the needs of the vast majority of practitioners who are and who will remain non-participants in research and evaluation (due in part to time, resource restraints and/or a lack of interest to engage in research activity directly). This latter group is often an overlooked resource in RCB, for while they may never directly conduct research projects, they provide essential links between research and practice.

It is important that the growing variety of peer-reviewed journals focusing on TCIM (including *Complementary Therapies in Medicine, Journal of Alternative and Complementary Medicine* and *BMC Complementary and Alternative Medicine*) are utilized and drawn on by practitioners to inform their clinical thinking and practice. Central to such utilization is producing a practitioner base that is research literate.

Early-career RCB
Building on research literacy training, a number of practitioners may desire to be more directly active in the research process (Farmer and Weston, 2002). In order to accommodate such practitioners and other early-career researchers (non-practitioners) focused on TCIM, NORPHCAM has devised a series of early-career research activities. This aspect of the NORPHCAM RCB programme includes one-on-one tuition and mentoring, a workshop series focused on a range of appropriate methodological training and substantive topics, and intensive pre-arranged group work (whereby a group or team of early-career researchers may work with NORPHCAM Executive member(s) to brainstorm and advance specific ideas, a project or a paper-writing process). Another innovative development that has been running for the

last couple of years is the NORPHCAM internship scheme, whereby early-career TCIM researchers (often from overseas) visit a number of NORPHCAM Executive members and work over a period of two to three weeks on a specific peer-reviewed journal article. The intern receives the mentoring and collaborative insights of one or more of the NORPHCAM Executive (relevant to the manuscript focus) and the short, intense visit also provides strategic training and insights to help encourage the future efficient production of quality research outputs (in terms of journal articles, books and external grant proposals).

Such early-career RCB work is also complemented by the NORPHCAM PhD Scholarship programme, which over the last three years has successfully recruited and funded six PhD students in topics across the public health/health services research of TCIM (including health economics and economic evaluations of CAM, TCIM and women's health and the interface between primary health care and CAM in rural health). NORPHCAM is also now focused on developing and establishing postdoctoral positions for these and other newly emerging PhD students so as to ensure that their skills and experiences are not later lost to other health research fields or topics.

Mid-career and leadership RCB

Finally, NORPHCAM is also focused on and actively addressing the challenges of RCB for mid-career researchers and more senior research leaders. Participants at these more advanced levels of TCIM research often require RCB activities that *accommodate* networking, working through the pressures of managing numerous projects and personnel (while remaining productive and effective in the field), and fine-tuning their research leadership qualities (while nurturing their responsibility to advance the field and their more junior colleagues along the way, which is vital for sustained growth and prosperity in the field). In response, NORPHCAM has developed a programme of expert retreats, whereby senior national and international TCIM researchers can explore leadership issues, plan collaborative programmes and exchange insights and experiences in a non-competitive, collegial environment. NORPHCAM activity at this advanced level of RCB also includes sponsoring, organizing and chairing symposiums and paper sessions at both national and international events (such as the Public Health Association of Australia Annual Conference and the American Public Health Association Annual Conference) as a means of promoting TCIM and its importance to leaders in other related health research fields.

Conclusion

The vision of the NORPHCAM Executive and network more generally is to generate future capacity that promotes *sustainable* growth in TCIM research. TCIM constitutes a significant element of health care provision and utilization around the world (whether officially recognized or not). To ignore the importance of RCB in TCIM would not only have serious implications for the immediate field, but would also deny the wider medical and health research community the opportunity of fully benefiting from insights gained from rigorous, scientific study on this broad and important health care topic. It is essential that RCB endeavours incorporate the input of a whole range of stakeholders, often beyond the confines of the immediate TCIM research field (including governments and other levels of policy and practice decision makers). Nevertheless, it is also important to acknowledge that TCIM research (like all health research fields) is now a multidisciplinary, collaborative venture and that 'the market for expansion in CAM research [may be] literally at our doorsteps, staring us in the face' (Andrews, 2006: 14).

The more complex challenge facing the field may not necessarily be attracting interest (the exponential growth in TCIM research journal articles over recent years illustrates the healthy progress made on this front), but ensuring that such interest and activity are sustainable over the mid to long term. The NORPHCAM RCB programme, like those of other relevant organizations, provides one initiative with which to work towards such a broader vision for the TCIM research community.

Further reading

Lasater, K., Salanti, S., Fleischman, S. *et al.* (2009) Learning activities to enhance research literacy in a CAM college curriculum. *Journal of Alternative and Complementary Medicine* 15(4): 46–54.

Network of Researchers in the Public Health of Complementary and Alternative Medicine (www.norphcam.org)

Willinsky, J. and Quint-Rappaport, M. (2007) How complementary and alternative medicine practitioners use PUBMED. *Journal of Medical Internet Research* 9(2): 19.

References

Adams, J. (ed.) (2007) *Researching Complementary and Alternative Medicine.* London: Routledge.

Adams, J. and Smith, A. (2003) Qualitative methods in radiography research: A proposed framework. *Radiography* 9(3): 193–9.

Andrews, G. (2006) Encouraging additional research capacity as an intellectual enterprise: Extending Ernst's engagement. *Complementary Therapies in Clinical Practice* 12: 13–17.

Cooke, J. (2005) A framework to evaluate research capacity building in health care. *BMC Family Practice* 6: 44.

Farmer, E. and Weston, K. (2002) A conceptual model for capacity building in Australian primary health care research. *Australian Family Physician* 31(12): 1139–42.

House of Lords (2000) *House of Lords Select Committee on Science and Technology Sixth Report on Complementary and Alternative Medicine.* London: HMSO.

Lansang, M. and Dennis, R. (2004) Building capacity in health research in the developing world. *Bulletin of the World Health Organization* 82: 764–70.

Lewith, G., Verhoef, M., Koithan, M. and Zick, S. (2006) Developing CAM research capacity for complementary medicine. *eCAM* 3(2): 283–9.

National Center for Complementary and Alternative Medicine (2011) *Exploring the Science of Complementary and Alternative Medicine: Third Strategic Plan 2011–2015.* Bethesda, MA: NIH.

Wye, L. and Digby, K. (2008) Building research capacity amongst kinesiologists: Results from a mixed methods study. *Complementary Therapies in Clinical Practice* 14: 65–72.

Index

acupressure   36, 38, 225
acupuncture   xvii, 1, 20, 36, 36, 38,
   41, 45, 54, 81, 84, 95, 110, 112,
   117, 160, 162, 164, 198–200,
   223–6, 233, 248, 250, 257–60,
   267
Adams, Denise   44–52
Adams, Jon   1–6, 9–17, 26–43, 61–70,
   105–6, 133–4, 150–8, 185–6, 212–
   19, 229–36, 255–6, 266–82
aromatherapy   1, 36, 38, 39, 45, 63,
   232, 233
ageing   53–9, 123
ageing population   81, 116
Andrews, Gavin J.   1–6, 9–17, 33–4,
   61–2, 105–6, 133–4, 157–8,
   185–6, 229–36, 255–6
anthropology   1, 114, 125–32, 190,
   191, 193
ayurveda/ayurvedic medicine   80, 116,
   117, 122, 125–32

Balneaves, Lynda   71–8
Barnes, Joanne   1–6, 33–4, 61–2,
   105–6, 133–4, 157–8, 185–6,
   229–30, 255–6
biofeedback   94–102
Broom, Alex   1–6, 9–10, 33–4, 61–2,
   103–4, 116–24, 133–4, 157–8,
   185–6, 229–30, 255–6, 275–82

cancer   12, 28, 44, 61, 71–8, 95–8,
   105, 116–24, 206, 208, 221, 258,
   262
Cartwright, Tina   53–60
children   44–52, 192
chiropractic   1, 36, 39, 45, 161, 164,
   188, 206, 215, 221–4, 227, 250,
   257–9, 260, 261
Connor, Linda   18–25
Coulter, Ian   159–67, 204–11, 257–66

dermatology   63–70
dietary supplements   38, 39, 45, 47,
   134, 142–9
doctors (biomedical/conventional)   21,
   22, 107, 110, 120, 128, 131, 173,
   223, 226, 238

economic analysis/methods   3, 229,
   230, 245–54
ethics   47, 48, 142–9, 233
Ernst, Edzard   29, 63, 66, 87, 217,
   245, 267
evidence based medicine (EBM)   185,
   187–95, 204–11

family physicians

geography   3, 30, 229, 231–6
general practitioners (GPs)   209, 277

Harvey, Richard   94–102
health services research   256, 268, 269,
   275, 276, 279
herbalism   2
Hollenberg, Daniel   237–44
homeopathy   2, 36, 63, 81, 117, 145,
   146, 190–3, 224, 227, 257, 258

Kemper, Kathi   44–52

Lake, James   79–86
Lewith, George   196–203
Lui, Chi Wai   11–17, 35–43, 231–6

Magin, Parker   1–6, 9–10, 33–4,
   61–70, 105–6, 133–4, 157–8,
   185–6, 229–30
massage   2, 37–9, 45, 66, 75, 154,
   166, 221–6, 250, 257, 258, 262
meditation   2, 39, 45, 117
midwifery   2, 41, 151

National Center for Complementary and
  Alternative Medicine (NCCAM)
  179, 180, 204, 247, 261, 276
naturopathy   2, 45, 82, 223, 224, 235,
  257, 258
Network of Researchers in the Public
  Health of Complementary and
  Alternative Medicine
  (NORPHCAM)   243, 271,
  275–81
nursing   2, 134, 150–6

osteopathy   2, 55, 223, 247, 248
older people   53–9

pharmacy/pharmacists   134, 142–9,
  158, 169, 172, 186, 213, 276
pregnancy   33, 35–43, 192, 207
primary health care   62, 111, 133–4,
  177, 237–44, 277, 279
public health   3, 23, 62, 84, 113, 114,
  186, 212, 214, 216, 229, 230,
  237–44
qualitative research   83, 119

randomized controlled trials (RCT)
  187–96, 207–9, 247–51, 267, 268,
  281, 283

regulation   109–11, 170, 173, 185,
  186, 213, 217, 220–7, 232, 233,
  235
reflexology   1, 45
research capacity building   275–81
risk 18–25, 41, 47, 48, 74, 90, 109,
  144, 185, 186, 199, 212–19, 222,
  267

Sarris, Jerome   79–86
Seely, Dugald   71–8, 266–74
Segrott, Jeremy   11–17, 231–6
Sibbritt, David   26–32

tai chi   81
traditional Chinese medicine (TCM)
  80, 161, 162, 166, 175, 225, 257,
  260

Verhoef, Marja   13, 82, 139, 270
Vohra, Sunita   44–52

Wardle, Jon   35–43, 212–19, 266–82
wellbeing   56, 62, 94–101
Weeks, Laura   71–8

yoga   2, 36, 37, 39, 45, 81, 117,
  260